T0324121

DRUGS, ADDICTION, AND THE BRAIN

DRUGS, ADDICTION, AND THE BRAIN

GEORGE F. KOOB
The Scripps Research Institute,
La Jolla, CA, USA

MICHAEL A. ARENDS
The Scripps Research Institute,
La Jolla, CA, USA

MICHEL LE MOAL
University of Bordeaux and Neurocentre Magendie Inserm U862,
Bordeaux, France

AMSTERDAM • BOSTON • HEIDELBERG • LONDON
NEW YORK • OXFORD • PARIS • SAN DIEGO
SAN FRANCISCO • SINGAPORE • SYDNEY • TOKYO
Academic Press is an imprint of Elsevier

Academic Press is an imprint of Elsevier
The Boulevard, Langford Lane, Kidlington, Oxford, OX5 1GB, UK
225 Wyman Street, Waltham, MA 02451, USA

First published 2014

British Library Cataloguing in Publication Data
A catalogue record for this book is available from the British Library

Library of Congress Cataloging in Publication Data
A catalog record for this book is available from the Library of Congress

ISBN: 978-0-12-386937-1

For information on all Academic Press publications visit
our website at store.elsevier.com

Printed and bound in the United States of America

15 16 17 18   10 9 8 7 6 5 4 3 2 1

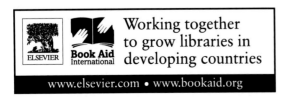

Working together
to grow libraries in
developing countries

www.elsevier.com • www.bookaid.org

Contents

Preface

Addiction is a brain disease that afflicts millions of individuals, costs society enormously in terms of medical and social expense, and causes an untold amount of suffering among those with the disease and their loved ones. One of the most compelling arguments that addiction is a biological disorder comes from advances in our understanding of the brain in the context of addiction. The study of the neurobiology of addiction has also taught us much about how the brain works, particularly in the domains of reward, motivation, and emotions.

This textbook is an effort to bring the neurobiology of addiction to a didactic level for university and college students. We envision this book as serving as material for upper-division college courses, Masters and Ph.D. graduate programs, and seminars on the neurobiology of addiction. We also envision this book as a resource for those in the medical field, including pharmacists and addiction treatment professionals, to help them to gain a basic understanding of the neurobiology of addiction. We are convinced that a better understanding of the disorder by both professionals and patients will allow them to better understand addiction processes and the challenges of recovery.

The book is organized on the basis of concepts that have guided our research in the field for some time, but particularly the concept that addiction is a chronically relapsing disorder characterized by:

(i) A compulsion to seek and take drugs,
(ii) Loss of control over drug intake, and
(iii) Emergence of a negative emotional state (e.g., dysphoria, anxiety, and irritability) that defines a motivational withdrawal syndrome when access to the drug is prevented.

In this context, we have conceptualized addiction as a three-stage cycle – *binge/intoxication*, *withdrawal/negative affect*, and *preoccupation/anticipation* – that worsens over time and involves allostatic-like changes in the brain incentive salience, reward, stress, and executive function systems. Allostasis is defined as stability with change and refers to a break with normal homeostatic processes that can lead to overt pathology and on the way generate prolonged pathophysiology known as addiction.

This book is divided into three major parts. Chapters 1–3 outline basic information that the reader will need to interpret and place in context the specific discussions of each major drug class. Chapter 1 defines the concept of addiction from a historical perspective and includes discussions of the new diagnostic criteria defined by the American Psychiatric Association's *Diagnostic and Statistical Manual of Mental Disorders*, 5th edition (DSM-V). Chapter 2 defines basic neurobiological concepts relevant to addiction and provides an overall summary of the neurobiology of addiction. Chapter 3 outlines animal models of various aspects of the addiction cycle and their reliability and validity.

Chapters 4–8 outline in detail the major classes of drugs of abuse using a standard format for each chapter: Definitions; History of Use; Use, Abuse and Addiction; Medical Uses; Behavioral and Physiological Effects; Pharmacokinetics; Behavioral Mechanism of Action; and Neurobiological Effects divided into the *binge/intoxication*, *withdrawal/negative affect*, and *preoccupation/anticipation* stages. The neurobiology section follows the outline of the three stages of the addiction cycle so readers can explore the similarities and differences between each drug class. Each chapter includes a history of how the use of the drug evolved. In addition to the neurobiological mechanism of action, a section on the behavioral mechanism of action is provided to demonstrate a unifying and integrating principle of order and predictability at the behavioral level for a given drug. Although the addiction process for each drug class has certain common neurobiological elements, each class of drugs is also unique and engages the addiction cycle at different points.

Finally, the third section of the book, represented by Chapter 9, is an attempt to translate the neurobiology of addiction to the realm of the pharmacotherapeutic treatment of addiction. This chapter explores the mechanisms of action of known approved treatments of addiction, again within the construct of the three stages of the addiction cycle.

We provide many opportunities for readers to relate the concepts herein with the real world of individuals with addiction by including various case histories and studies of addiction. We also provide references for the data presented in the figures and tables and various suggestions for further reading so that students may pursue certain topics of interest in more depth. This book takes a unique approach to the study of the neurobiology of addiction, guided by a conceptual framework honed from over 40 years of different but complementary basic research from the Koob and Le Moal laboratories in the domains of the motivation and pathophysiology of motivation. Students will receive a rich but catholic view of the neurobiology of addiction that will stimulate future interest in the field and hopefully drive excitement to gain further knowledge.

ACKNOWLEDGMENTS

All of the figures in this book were redrawn from their original sources by Janet Hightower of The Scripps Research Institute Biomedical Graphics department. We are always grateful for her efforts. We thank Lisa Romero for assistance with proof processing. We would also like to extend our deep appreciation to the following colleagues for providing encouragement, suggestions, references, figures, and their own personal interpretations: R. Adron Harris, Barbara Mason, Mandy McCracken, Elizabeth D'Amico, Joel Schlosburg, Ami Cohen, Tom Eissenberg, Scott Edwards, Ken Warren, Antonio Noronha, Olivier George, and Pietro Sanna.

George F. Koob
Michael A. Arends
Michel Le Moal

What is Addiction?

DEFINITIONS OF ADDICTION

Drug Use, Drug Abuse, and Drug Addiction

Drug addiction, formerly known as substance dependence (American Psychiatric Association, 1994), is a chronically relapsing disorder that is characterized by:

1) A compulsion to seek and take a drug,
2) Loss of control in limiting intake, and
3) Emergence of a negative emotional state (e.g., dysphoria, anxiety, irritability) when access to the drug is prevented.

The occasional but limited use of an abusable drug is clinically distinct from escalated drug use, the loss of control over limiting drug intake, and the emergence of chronic compulsive drug seeking that characterize addiction. Historically, three types of drug use have been delineated:

1) Occasional, controlled, or social use,
2) Drug abuse or harmful use, and
3) Drug addiction as characterized as either Substance Dependence (*Diagnostic and Statistical Manual of Mental Disorders*, 4th edition [DSM-IV]) or Dependence (see below, and Tables 1.1 and 1.2).

More current descriptions have elaborated a continuum of behavioral pathology, from drug use to addiction, in the context of substance use disorders.

TABLE 1.1   DSM-5, DSM-IV, and ICD-10 Diagnostic Criteria for Abuse and Dependence

DSM-5	DSM-IV	ICD-10
DEPENDENCE		
A problematic pattern of substance use leading to clinically significant impairment or distress, as manifested by at least two of the following occurring within a 12 month period	*A maladaptive pattern of substance use, leading to clinically significant impairment or distress as manifested by three or more of the following occurring at any time in the same 12-month period*	*Three or more of the following have been experienced or exhibited at some time during the previous year*
1. Tolerance is defined by either of the following: a) a need for markedly increased amounts of substance to achieve intoxication or desired effect b) a markedly diminished effect with continued use of the same amount of substance.	1. Need for markedly increased amounts of a substance to achieve intoxication or desired effect; or markedly diminished effect with continued use of the same amount of the substance.	1. Evidence of tolerance, such that increased doses are required in order to achieve effects originally produced by lower doses.
2. Withdrawal is manifested by either of the following: a) the characteristic withdrawal syndrome for substance or b) substance is taken to relieve or avoid withdrawal symptoms.	2. The characteristic withdrawal syndrome for a substance or use of a substance (or a closely related substance) to relieve or avoid withdrawal symptoms.	2. A physiological withdrawal state when substance use has ceased or been reduced as evidenced by: the characteristic substance withdrawal syndrome, or use of substance (or a closely related substance) to relieve or avoid withdrawal symptoms.
3. There is persistent desire or unsuccessful efforts to cut down or control substance use.	3. Persistent desire or one or more unsuccessful efforts to cut down or control substance use.	3. Difficulties in controlling substance use in terms of onset, termination, or levels of use.
4. Substance is often taken in larger amounts or over a longer period than was intended.	4. Substance used in larger amounts or over a longer period than the person intended.	None
5. Important social, occupational, or recreational activities are given up or reduced because of substance use.	5. Important social, occupational, or recreational activities given up or reduced because of substance use.	4. Progressive neglect of alternative pleasures or interests in favor of substance use; or A great deal of time spent in activities necessary to obtain, to use, or to recover from the effects of substance use.
6. A great deal of time is spent in activities necessary to obtain substance, use substance, or recover from its effects.	6. A great deal of time spent in activities necessary to obtain, to use, or to recover from the effects of substance used.	
7. Continued substance use despite having persistent or recurrent social or interpersonal problems caused or exacerbated by the effects of substance.	7. Continued substance use despite knowledge of having a persistent or recurrent physical or psychological problem that is likely to be caused or exacerbated by use.	5. Continued substance use despite clear evidence of overtly harmful physical or psychological consequences.
None	None	6. A strong desire or sense of compulsion to use substance.

Continued

TABLE 1.1   DSM-5, DSM-IV, and ICD-10 Diagnostic Criteria for Abuse and Dependence—cont'd

DSM-5	DSM-IV	ICD-10
ABUSE		
	A maladaptive pattern of substance use leading to clinically significant impairment or distress, as manifested by one (or more) of the following occurring with a 12 month period	*A pattern of substance use that is causing damage to health.*
8. Substance use is continued despite knowledge of having a persistent or recurrent physical or psychological problem that is likely to have been caused or exacerbated by substance	1. Recurrent substance use resulting in a failure to fulfill major role obligations at work, school, or home.	*The damage may be physical or mental. The diagnosis requires that actual damage should have been caused to the mental or physical health of the user*
9. Recurrent use in situations in which it is physically hazardous	2. Recurrent substance use in situations in which use is physically hazardous.	
None	3. Recurrent substance-related legal problems.	
10. Recurrent substance use resulting in a failure to fulfill major role obligations at work, school or home	4. Continued substance use despite having persistent or recurrent social or interpersonal problems caused or exacerbated by the effects of the drug.	
11. Craving or a strong desire or urge to use alcohol (or other substance)	None	None

TABLE 1.2   Estimated Number and Percentage of Persons of the US Population Aged 12 and Older (N = 258 Million) Who Ever Used Alcohol, Tobacco, Cannabis, Cocaine, Heroin, or Prescription Opioids, the Number and Percentage Who Used these Drugs in the Last Year, the Number and Percentage Who Ever Showed Dependence (DSM-IV Criteria; See Text) in the Last Year, and the Number and Percentage Who Showed Abuse or Dependence (DSM-5 Criteria; See Text) in the Last Year

	Ever Used		Last-Year Use		Last-Year Use with Dependence		Last-Year Use with Abuse or Dependence	
Drug	Millions	%	Millions	%	Millions	%	Millions	%
Cocaine	36.9	14.6	3.9	1.5	0.58	14.5	0.82	21.1
Stimulants	20.4	7.2	2.7	1.0	0.25	9.3	0.33	12.9
Methamphetamine	11.9	4.6	1.0	0.4	–	–	–	–
Heroin	4.2	1.7	0.6	0.2	0.37	57.0	0.43	65.5
Analgesics	34.2	13.5	11.1	4.3	1.4	12.7	1.8	16.5
Alcohol	211.7	82.1	170.4	65.9	7.8	4.6	16.7	9.8
Tobacco	173.9	67.5	81.9	31.8	–	–	–	–
Cigarettes*	161.8	62.8	67.1	26.1	22.9	34.2	22.9	34.2
Cannabis	107.8	42.0	29.7	11.5	2.6	8.8	4.2	13.9

There is no abuse category for cigarettes, so the third and fourth columns of the table are identical.
Data from Substance Abuse and Mental Health Services Administration, National Survey on Drug Use and Health, *2011*

Diagnostic Criteria for Addiction

The diagnostic criteria for addiction, as described in the DSM, have evolved from the first edition published in 1952 to DSM-IV, with a shift from an emphasis on the criteria of tolerance and withdrawal to other criteria which are more directed at compulsive use. The criteria for Substance Use Disorders outlined in the DSM-IV closely resemble those outlined in the *International Statistical Classification of Diseases and Related Health Problems* (ICD-10) for Drug Dependence (World Health Organization, 1992; Table 1.1). The DSM-5 was published in 2013 (American Psychiatric Association, 2013). In this, the criteria for drug addiction have changed both conceptually and diagnostically. The new diagnostic criteria for addiction merge the abuse and dependence constructs (i.e., substance abuse and substance dependence) into one continuum that defines "substance use disorders" on a range of severity, from mild to moderate to severe, based on the number of criteria that are met out of a total of 11. The severity of a substance use disorder (addiction) depends on how many of the established criteria are met by an individual. Mild Substance Use Disorder is the presence of 2–3 criteria, moderate is 4–5 criteria, and severe is six or more criteria. These criteria remain basically the same as in the previous edition of the DSM (DSM-IV) and ICD-10, with the exception of the removal of "committing illegal acts" and the addition of a new "craving" criterion. For example, rather than differentiating "alcoholics" and "alcohol abusers," the new classification Substance Use Disorder on Alcohol encompasses individuals who are afflicted by the disorder to different degrees, from "mild" (e.g., a typical college binge drinker who meets two criteria, such as alcohol is often taken in larger amounts or over a longer period than was intended and there is a persistent desire or unsuccessful efforts to cut down or control alcohol use) to "severe" (e.g., a classic person with alcoholism who meets six or more criteria, such as a great deal of time spent in activities necessary to obtain alcohol, use alcohol, or recover from its effects, recurrent alcohol use resulting in a failure to fulfill major role obligations at work, school, or home, alcohol use despite knowledge of having a persistent or recurrent physical or psychological problem, continued alcohol use despite persistent social or interpersonal problems, tolerance, and withdrawal).

The terms *Substance Use Disorder* and *Addiction* will be used interchangeably throughout this book to refer to a usage process that moves from drug use to addiction as defined above. Drug addiction is a disease and, more precisely, a *chronic* relapsing disease (Figures 1.1 and 1.2).

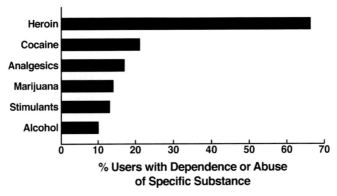

FIGURE 1.1 **Last-year use with abuse or dependence** *(data from Substance Abuse and Mental Health Services Administration, National Survey on Drug Use and Health, 2011; see Table 1.2).*

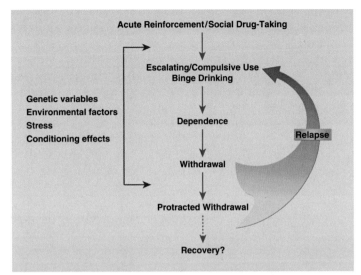

FIGURE 1.2 **Stages of addiction to drugs of abuse.** Drug taking invariably begins with social drug taking and acute reinforcement and often, but not exclusively, moves in a pattern of use from escalating compulsive use to dependence, withdrawal, and protracted abstinence. During withdrawal and protracted abstinence, relapse to compulsive use is likely to occur with a repeat of the cycle. Genetic factors, environmental factors, stress, and conditioning all contribute to the vulnerability to enter the cycle of abuse/dependence and relapse within the cycle. [*Taken with permission from Koob GF, Le Moal M.* Neurobiology of Addiction. *Academic Press, London, 2006.*]

The associated medical, social, and occupational difficulties that usually develop during the course of addiction do not disappear after detoxification. Addictive drugs produce changes in brain circuits that endure long after the person stops taking them. These prolonged neurochemical and neurocircuitry changes and the associated personal and social difficulties put former patients at risk of relapse, a risk that is >60% within the first year after discharge.

Frequency and Cost of Addiction

A shortcut for examining the frequency of substance use disorders is to utilize a combination of the percentage of individuals who have drug abuse and drug dependence as defined by the DSM-IV, since no data are yet available for the frequency of substance use disorders based on the DSM-5 criteria. Combining the old drug abuse and dependence criteria yields an approximate percentage of 15% (38.6 million people as of 2011) for the U.S. population who are 12 or older who suffered from Substance Use Disorders for alcohol, tobacco, or illicit drugs in the last year (Table 1.2). For alcohol, 9.8% of last-year users met the criteria for Substance Abuse or Dependence on Alcohol. For

tobacco, 32% of the population used tobacco in the last year. For cannabis, 13.9% of last-year users met the criteria for Substance Abuse or Dependence on cannabis. For cocaine, 21.1% of last-year users met the criteria for Substance Abuse or Dependence on cocaine. For heroin, 65.5% of last-year users met the criteria for Substance Abuse or Dependence on heroin.

The cost to society of drug abuse and drug addiction is prodigious in terms of both the direct costs and indirect costs associated with secondary medical events, social problems, and loss of productivity. In the United States alone, illicit drug use and addiction cost society $161 billion per year in 2011. Alcoholism cost society $223 billion per year in 2012, and nicotine addiction costs society $155 billion. In terms of health burden, alcohol and tobacco use are in the top 10 greatest risk factors for loss of years to disease and disability.

Much of the initial research into the neurobiology of drug addiction focused on the acute impact of drugs of abuse (analogous to comparing no drug use to drug use). The focus has shifted to chronic administration and the acute and long-term neuroadaptive changes that occur in the brain. Sound arguments have been made to support the hypothesis that addictions are similar to other chronic relapsing disorders, such as diabetes, asthma, and hypertension, in their chronic relapsing nature and treatment efficacy (for further reading, see McLellan et al., 2000). Current neuroscientific drug abuse research seeks to understand the cellular and molecular mechanisms that mediate the transition from occasional, controlled drug use to the loss of behavioral control over drug seeking and drug taking that defines chronic addiction.

Patterns of Addiction

Different drugs produce different patterns of addiction, with an emphasis on different components of the addiction cycle. Opioids are a classic drug of addiction, in which an evolving pattern of use includes intravenous or smoked drug taking, intense initial intoxication, the development of profound tolerance, escalation in intake, and profound dysphoria, physical discomfort, and somatic withdrawal signs during abstinence (Box 1.1). Intense preoccupation with obtaining opioids (craving) develops and often precedes the somatic signs of withdrawal. This preoccupation is linked to stimuli associated with obtaining the drug, stimuli associated with withdrawal, and internal and external states of stress. A pattern develops in which the drug must be administered to avoid the severe dysphoria and discomfort of abstinence.

Alcohol substance use disorder or alcoholism follows a somewhat different pattern of drug taking that depends on the severity of the disorder. The initial intoxication is less intense than opioids, and the pattern of drug taking often is characterized by binges of alcohol intake that can be daily episodes or

---

BOX 1.1

Jimmy pulls out of the graveled driveway onto the smooth asphalt surface of the road. It feels so good to drive again after the long months in "rehab." No heroin use in over 6 months. "Not bad," he congratulates himself. But as he takes the exit to the old neighborhood, his bowels begin to growl. He breaks out in sweat, gripping the steering wheel and trying to ignore the raw, acid taste in the back of his throat. Yawning, eyes watering, he feels mounting panic, and the desire for drugs begins to burn in the pit of his stomach, "So much for good intentions," be mutters, turning toward a familiar alley and the drug that will make everything right again.

Dennis leaves his cocaine therapy group full of energy. "I've got 30 days clean, and now I'm going for 90!" he yells to a buddy as they enter their cars. As he leaves the parking lot, a familiar white sedan is pulling in – Diana's car;

she probably is going to the next group session. Dennis' heart begins to pound – gripped by a flood of memories about the car, where he and Diana had shared so much cocaine. A wave of intense feeling rushes from the tip of his toes, up to his head and back down again. Thoughts racing, desire coursing through his body, he turns away from the road home, into the night. As he approaches the familiar buying corner, he can taste the cocaine in the back of his throat. He is sweating heavily now, ears ringing. "Just a taste," he bargains with himself, "just a taste is all I'm going to buy."

From: Childress AR, Hole AV, Ehrman RN, Robbins SJ, McLellan AT, O'Brien CP, Cue reactivity and cue reactivity interventions in drug dependence. In: Onken LS, Blaine JD, Boren JJ (Eds.), Behavioral Treatments for Drug Abuse and Dependence (series title: NIDA Research Monograph, vol. 137), National Institute on Drug Abuse, Rockville MD, 1993, pp. 73–95.

prolonged days of heavy drinking. A binge is currently defined by the US National Institute on Alcohol Abuse and Alcoholism as consuming five standard drinks for males and four standard drinks for females in a two hour period, or obtaining a blood alcohol level of 0.08 gram percent. Alcoholism is characterized by a severe emotional and somatic withdrawal syndrome and intense craving for the drug that is often driven by negative emotional states but also by positive emotional states. Many individuals with alcoholism continue with such a binge/withdrawal pattern for extended periods; for others, the pattern evolves into opioid-like addiction, in which they must have alcohol available at all times to avoid the consequences of abstinence.

Tobacco addiction contrasts with the above patterns. Tobacco is associated with virtually no binge-like behavior in the *binge/intoxication* stage of the addiction cycle. Cigarette smokers who met the criteria for substance dependence or dependence under the DSM-IV and ICD 10 criteria are likely to smoke throughout their waking hours and experience negative emotional states (dysphoria, irritability, and intense craving) during abstinence. The pattern of intake is one of highly titrated intake of the drug during waking hours.

Psychostimulants, such as cocaine and amphetamines, show a pattern that has a greater emphasis on the *binge/intoxication* stage. Such binges can last hours or days, often followed by a crash that is characterized by extreme dysphoria and inactivity. Intense craving and anxiety occur later and are driven by both environmental cues that signify the availability of the drug, and internal states that are often linked to negative emotional states and stress.

Marijuana substance use disorder follows a pattern similar to opioids and tobacco, with a significant intoxication stage. As chronic use continues, subjects begin to show a pattern of chronic intoxication during waking hours. Withdrawal is characterized by dysphoria, irritability, and sleep disturbances. Although marijuana craving has been less studied to date, it is most likely linked to both cues and internal states often associated with negative emotional states and stress, similarly to other drugs of abuse.

The "Dependence" View of Addiction

The term "dependence" within the conceptual framework of addiction has a confused history. However, discussing the evolution of the term is instructive. Historically, definitions of addiction began with definitions of dependence. Himmelsbach defined physical dependence as:

> "...an arbitrary term used to denote the presence of an acquired abnormal state wherein the regular administration of adequate amounts of a drug has, through previous prolonged use, become requisite to physiologic equilibrium. Since it is not yet possible to diagnose physical dependence objectively without withholding drugs, the *sine qua non* of physical dependence remains the demonstration of a characteristic abstinence syndrome."
>
> (Himmelsbach CK. Can the euphoric, analgetic, and physical dependence effects of drugs be separated? IV. With reference to physical dependence. Federation Proceedings, 1943, (2), 201–203).

This definition eventually evolved into the definition for physical dependence: "intense physical disturbances when the administration of a drug is suspended" (Eddy NB, Halbach H, Isbell H, Seevers MH. Drug dependence: its significance and characteristics. Bulletin of the World Health Organization, 1965, (32), 721–733). However, this terminology clearly did not capture many of the aspects of an addictive process that do not show physical signs, necessitating the creation of the term *psychic dependence* to capture the behavioral aspects of the symptoms of addiction:

> "A condition in which a drug produces 'a feeling of satisfaction and a psychic drive that require periodic or continuous administration of the drug to produce pleasure or to avoid discomfort'..."
>
> (Eddy NB, Halbach H, Isbell H, Seevers MH. Drug dependence: its significance and characteristics. Bulletin of the World Health Organization, 1965, (32), 721–733).

Later definitions of addiction resembled a combination of physical and psychic dependence, with more of an emphasis on the psychic or motivational aspects of withdrawal, rather than on the physical symptoms of withdrawal:

> "*Addiction;* from the Latin verb 'addicere,' to give or bind a person to one thing or another. Generally used in the drug field to refer to chronic, compulsive, or uncontrollable drug use, to the extent that a person (referred to as an 'addict') cannot or will not stop the use of some drugs. It usually implies a strong (Psychological) Dependence and (Physical) Dependence resulting in a Withdrawal Syndrome when use of the drug is stopped. Many definitions place primary stress on psychological factors, such as loss of self-control and overpowering desires; i.e., addiction is any state in which one craves the use of a drug and uses it frequently. Others use the term as a synonym for physiological dependence; still others see it as a combination (of the two)."
>
> (Nelson JE, Pearson HW, Sayers M, Glynn TJ (eds.) Guide to Drug Abuse Research Terminology. *National Institute on Drug Abuse, Rockville MD, 1982*).

Unfortunately, the word *dependence* in this process has multiple meanings. Any drug can produce dependence if dependence is defined as the manifestation of a withdrawal syndrome upon the cessation of drug use, see above. Meeting the ICD-10 criteria for *Dependence* or the DSM-5 criteria for Substance Use Disorder requires much more than simply manifesting a withdrawal syndrome. For the purposes of this book, *dependence* (with a lowercase "d") will refer to the manifestation of a withdrawal syndrome, and *addiction* will refer to Dependence as defined by the ICD-10. The terms *Dependence* (with a capital "D"), *addiction*, and *alcoholism* will be held equivalent for this book. The term Substance Use Disorder is defined as a problematic pattern of drug use that leads to clinically significant impairment or distress, reflected by at least two the 11 criteria within a 12 month period (see above). How this cluster of cognitive, behavioral, and physiological symptoms will be considered equivalent to "addiction" remains to be determined.

Psychiatric View of Addiction

From a psychiatric perspective, drug addiction has aspects of both impulse control disorders and compulsive disorders. Impulse control disorders are characterized by an increasing sense of tension or arousal before committing an impulsive act, pleasure, gratification, or relief at the time of committing the act, and regret, self-reproach, or guilt following the act (see early versions of the DSM of the American Psychiatric Association). In contrast, compulsive disorders are characterized by anxiety and stress before committing a compulsive repetitive behavior and relief from the stress by performing the compulsive behavior. As an individual moves from an impulsive disorder to a compulsive disorder, a shift occurs from positive reinforcement to negative reinforcement that drives the motivated behavior (Figure 1.3). Drug addiction progresses from impulsivity to compulsivity in a collapsed cycle of addiction that consists of three stages: *preoccupation/anticipation, binge/intoxication,* and *withdrawal/negative affect.* Different theoretical perspectives from experimental psychology, social psychology, and neurobiology can be superimposed on these three stages, which are conceptualized as feeding into each other, becoming more intense, and ultimately leading to the pathological state known as addiction (Figure 1.4; for further reading, see Koob and Le Moal, 1997).

Psychodynamic View of Addiction

A psychodynamic view of addiction that integrates the neurobiology of addiction was elaborated by Khantzian and colleagues (for further reading, see Khantzian, 1997) with a focus on the factors that produce vulnerability to addiction. This perspective is deeply rooted in the psychodynamic aspects of clinical practice developed

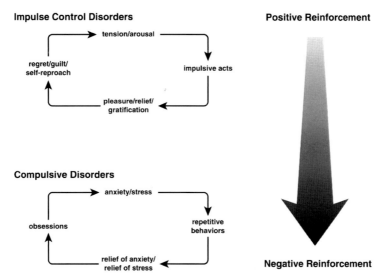

FIGURE 1.3 **Diagram showing stages of impulse control disorder and compulsive disorder cycles related to the sources of reinforcement.** In impulse control disorders, increasing tension and arousal occur before the impulsive act, with pleasure, gratification or relief during the act, and regret or guilt following the act. In compulsive disorders, recurrent and persistent thoughts (obsessions) cause marked anxiety and stress followed by repetitive behaviors (compulsions) that are aimed at preventing or reducing distress. Positive reinforcement (pleasure/gratification) is more closely associated with impulse control disorders. Negative reinforcement (relief of anxiety or relief of stress) is more closely associated with compulsive disorders. *[Taken with permission from Koob GF. Allostatic view of motivation: implications for psychopathology. In: Bevins RA, Bardo MT (eds.)* Motivational Factors in the Etiology of Drug Abuse *(series title:* Nebraska Symposium on Motivation, *vol 50). University of Nebraska Press, Lincoln NE, 2004, pp. 1–18.]*

from a contemporary perspective with regard to substance use disorders. The focus of this approach is on developmental difficulties, emotional disturbances, structural (ego) factors, personality organization, and the building of the "self."

Two critical elements (disordered emotions and disordered self-care) and two contributory elements (disordered self-esteem and disordered relationships) were identified. These evolved into a self-medication hypothesis, in which individuals with substance use disorders take drugs as a means to cope with painful and threatening emotions. In this conceptualization, individuals with addiction experience states of subjective distress and suffering that may or may not be sufficient in meeting DSM-5 criteria for a psychiatric diagnosis. Individuals with addiction have feelings that are

overwhelming and unbearable and may consist of an affective life that is absent and nameless. From this perspective, drug addiction is viewed as an attempt to medicate such a dysregulated affective state. Patient suffering is deeply rooted in disordered emotions, characterized at their extremes by unbearable painful affect or a painful sense of emptiness. Others cannot express personal feelings or cannot access emotions and may suffer from alexithymia, defined as "a marked difficulty to use appropriate language to express and describe feelings and to differentiate them from bodily sensation" (*Sifneos PE. Alexithymia, clinical issues, politics and crime.* Psychotherapy and Psychosomatics, *2000, (69) 113–116).*

Such self-medication may be drug-specific. Patients may preferentially use drugs that fit the nature of their painful affective states. Opiates

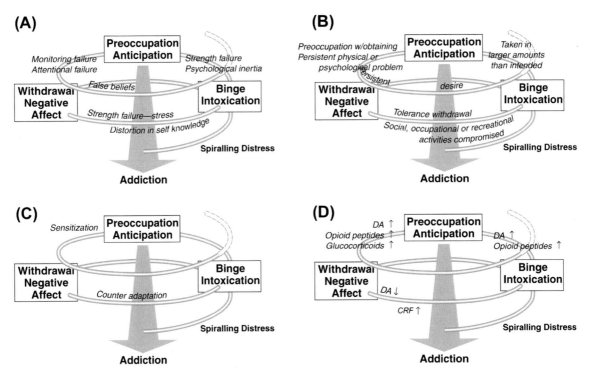

FIGURE 1.4   **Diagram describing the spiraling distress/addiction cycle from four conceptual perspectives: social psychological, psychiatric, dysadaptational, and neurobiological.** Notice that the addiction cycle is conceptualized as a spiral that increases in amplitude with repeated experience, ultimately resulting in the pathological state known as addiction. (A) The three major components of the addiction cycle – *preoccupation/anticipation, binge/intoxication,* and *withdrawal/negative affect* – and some of the sources of potential self-regulation failure in the form of underregulation and misregulation. (B) The same three major components of the addiction cycle with the different criteria for substance dependence incorporated from the DSM-IV. (C) The places of emphasis for the theoretical constructs of sensitization and counteradaptation. (D) The hypothetical role of different neurochemical and endocrine systems in the addiction cycle. Small arrows refer to increased or decreased functional activity. DA, dopamine; CRF, corticotropin-releasing factor. *[Taken with permission from Koob GF, Le Moal M. Drug abuse: hedonic homeostatic dysregulation. Science, 1997, (278), 52–58.]*

might effectively reduce psychopathological states of violent anger or rage. Others who suffer from hypohedonia, anergia, or lack of feelings might prefer the activating properties of psychostimulants. Still others who sense themselves as being flooded by their feelings, or cut off from their feelings entirely, may opt for repeated moderate doses of alcohol or depressants in a medicinal effort to express feelings that they are unable to communicate. The common element of the self-medication hypothesis is that each drug class serves as an antidote or "replacement for a defect in the psychological structure" (Kohut H.

The Analysis of the Self: A Systematic Approach to the Psychoanalytic Treatment of Narcissistic Personality Disorders [series title: *The Psychoanalytic Study of the Child,* vol 4]. International Universities Press, New York, 1971). The paradox is that using drugs to self-medicate emotional pain will eventually perpetuate it by perpetuating a life that revolves around drugs.

Self-care deficits reflect an inability to ensure one's self-preservation and are characterized by an inability to anticipate or avoid harmful or dangerous situations and an inability to use appropriate judgment and feeling as guides in the face of adversity. Thus, self-care deficits reflect an inability to appropriately experience emotions and fully recognize the consequences of dangerous behaviors. Disordered self-care combines with a disordered emotional life to become a principal determinant of substance use disorders. The core element of this psychodynamic perspective is a dysregulated emotional system in individuals who are vulnerable to addiction.

This psychodynamic approach integrates well with the critical role of dysregulated brain reward and stress systems that are revealed by studies of the neurobiology of addiction. From a neurobiological perspective, additional harm to the personality can by produced by the direct effects of the drugs themselves, thus perpetuating or actually *creating* such character flaws.

Social Psychological and Self-Regulation Views of Addiction

At the social psychology level, failures in self-regulation have been argued to be the root of major social pathologies (for further reading, see Baumeister et al., 1994). Important self-regulation elements are involved in different stages of addiction, including other pathological behaviors, such as compulsive gambling and binge eating. Failures in self-regulation can lead to addiction in the case of drug use or an addiction-like pattern with nondrug behaviors. Underregulation, reflected by strength deficits, a failure to establish standards, conflicting standards, attentional failures, and misregulation (misdirected attempts to self-regulate) can contribute to the development of addiction-like behavioral patterns (Figure 1.4, Box 1.2). The transition to addiction can be facilitated by lapse-activated causal patterns (patterns of behavior that contribute to the transition from an initial lapse in self-regulation to a large-scale breakdown), thus leading to spiraling distress. In some cases, the first self-regulation failure can lead to emotional distress, setting the stage for a cycle of repeated failures to self-regulate and

where each violation brings additional negative affect, resulting in spiraling distress. For example, a failure of strength may lead to initial drug use or relapse, and other self-regulation failures can be recruited to provide entry into or prevent exit from the addiction cycle (Box 1.3).

At the neurobehavioral level, such dysregulation may be reflected by deficits in information-processing, attention, planning, reasoning, self-monitoring, inhibition, and self-regulation, many of which involve functioning of the frontal lobe. Executive function deficits, self-regulation problems, and frontal lobe dysfunction or pathology constitute risk factors for biobehavioral disorders, including drug abuse. Deficits in frontal cortex regulation in children or young adolescents predict later drug and alcohol consumption, especially in children raised in families with histories of drug and biobehavioral problems.

Vulnerability to Addiction

A wide range of factors may predispose individuals to addiction, many of which provide insights into the etiology of the disorder. These include comorbidity with other psychiatric disorders, including anxiety, affective, personality, and psychotic disorders, and neurobehavioral traits, such as impulsivity, development (adolescence), psychosocial stress, and gender (see Table 1.3). The neurobiological differences in predisposing factors which are common to the neurobiological changes associated with addiction provide insights into the neuropathology associated with the development of addiction. Individual differences in temperament, social development, comorbidity, protective factors, and genetics are areas of intense research, and a detailed discussion of these contributions to addiction is beyond the scope of this book. Each of these factors presumably interacts with the neurobiological processes discussed in this book. A reasonable assertion is that the initiation of drug abuse is more associated with social and environmental factors, whereas the

BOX 1.2

When Heather Brooks entered high school in 1991, her guidance counselor pegged her as someone with high potential. In her first semester, she earned top grades, She participated in many extracurricular activities.

A student of classical piano, Heather filled her family's suburban Chicago home with Chopin and Beethoven.

During her freshman year, 14-year-old Heather made friends with some older kids, and her life took a sudden turn. One evening while she was with them in a neighborhood park, a tall, good-looking junior handed her a marijuana cigarette. "Take a drag," he urged, "it'll mellow you out."

At first Heather held off. She'd always disapproved of drugs. But Justin reassured her. "It's not a drug," he said, "it's only pot."

Heather decided to give it a try. "Okay," she conceded, "just one puff."

With instructions from her friends, she pulled the sweet-smelling smoke into her lungs and held it there until she thought she'd burst. Then came more puffs. As she blew out the wispy remnants of smoke, she felt dizzy – and euphoric. "Give me another drag," she begged, tugging on Justin's arm.

After a few more drags on the joint, Heather felt a deepening glow of contentment. Time slowed to a crawl. Colors and sounds seemed more intense. *"Wow!"* she thought, *"This stuff is fantastic!"*.

Her high lasted four hours. Heather couldn't wait for the next invitation from her new friends. Because she'd taken the big step and smoked a joint, she felt a strong bond with them. She was confident someone would bring more pot to share.

She wasn't disappointed. The next weekend, when Justin offered her a joint, Heather took it eagerly. *"Why do adults get so bent cut of shape over a little pot?"* she wondered. All she knew was that

the more she smoked, the more outrageously fabulous she felt.

As Heather's freshman year – and her use of marijuana – progressed, pot was no longer just a social drug. First thing in the morning, she smoked a joint to get herself out of bed. She smoked in a friend's car on the way to school. Between classes she smoked in the bathroom. She was even stoned when she sang in a school choir concert.

To achieve a high, meanwhile, required ever increasing amounts of the substance. She graduated to using a bong, or water pipe, which concentrates the smoke inside a chamber so none is lost into the air. "The only thing wasted," a bong purveyor promised, "is you."

Heather didn't worry that she needed more and more of the stuff. To her, this was a sign of prowess. "Look how much I can smoke and not get loaded," she bragged. And she downplayed thoughts of addiction. Pot, her friends kept reminding her, wasn't any more habit-forming than milk. She was sure she could quit any time.

When Heather's parents asked how school was going, she always flashed a big smile. "Everything's fine," she'd say. Because she'd always been such a good daughter, Frank and Diana Brooks had every reason to believe her. Gradually, though, Heather had become a highly accomplished liar.

"I'll be at Amy's house after school," she said one morning, looking her mother squarely in the eye. Instead, Heather drove with her friends to a dead-end dirt road where they smoked pot until it was time to go home for dinner.

On Friday nights, Heather came home promptly at her eleven o'clock curfew and said good-night to her parents. After the sliver of light under their door went out, she waited ten minutes, then tiptoed downstairs and slipped out the door to go party.

BOX 1.2   *(cont'd)*

When Heather's gang smoked pot, they also always drank – beer or tumblers of vodka and cranberry juice. The alcohol made Heather feel more mellow than ever. It also amazed her how much she could drink without ever getting sick.

At school Heather's absences began to mount and her grades took a nose dive. Yet for a while she continued to fool her parents. When report cards were mailed, she intercepted them at home and, with skillful use of correction fluid and a photocopying machine, turned Ds and Fs to As and Bs. She even added some nice comments: "Heather is a pleasure to have in class," she wrote, imitating the handwriting of one of her teachers.

By the end of Heather's freshman year, her grade-point average had plummeted from 4.0 to 1.2, and she'd tallied up a staggering 39 absences.

Meanwhile, Heather dropped many of her extracurricular activities. When her parents asked why, she said she just needed some "space." Diana and Frank Brooks pinned this on normal teenage turmoil.

By now, Heather no longer cared about anyone or anything – except her next high. Her drive and motivation were gone, replaced by total apathy.

Drugs had become her life. She couldn't stop. In her journal she wrote: "Pot is a motionless sea of destruction. I'm drowning."

Indeed, always in excellent health, Heather now felt sick much of the time. Her hands and feet were constantly cold. She woke up coughing and pushed her face deep into her pillow so her parents wouldn't hear her. She also noticed that her menstrual cycle had become irregular.

Heather's parents saw the changes in their daughter. But their questions turned up nothing, and they were worried. By her sophomore year, Heather knew all the tricks. To hide the smell of pot in her room, she stuffed an empty paper-towel roll with a sheet of fabric softener and exhaled into the tube. She carried eye drops to clear up bloodshot eyes. Before heading home, she gargled with mouthwash or chewed cinnamon-flavored gum. Often she brought a clean shirt to a party and left the smoke saturated one behind.

As Heather's pot intake increased, she wanted even more. Encouraged by her friends, she experimented with a variety of mind-altering substances: LSD, mescaline, crack, codeine, cocaine and amphetamines. Through it all, however, marijuana remained her "drug of choice." It was what she started out with, and what she ended up with.

One warm night toward the end of Heather's sophomore year, she attended what had become a typical party for her: the host's parents were away, and there was plenty of liquor along with a variety of drugs. Heather wasn't supposed to be there. Through conferences with her guidance counselor, her parents had found out about her doctored grades and her frequent absences. They now suspected alcohol or drugs and grounded her. But that evening her parents had gone out. Heather figured she could slip out and be back before they returned.

Around 10 p.m., she hopped in the back seat of a car with four others for a ride home. Ryan, the driver, was both drunk and stoned. As he stomped on the accelerator on a straight stretch of highway, Heather saw the speedometer pass 100 m.p.h.

Moments later, the car slammed into a guardrail, rolled down an embankment and came to rest on its roof. Miraculously, everyone survived. Ryan's face was jammed onto the steering-wheel horn, which blared loudly. Others bled from their faces and dangled broken limbs. Numbed

Continued

BOX 1.2   (cont'd)

by alcohol, marijuana and cocaine, Heather was oblivious of her own injuries as she helped one of her friends from the tangled wreck.

Heather had suffered severe injuries to her back and neck, and would need a year of physical therapy.

"I didn't know Ryan had been drinking," Heather lied to her parents. They wanted desperately to believe her. Relieved that she was alive, they forgave her "just this once" for sneaking out. From then on, they warned, they were tightening their watch. But while she recuperated at home, Heather smoked pot secretly.

Heather had been dating Charlie Evans. He was handsome, athletic and popular with the girls. He was also heavily into marijuana and cocaine.

One evening three months after her accident, Charlie appeared at the front door with an eight-ball of cocaine (about an eighth of an ounce). Her parents were out to dinner. Soon Heather and Charlie were sniffing the white powder through straws.

After several lines, her heart began to race, something that had never happened before. She smoked a few joints to "mellow out," but instead she became more jumpy. Looking down, she saw her shirt move with the heavy pounding of her heart. Terrified, she told Charlie to call for help.

He dialed 911. "Send someone quick," he yelled. He didn't wait around. "I've got to split before the cops get here," he said, going out the back door.

En route to the hospital, Heather's heart rate soared to 196 beats a minute. "Talk to us," a paramedic urged, "we don't want to lose you." Finding Heather in intensive care and learning that she'd overdosed on cocaine, Diana Brooks broke

into anguished cries. This was the wake-up call that Heather had long needed – and her parents too. "You've hit rock bottom," Frank told his daughter later, "we're still your best friends – but we're going to be watching you every minute."

Each morning, Frank Brooks waited to leave for work until Heather was on her bus. When she returned, a parent was waiting for her. No more rides with friends. No more parties.

That summer, her parents took her to a La Jolla, Calif., beach house to get her away from her "friends." For four full weeks, Heather was shaky, nervous and sweaty as her body adjusted to a healthier lifestyle. She had so much difficulty adapting to any kind of schedule that she wasn't sure when to eat or sleep. Slowly, however, her numbed brain began to function. Frequently, she thought about the time she spent in the hospital: "*I almost died, and none of my friends even came to visit.*"

Returning to Chicago, Heather was as determined to turn her life around as she once seemed determined to destroy it. She doubled up on courses she had failed as a sophomore. The sounds of her piano once again filled the Brooks home.

As a senior, Heather traveled to Europe with the school choir. As she stood in an ancient cathedral, her soprano voice joining the others, she recalled the concert when she'd shown up stoned.

"*Just three years ago,*" she thought, "*What a different person I am now.*"

From: Ola P, D'Aulaire E. Here's what marijuana can do inside a teenager's body: "But It's Only Pot." Reader's Digest, 1997, Jan:83–89.

---

progression to a substance use disorder (addiction) is more associated with neurobiological factors. Temperament and personality traits and some temperament clusters have been identified as vulnerability factors, including impulsivity, novelty- and sensation-seeking, conduct disorder, and negative affect. From the perspective of comorbid psychiatric disorders,

BOX 1.3

We head north to the cabin. Along the way I learn that my parents, who live in Tokyo, have been in the States for the last two weeks on business. At four a.m. they received a call from a friend of mine who was with me at a hospital and had tracked them down in a hotel in Michigan. He told them that I had fallen face first down a fire escape and that he thought they should find me some help. He didn't know what I was on, but he knew there was a lot of it and he knew it was bad. They had driven to Chicago during the night.

We drive on and after a few hard silent minutes we arrive. We get out of the car and we go into the house and I take a shower because I need it. When I get out there are some fresh clothes sitting on my bed. I put them on and I go to my parents' room. They are up drinking coffee and talking but when I come in they stop.

"Hi."

Mom starts crying again and she looks away. Dad looks at me.

"Feeling better?"

"No."

"You should get some sleep."

"I'm gonna."

"Good."

I look at my Mom. She can't look back. I breathe.

"I just."

I look away.

"I just, you know."

I look away. I can't look at them.

"I just wanted to say thanks for picking me up."

Dad smiles. He takes my Mother by the hand and they stand and they come over to me and they give me a hug. I don't like it when they touch me so I pull away.

"Good night."

"Good night, James. We love you."

I turn and I leave their room and I close their door and I go to the kitchen. I look through the cabinets and I find an unopened half-gallon bottle of whiskey. The first sip brings my stomach back up, but after that it's all right. I go to my room and I drink and I smoke some cigarettes and I think about her. I drink and I smoke and I think about her and at a certain point blackness comes and my memory fails me.

Back in the car with a headache and bad breath. We're heading north and west to Minnesota. My Father made some calls and got me into a clinic and I don't have any other options, so I agree to spend some time there and for now I'm fine with it. It's getting colder.

I want to run or die or get fucked up. I want to he blind and dumb and have no heart. I want to crawl in a hole and never come out. I want to wipe my existence straight off the map. Straight off the fucking map. I take a deep breath.

We enter a small waiting room.

They're gonna check you in now.

We stand and we move toward a small room where a man sits behind a desk with a computer. He meets us at the door.

"You ready to get started?"

I don't smile.

"Sure."

He gets up and I get up and we walk down a hall. He talks and I don't. "The doors are always open here, so if you want to leave, you can. Substance use is not allowed and if you're caught using or possessing, you will be sent home. You are not allowed to say anything more than hello to any women aside from doctors, nurses, or staff members. If you violate this rule, you will be sent home. There are other rules, but those are the only ones you need to know right now."

We walk through a door into the medical wing. There are small rooms and doctors and nurses and a pharmacy. The cabinets have large

Continued

BOX 1.3 *(cont'd)*

steel locks. He shows me to a room. It has a bed and a desk and a chair and a closet and a window. Everything is white.

He stands at the door and I sit on the bed.

"A nurse will be here in a few minutes to talk with you."

"'Fine."

"You feel okay?"

"No, I feel like shit."

"It'll get better."

"Yeah."

"'Trust me."

"Yeah."

The man leaves and he shuts the door and I'm alone. My feet bounce, I touch my face, I run my tongue along my gums. I'm cold and getting colder. I hear someone scream.

The door opens and a nurse walks into the room. She wears white, all white, and she is carrying a clipboard. She sits in the chair by the desk.

"Hi James."

"Hi."

"I need to ask you some questions."

"All right."

"I also need to check your blood pressure and your pulse."

"All right."

"What type of substances do you normally use?"

"Alcohol."

"Every day?"

"Yes."

"What time do you start drinking?"

"When I wake up."

She marks it down.

"How much per day?"

"As much as I can."

"How much is that?"

"Enough to make myself look like I do."

She looks at me. She marks it down.

"Do you use anything else?"

"Cocaine."

"How often?"

"'Every day."

She marks it down.

"How much?"

"As much as I can."

She marks it down.

"In what form?"

"Lately crack, but over the years, in every form that it exists."

She marks it down.

"Anything else."

"Pills, acid, mushrooms, meth, PCP and glue."

Marks it down.

"How often?"

"When I have it."

"How often?"

"A few times a week."

Marks it down.

She moves forward and draws out a stethoscope.

"How are you feeling."

"Terrible."

"In what way?"

"In every way."

She reaches for my shirt.

"Do you mind?"

"No."

She lifts my shirt and she puts the stethoscope to my chest. She listens.

"Breathe deeply."

She listens.

"Good. Do it again."

She lowers my shirt and she pulls away and she marks it down.

"Thank you."

I smile.

"Are you cold?"

"Yes."

She has a blood pressure gauge.

BOX 1.3   *(cont'd)*

"Do you feel nauseous?"

"Yes."

She straps it on my arm and it hurts.

"When was the last time you used?"

She pumps it up.

"A little while ago."

"What and how much?"

"I drank a bottle of vodka."

"How does that compare to your normal daily dosage?"

"It doesn't."

She watches the gauge and the dials move and she marks it down and she removes the gauge.

"I'm gonna leave for a little while, but I'll be back."

I stare at the wall.

"We need to monitor you carefully and we will probably need to give you some detoxification drugs."

I see a shadow and I think it moves but I'm not sure.

"You're fine right now, but I think you'll start to feel some things."

I see another one. I hate it.

"If you need me, just call."

I hate it.

She stands up and she smiles and she puts the chair back and she leaves. I take off my shoes and I lie under the blankets and I close my eyes and I fall asleep.

I wake and I start to shiver and I curl up and I clench my fists. Sweat runs down my chest, my arms, the backs of my legs. It stings my face.

I sit up and I hear someone moan. I see a bug in the corner, but I know it's not there. The walls close in and expand. They close in and expand and I can hear them. I cover my ears but it's not enough.

I stand. I look around me. I don't know anything. Where I am, why, what happened, how to escape. My name, my life.

I curl up on the floor and I am crushed by images and sounds. Things I have never seen or heard or even knew existed. They come from the ceiling, the door, the window, the desk, the chair, the bed, the closet. They're coming from the fucking closet. Dark shadows and bright lights and flashes of blue and yellow and red as deep as the red of my blood. They move toward me and they scream at me and I don't know what they are but I know they're helping the bugs. They're screaming at me.

I start shaking – shaking and shaking and shaking. My entire body is shaking and my heart is racing and I can see it pounding through my chest and I'm sweating and it stings. The bugs crawl onto my skin, and they start biting me and I try to kill them. I claw at my skin, tear at my hair, start biting myself. I don't have any teeth and I'm biting myself and there are shadows and bright lights and flashes and screams and bugs, bugs, bugs. I am lost. I am completely fucking lost.

I scream.

I piss on myself.

I shit my pants.

The nurse returns and she calls for help and men in white come in and they put me on the bed and they hold me there. I try to kill the bugs but I can't move so they live. In me. On me. I feel the stethoscope and the gauge and they stick a needle in my arm and they hold me down.

I am blinded by blackness.

I am gone.

TABLE 1.3   12-Month Prevalence of Comorbid Disorders among Respondents with Nicotine Dependence, Alcohol
             Dependence, or any Substance Use Disorder

	Mood	Anxiety	Personality
Alcohol	27.6%	23.5%	39.5%
Nicotine	21.1%	22.0%	31.7%
Substance Dependence (including alcohol but not nicotine)	29.2%	24.5%	69.5%

Data from:

Grant BF, Hasin DS, Chou SP, Stinson FS, Dawson DA, *Nicotine dependence and psychiatric disorders in the United States: results from the National Epidemiologic Survey on Alcohol and Related Conditions,* Archives of General Psychiatry, 2004, (61), 1107–1115.

Grant BF, Stinson FS, Dawson DA, Chou SP, Dufour MC, Compton W, Pickering RP, Kaplan K, *Prevalence and co-occurrence of substance use disorders and independent mood and anxiety disorders: results from the National Epidemiologic Survey on Alcohol and Related Conditions,* Archives of General Psychiatry, 2004, (61), 807–816.

Grant BF, Stinson FS, Dawson DA, Chou SP, Ruan WJ, Pickering RP *Co-occurrence of 12-month alcohol and drug use disorders and personality disorders in the United States: results from the National Epidemiologic Survey on Alcohol and Related Conditions,* Archives of General Psychiatry, 2004, (61), 361–368.

the strongest associations are found with mood disorders, anxiety disorders, antisocial personality disorders, and conduct disorders. The association between attention-deficit/hyperactivity disorder (ADHD) and drug abuse can be explained largely by the higher comorbidity with conduct disorder in these individuals. Independent of this association, little firm data indicate a higher risk caused by the pharmacological treatment of ADHD with stimulants, and no preference for stimulants over other drugs of abuse has been noted. In fact, children with ADHD who are treated with psychostimulants are less likely to develop a substance use disorder.

Developmental factors are important components of vulnerability, with strong evidence that adolescent exposure to alcohol, tobacco, and drugs of abuse leads to a significantly higher likelihood of drug dependence and drug-related problems in adulthood. Individuals who experience their first intoxication at 16 or younger are more likely to drink and drive, ride with an intoxicated driver, be seriously injured when drinking, become heavy drinkers, and develop substance dependence on alcohol (Figure 1.5). Similarly, people who smoke their first cigarette at 14–16 years of age

are 1.6 times more likely to become dependent than people who begin to smoke when they are older. Others have argued that regular smoking during adolescence raises the risk of adult smoking by a factor of 16 compared with nonsmoking during adolescence. The age at which smoking begins influences the total years of smoking, the number of cigarettes smoked, and the likelihood of quitting (Figure 1.6). When the prevalence of lifetime illicit or nonmedical drug use and dependence was estimated for each year of onset of drug use from ages ≤13 and ≥21, the early onset of drug use was a significant predictor of the subsequent development of drug abuse (Figure 1.7). Overall, the lifetime prevalence of substance dependence (measured by the DSM-IV criteria) among people who began using drugs under the age of 14 was 34%. This percentage dropped to 14% for those who began using at age 21 or older.

The adolescent period is associated with specific stages and pathways of drug involvement. Initiation usually begins with legal drugs (alcohol and tobacco). Involvement with illicit drugs occurs later in the developmental sequence, and marijuana is often the bridge between licit and illicit drugs. However, although this sequence is common, it does not represent an inevitable

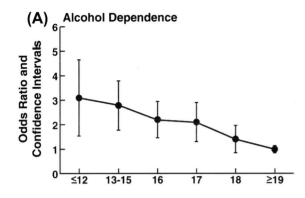

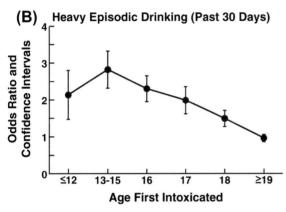

FIGURE 1.5 **Representative college alcohol survey.** (A) Alcohol dependence according to age first intoxicated. (B) Past 30 days of heavy episodic drinking according to age first intoxicated. After controlling for personal and demographic characteristics and respondent age, the odds of meeting alcohol dependence criteria were 3.1 times greater for those who were first drunk at or prior to age 12 compared with drinkers who were first drunk at age 19 or older. The relationship between early onset of being drunk and heavy episodic drinking in college persisted even after further controlling for alcohol dependence. Respondents who were first drunk at or prior to age 12 were 2.1 times to report recent heavy episodic drinking than college drinkers who were first drunk at age 19 or older. *[Taken with permission from Hingson R, Heeren T, Zakocs R, Winter M, Wechsler H. Age of first intoxication, heavy drinking, driving after drinking and risk of unintentional injury among US college students.* Journal of Studies on Alcohol, *2003, (64), 23–31.]*

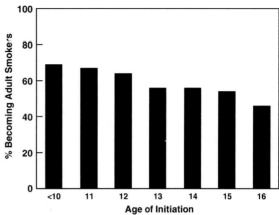

FIGURE 1.6 **Percentage of adolescent regular smokers who became adult regular smokers as a function of grade of smoking initiation.** The subjects consisted of all consenting 6th to 12th graders in a Midwestern county school system in the United States who were present in school on the day of testing. All 6th to 12th grade classrooms (excluding special education) were surveyed annually between 1980 and 1983. A potential pool of 5,799 individuals had been assessed at least once during adolescence between 1980 and 1983. At the time of follow-up, 25 of these subjects were deceased, 175 refused participation, and 4,156 provided data (72%). The subjects were predominantly Caucasian (96%), equally divided by sex (49% male, 51% female), and an average of 21.8 years old. Of the respondents, 71% had never been married, and 26% were currently married; 58% had completed at least some college by the time of follow-up; 32% were still students; and 43% had a high school education. For nonstudents, occupational status ranged from 29% in factory, crafts, and labor occupations, to 39% in professional, technical, and managerial occupations. At follow-up, the overall rate of smoking at least weekly was 26.7%. *[Taken with permission from Chassin L, Presson CC, Sherman SJ, Edwards DA. The natural history of cigarette smoking: predicting young-adult smoking outcomes from adolescent smoking patterns.* Health Psychology, *1990, (9), 701–716.]*

progression. Only a very small percentage of young people progress from one stage to the next and on to late-stage illicit drug use or dependence (for further reading, see Kandel, 1975).

Genetic contributions to addiction can result from complex genetic differences that range from alleles that control drug metabolism to hypothesized genetic control over drug sensitivity and environmental influences. The classic approach to studying complex genetic traits is to examine co-occurrence or comorbidity in monozygotic vs. dizygotic twins who are reared together or apart or in family studies with biological relatives. Twin and adoption studies

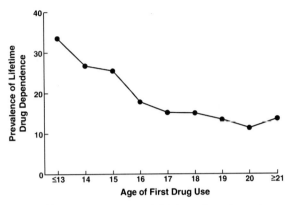

FIGURE 1.7 Prevalence of lifetime drug dependence by age at first drug use. The prevalence of lifetime dependence decreased steeply with increasing age of onset of drug use. Overall, the prevalence of lifetime dependence among those who started using drugs under the age of 14 years was approximately 34%, dropping sharply to 15.1% for those who initiated use at age 17, to approximately 14% among those who initiated use at age 21 or older. *[Taken with permission from Grant BF, Dawson DA. Age of onset of drug use and its association with DSM-IV drug abuse and dependence: results from the National Longitudinal Alcohol Epidemiologic Survey.* Journal of Substance Abuse, *1998, (10), 163–173.]*

TABLE 1.4 Heritability Estimates for Drug Dependence

	Males	Females
Cocaine	44%	65%
Heroin (opiates)	43%	–
Marijuana	33%	79%
Tobacco	53%	62%
Alcohol	49% (40–60%)	64%
Addiction overall	40%	

Male cocaine, heroin, marijuana: *Tsuang MT, Lyons MJ, Eisen SA, Goldberg J, True W, Lin N, Meyer JM, Toomey R, Faraone SV, Eaves L, Genetic influences on DSM-III-R drug abuse and dependence: a study of 3,372 twin pairs,* American Journal of Medical Genetics, *1996, (67), 473–477.*
Male nicotine: *Carmelli D, Swan GE, Robinette D, Fabsitz RR, Heritability of substance use in the NAS-NRC Twin Registry,* Acta Geneticae Medicae et Gemellologiae, *1990, (39), 91–98.*
Female cocaine: *Kendler KS, Prescott CA, Cocaine use, abuse and dependence in a population-based sample of female twins,* British Journal of Psychiatry, *1998, (173), 345–350.*
Female marijuana: *Kendler KS, Prescott CA, Cannabis use, abuse, and dependence in a population-based sample of female twins,* American Journal of Psychiatry, *1998, (155), 1016–1022.*
Female nicotine: *Kendler KS, Neale MC, Sullivan P, Corey LA, Gardner CO, Prescott CA, A population-based twin study in women of smoking initiation and nicotine dependence,* Psychological Medicine, *1999, (29), 299–308.*
Male alcohol: *Liu IC, Blacker DL, Xu R, Fitzmaurice G, Lyons MJ, Tsuang MT, Genetic and environmental contributions to the development of alcohol dependence in male twins,* Archives of General Psychiatry, *2004, (61), 897–903; Prescott CA, Kendler KS, Genetic and environmental contributions to alcohol abuse and dependence in a population-based sample of male twins,* American Journal of Psychiatry, *1999, (156), 34–40; McGue M, Pickens RW, Svikis DS, Sex and age effects on the inheritance of alcohol problems: a twin study,* Journal of Abnormal Psychology, *1992, (101), 3–17.*
Female alcohol: *McGue M, Pickens RW, Svikis DS, Sex and age effects on the inheritance of alcohol problems: a twin study,* Journal of Abnormal Psychology, *1992, (101), 3–17.*
Addiction overall: *Uhl GR, Grow RW, The burden of complex genetics in brain disorders,* Archives of General Psychiatry, *2004, (61), 223–229.*

provide researchers with estimates of the extent to which genetics influence a given phenotype, termed *heritability*. Genetic factors may account for approximately 40% of the total variability of the phenotype (Table 1.4). In no case does heritability account for 100% of the variability, which argues strongly for gene–environment interactions, including the specific stages of the addiction cycle, developmental factors, and social factors.

Genetic factors can also convey protection against drug abuse. For example, certain Asian populations who lack one or more alleles for the acetaldehyde dehydrogenase gene show significantly less vulnerability to alcoholism. A similar genetic defect in metabolizing nicotine has been discovered, in which those who metabolize nicotine more quickly have higher smoking rates and may also have a higher vulnerability to dependence (for further reading, see Tyndale et al., 2001).

NEUROADAPTATIONAL VIEWS OF ADDICTION

Behavioral Sensitization

Repeated exposure to many drugs of abuse results in progressive and enduring enhancement of the motor stimulant effect elicited by subsequent exposure to the drug. This phenomenon of *behavioral sensitization* was hypothesized to underlie some aspects of the neuroplasticity of drug addiction (for further reading, see Vanderschuren and Kalivas, 2000; Robinson and Berridge, 1993). Behavioral or psychomotor sensitization, defined as increased locomotor activation produced by repeated administration of a drug, is more likely to occur with intermittent drug exposure, whereas tolerance is more likely to occur with continuous exposure. Sensitization may also grow with the passage of time. Stress and stimulant sensitization show cross-sensitization. This phenomenon was observed and characterized in the 1970s and 1980s for various drugs and helped identify some of the early neuroadaptations and neuroplasticity associated with repeated drug administration that can lead to substance use disorders. Psychomotor sensitization was invariably linked to sensitization of the activity of the mesolimbic dopamine system.

The conceptualization of a role for psychomotor sensitization in drug addiction was proposed, in which a shift in an incentive salience state, described as *wanting* (as opposed to *liking*), progressively increases with repeated drug exposure. Pathologically strong *wanting* or craving was proposed to define compulsive use. This theory also stated that there is no causal relationship between the subjective pleasurable effects of the drug (drug *liking*) and the motivation to take it (drug *wanting*). The systems of the brain that are sensitized were argued to mediate a subcomponent of reward, termed *incentive salience* (that is, the motivation to take the drug or drug *wanting*), rather than the pleasurable or euphoric effects of drugs. The psychological process of incentive salience was theorized to be responsible for instrumental drug seeking and drug taking behavior (*wanting*). This sensitized incentive salience process then produces compulsive patterns of drug use. Through associative learning, the enhanced incentive value becomes oriented specifically toward drug-related stimuli, leading to escalated drug seeking and taking. This theory further argued that the underlying sensitization of neural structures persists, making individuals with addiction vulnerable to long-term relapse. As detailed as this theory is in terms of its attempts to explain the transition from initial drug use to compulsive use, it has been undermined by multiple scientific observations. Individuals with addiction invariably show tolerance to the rewarding effects of drugs of abuse – *not* sensitization. Animal models of compulsive-like responses to drugs also show tolerance, not sensitization, and millions of individuals take psychostimulants as medications for ADHD; they do not show sensitization. Nonetheless, the one redeeming feature of the sensitization model is its focus on the incentive salience of drugs, which has both empirical and conceptual merit but may involve other mechanisms than those reflected in behavioral (locomotor) sensitization as outlined by the Robinson and Berridge theory.

Counteradaptation and Opponent Process

Counteradaptation hypotheses have long been proposed in an attempt to explain tolerance and withdrawal and the motivational changes that occur with the development of addiction. The initial acute effects of a drug are opposed or counteracted by homeostatic changes in systems that mediate the primary drug effects. The origins of the counteradaptive hypotheses can be traced back to much earlier work on physical dependence (for further reading of early formulations, see Himmelsbach, 1943) and the counteradaptive changes in physiological measures associated with acute and chronic opioid administration.

The opponent-process theory was developed in the 1970s (for further reading, see Solomon and Corbit, 1974; Solomon, 1980). Since then, it has been applied by many researchers to various situations, including drugs of abuse, fear conditioning, tonic immobility, ulcer formation, eating disorders, jogging, peer separation, glucose preference, and even parachuting.

The theory assumes that the brain contains many affect control mechanisms that serve as a kind of emotional immunization system that counteracts or opposes departures from emotional neutrality or equilibrium, regardless of whether they are aversive or pleasant. The theory is basically a negative feed-forward control construct designed to keep mood in check even though stimulation is strong. The system is conceptualized as being composed of three subparts organized in a temporal manner. Two opposing processes control a *summator*, which determines the controlling affect at a given moment. First, an unconditioned arousing stimulus triggers a primary affective process, termed the *a-process*; an unconditional reaction that translates the intensity, quality, and duration of the stimulus (for example, the first, initial use of an opiate). Second, as a consequence of the *a-process*, the opposing *b-process* is evoked after a short delay, thus defining the opponent process. The *b-process* feeds a negative signal into the summator, subtracting the impact of the already existing *a-process* in the summator. These two responses are consequently and temporally linked (*a* triggers *b*) and depend on different neurobiological mechanisms. The *b-process* has a longer latency, but some data show that it may appear soon after the beginning of the stimulus in the course of the stimulus action and have more inertia, slower recruitment, and a more sluggish decay. At any given moment, the pattern of affect will be simply the algebraic sum of these opposite influences, yielding the net product of the opponent process with the passage of time (Figure 1.8).

Importantly, with repetition of the stimulus, the dynamics or net product is a result of a progressive increase in the *b-process*. In other words, the *b-process* itself is sensitized with repeated drug use and appears more and more rapidly after the unconditional stimulus onset. It then persists longer after its initial, intended action (the unconditioned effect) and eventually masks the unconditioned effect (*a-process*), resulting in apparent tolerance (for further reading, see Colpaert, 1996). Experimental data show that if the development of the *b-process* is blocked, then no tolerance can develop with drugs. The unconditioned effect of the drug does not change with repeated drug administration. The development of the *b-process* equals the development of a negative affective state and withdrawal symptoms, in opposition to the hedonic quality of the unconditioned stimulus. Importantly, the nature of the acquired motivation is specified by the nature of the *b-process* (that is, an aversive affect in the case of drug abuse). The individual will work to reduce, terminate, or prevent the negative affect.

In this opponent-process theory from a drug addiction perspective, tolerance and dependence are inextricably linked. Solomon argued that the first few self-administrations of an opiate drug produce a pattern of motivational changes. The onset of the drug effect produces euphoria (*a-process*), followed by a subsequent decline in intensity. After the effects of the drug wear off, the *b-process* emerges as an aversive craving state. The *b-process* gets progressively stronger over time, in effect contributing to or producing more complete tolerance to the initial euphoric effects of the drug (Figure 1.8).

Motivational View of Addiction

Rather than focusing on the *physical* signs of dependence, our conceptual framework has focused on the *motivational* aspects of addiction. The emergence of a negative emotional state (dysphoria, anxiety, irritability) when access to the drug is prevented is associated with the transition from drug use to addiction. The development of such a negative affective state can define dependence as it relates to addiction:

"The notion of dependence on a drug, object, role, activity or any other stimulus-source requires the crucial feature of negative affect experienced in its

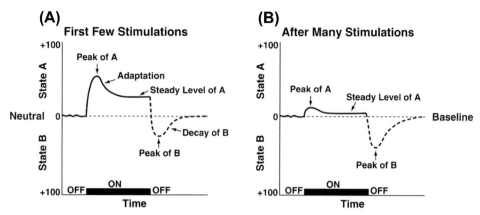

FIGURE 1.8 (A) The standard pattern of affective dynamics produced by a relatively novel unconditioned stimulus. (B) The standard pattern of affective dynamics produced by a familiar, frequently repeated unconditioned stimulus. *[Taken with permission from Solomon RL. The opponent-process theory of acquired motivation: the costs of pleasure and the benefits of pain. American Psychologist, 1980, (35), 691–712.]*

absence. The degree of dependence can be equated with the amount of this negative affect, which may range from mild discomfort to extreme distress, or it may be equated with the amount of difficulty or effort required to do without the drug, object, etc."

(Russell MAH. What is dependence? In: Edwards G (ed) Drugs and Drug Dependence. Lexington Books, Lexington MA, 1976, pp. 182–187).

A key common element of all drugs of abuse in animal models is dysregulation of brain reward function associated with the cessation of chronic drug administration. Rapid acute tolerance and opponent-process-like actions against the hedonic effects of cocaine have been reported in humans who smoke coca paste (Figure 1.9). After a single cocaine smoking bout, the onset and intensity of the "high" are very rapid via the smoked route of administration. Rapid tolerance is evident, in which the "high" decreases rapidly despite significant blood levels of cocaine. Human subjects also report subsequent dysphoria, again despite significant blood levels of cocaine. Intravenous cocaine produces similar patterns (a rapid "rush" followed by an increased "low") (Figure 1.10).

The hypothesis that the compulsive use of cocaine is accompanied by the chronic perturbation of brain reward homeostasis has been tested in an animal model of escalation in drug intake with prolonged access. Animals that have access to intravenous cocaine self-administration show increases in cocaine self-administration over days when given prolonged access (long-access [LgA] for 6h) compared with short-access (ShA; 1h access). This differential exposure to cocaine also has dramatic effects on intracranial self-stimulation (ICSS) reward thresholds. ICSS thresholds progressively increase in LgA rats but not ShA or control rats across successive self-administration sessions (see Chapter 4, Psychostimulants). Elevations in baseline ICSS thresholds temporally precede and are highly correlated with escalated cocaine intake. Post-session elevations in ICSS reward thresholds then fail to return to baseline levels before the onset of subsequent self-administration sessions, thereby deviating more and more from control levels. The progressive elevation in reward thresholds is associated with a dramatic escalation in cocaine consumption. After escalation occurs, an acute cocaine challenge facilitates brain reward responsiveness to the same degree as before but results in higher absolute brain reward thresholds in LgA rats than in ShA rats.

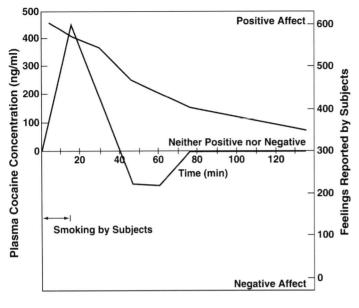

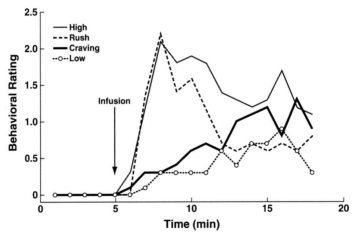

FIGURE 1.10 **Average behavioral ratings after an infusion of cocaine (0.6 mg/kg over 30 s; n = 9).** The rush, high, low, and craving ratings were averaged within each category for the subjects who had interpretable cocaine functional magnetic resonance imaging data after motion correction and behavioral ratings time-locked to the scanner. Both peak rush and peak high occurred 3 min post-infusion. Peak low (primary reports of dysphoria and paranoia) occurred 11 min post-infusion. Peak craving occurred 12 min post-infusion. No subject reported effects from the saline infusion on any of the four measures. Ratings obtained for rush, high, low, and craving measures were higher in subjects blinded to the 0.6 mg/kg cocaine dose compared with subjects unblinded to a 0.2 mg/kg cocaine dose. [*Taken with permission from Breiter HC, Gollub RL, Weisskoff RM, Kennedy DN, Makris N, Berke JD, Goodman JM, Kantor HL, Gastfriend DR, Riorden JP, Mathew RT, Rosen BR, Hyman SE. Acute effects of cocaine on human brain activity and emotion. Neuron, 1997, (19), 591–611.*]

With intravenous cocaine self-administration in animal models, such elevations in reward threshold begin rapidly and can be observed within a single self-administration session (Figure 1.11), bearing a striking resemblance to human subjective reports. These results demonstrate that the elevated brain reward thresholds following prolonged access to cocaine fail

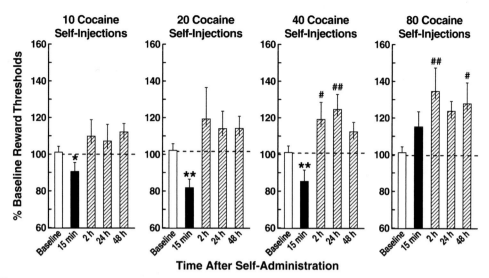

FIGURE 1.11 Rats (n = 11) were allowed to self-administer 10, 20, 40, and 80 injections of cocaine (0.25 mg per injection), and intracranial self-stimulation thresholds were measured 15 min, 2 h, 24 h, and 48 h after the end of each intravenous cocaine self-administration session. The horizontal dotted line in each plot represents 100% of baseline levels. The data are expressed as the mean percentage of baseline intracranial self-stimulation thresholds. $*p < 0.05$, $**p < 0.01$, compared with baseline; $\#p < 0.05$, $\#\#p < 0.01$, compared with baseline. [*Taken with permission from Kenny PJ, Polis I, Koob GF, Markou A. Low dose cocaine self-administration transiently increases but high dose cocaine persistently decreases brain reward function in rats.* European Journal of Neuroscience, 2003, (17), 191–195.]

to return to baseline levels, thus creating a progressive elevation in "baseline" ICSS thresholds and defining a new *set point*. These data provide compelling evidence for brain reward dysfunction in escalated cocaine self-administration and strong support for a hedonic allostasis model of drug addiction.

Allostasis and Neuroadaptation

More recently, opponent process theory has been expanded into the domains of the neurocircuitry and neurobiology of drug addiction from a physiological perspective. An allostatic model of the brain motivational systems has been proposed to explain the persistent changes in motivation that are associated with vulnerability to relapse in addiction, and this model may generalize to other psychopathologies associated with dysregulated motivational systems. Allostasis from the addiction perspective has been defined as the process of maintaining apparent

reward function stability through changes in brain reward mechanisms (Koob and Le Moal, 2001). The allostatic state represents a chronic deviation of brain reward set point that is often *not* overtly observed while the individual is actively taking the drug. Thus, the allostatic view is that not only does the *b-process* get larger with repeated drug taking, but the reward set point from which the *a-process* and *b-process* are anchored gradually moves downward, creating an allostatic state (Figure 1.12).

The allostatic state is fueled by the dysregulation of neurochemical elements of brain reward circuits and activation of brain and hormonal stress responses. It is currently unknown whether this hypothesized reward dysfunction is drug-specific and common to all addictions. The established anatomical connections and manifestation of this allostatic state as compulsive drug taking and loss of control over drug intake are critically based on dysregulation of specific neurotransmitter function in the neurocircuits of the ventral

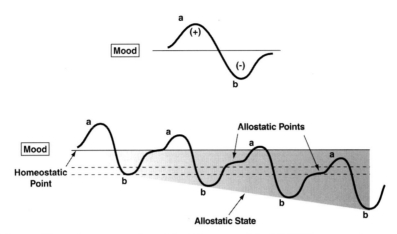

FIGURE 1.12 **Diagram illustrating an extension of the Solomon and Corbit (1974) opponent-process model of motivation to outline the conceptual framework of the allostatic hypothesis.** Both panels represent the affective response to the presentation of a drug. (Top) This diagram represents the initial experience of a drug with no prior drug history. The *a-process* represents a positive hedonic or positive mood state, and the *b-process* represents the negative hedonic or negative mood state. The affective stimulus (state) has been argued to be a sum of both an *a-process* and a *b-process*. An individual who experiences a positive hedonic mood state from a drug of abuse with sufficient time between re-administering the drug is hypothesized to retain the *a-process*. In other words, an appropriate counteradaptive opponent-process (*b-process*) that balances the activational process (*a-process*) does not lead to an allostatic state. (Bottom) The changes in the affective stimulus (state) in an individual with repeated frequent drug use that may represent a transition to an allostatic state in the brain reward systems and, by extrapolation, a transition to addiction. The apparent *b-process* never returns to the original homeostatic level before drug taking is reinitiated, thus creating a greater and greater allostatic state in the brain reward system. The counteradaptive opponent-process (*b-process*) does not balance the activational process (*a-process*) but in fact shows residual hysteresis. Although these changes are exaggerated and condensed over time in the present conceptualization, the hypothesis is that even after detoxification during a period of prolonged abstinence, the reward system is still bearing allostatic changes. In the nondependent state, reward experiences are normal, and the brain stress systems are not greatly engaged. During the transition to the state known as addiction, the brain reward system is in a major underactivated state while the brain stress system is highly activated. The following definitions apply: *allostasis*, the process of achieving stability through change; *allostatic state*, a state of chronic deviation of the regulatory system from its normal (homeostatic) operating level; *allostatic load*, the cost to the brain and body of the deviation, accumulating over time, and reflecting in many cases pathological states and accumulation of damage. *[Taken with permission from Koob GF, Le Moal M. Drug addiction, dysregulation of reward, and allostasis.* Neuropsychopharmacology, 2001, (24), 97–129.]

striatum and extended amygdala (see Chapter 2). Chronic elevation in reward thresholds is viewed as a key element in the development of addiction that sets up other self-regulation failures and persistent vulnerability to relapse during protracted abstinence. The view that drug addiction and alcoholism are the pathology that results from an allostatic mechanism that usurps the circuits established for natural rewards provides an approach to identifying the neurobiological factors that produce the vulnerability to addiction and relapse.

SUMMARY

This chapter defines addiction as a chronic relapsing disorder characterized by compulsive drug seeking, a loss of control in limiting intake, and emergence of a negative emotional state when access to the drug is prevented. The definition of addiction is derived from the evolution of the concept of dependence and the nosology of addiction diagnosis. A distinction is made between drug use and substance use disorders (formerly abuse and dependence). Addiction affects a large percentage of society and has enormous monetary costs. Addiction evolves over time, moving from impulsivity to compulsivity and ultimately being composed of three stages: *preoccupation/anticipation*, *binge/intoxication*, and *withdrawal/negative affect*. Motivational, psychodynamic, social psychological, and vulnerability factors all contribute to the etiology of addiction, but this book focuses on the neuroadaptational changes that occur during the addiction cycle. A theoretical construct is described that derives from early homeostatic theories and subsequent opponent process theories to provide a basis for understanding the neurobiology of addiction. This three-stage cycle framework is followed in each chapter for each major drug class (Psychostimulants, Opioids, Alcohol, Nicotine, and Cannabis).

Suggested Reading

American Psychiatric Association, 2013. Diagnostic and Statistical Manual of Mental Disorders, fifth ed. American Psychiatric Publishing, Washington DC.

American Psychiatric Association, 1994. Diagnostic and Statistical Manual of Mental Disorders, fourth ed. American Psychiatric Press, Washington DC.

Baumeister, R.F., Heatherton, T.F., Tice, D.M. (Eds.), 1994. Losing Control: How and Why People Fail at Self-Regulation. Academic Press, San Diego.

Colpaert, F.C., 1996. System theory of pain and of opiate analgesia: no tolerance to opiates. Pharmacol. Rev. 48, 355–402.

Himmelsbach, C.K., 1943. Can the euphoric, analgetic, and physical dependence effects of drugs be separated? IV. With reference to physical dependence. Fed. Proc. 2, 201–203.

Kandel, D.B., 1975. Stages in adolescent involvement in drug use. Science 190, 912–914.

Khantzian, E.J., 1997. The self-medication hypothesis of substance use disorders: a reconsideration and recent applications. Harv. Rev. Psychiatry. 4, 231–244.

Koob, G.F., Le Moal, M., 1997. Drug abuse: hedonic homeostatic dysregulation. Science 278, 52–58.

Koob, G.F., Le Moal, M., 2001. Drug addiction, dysregulation of reward, and allostasis. Neuropsychopharmacology 24, 97–129.

McLellan, A.T., Lewis, D.C., O'Brien, C.P., Kleber, H.D., 2000. Drug dependence, a chronic medical illness: implications for treatment, insurance, and outcomes evaluation. J. Am. Med. Assoc. 284, 1689–1695.

Robinson, T.E., Berridge, K.C., 1993. The neural basis of drug craving: an incentive-sensitization theory of addiction. Brain Res. Rev. 18, 247–291.

Solomon, R.L., Corbit, J.D., 1974. An opponent-process theory of motivation: 1. Temporal dynamics of affect. Psychol. Rev. 81, 119–145.

Solomon, R.L., 1980. The opponent-process theory of acquired motivation: the costs of pleasure and the benefits of pain. Am. Psychol. 35, 691–712.

Tyndale, R.F., Sellers, E.M., 2001. Variable CYP2A6-mediated nicotine metabolism alters smoking behavior and risk. Drug. Metab. Dispos. 29, 548–552.

Vanderschuren, L.J., Kalivas, P.W., 2000. Alterations in dopaminergic and glutamatergic transmission in the induction and expression of behavioral sensitization: a critical review of preclinical studies. Psychopharmacology 151, 99–120.

World Health Organization, 1992. International Statistical Classification of Diseases and Related Health Problems, 10th revision. World Health Organization, Geneva.

Introduction to the Neuropsychopharmacology of Drug Addiction

"Neuro-," of or relating to the brain

The brain is not simply an amorphous mass of grayish tissue. It courses with blood and electrical impulses. It regulates the body's temperature. It tells us how we feel. It allows us to interact with others and the world. It says when to wake up and when to fall asleep. It helps us put our shoes on in the morning. It also is susceptible to a host of external influences, including drugs. To better understand the subsequent chapters in this book and to put the medical, biological, and neurobiological mechanisms of drug addiction into context, we must take a step back to define and explain the common components of the body's central nervous system, from the macro (brain regions) to the micro (neurons, neurotransmitters). Armed with this information, students will be able to appreciate the in-depth knowledge that has been gained from extensive scientific research during the past 100 years, with the hope that they, too, will be able to discover greater intricacies to explain why many individuals succumb to drug addiction.

THE CENTRAL NERVOUS SYSTEM

The human brain consists of two types of cells: roughly 100 billion neurons and a greater number of glia. Neurons are highly specialized cells that have an important and unique functional property that is not shared with any other cells in the body. Neurons communicate with each other through both electrical and chemical mechanisms. More importantly for the theme of this book, neurons communicate through circuits, and these circuits form the structural bases of feelings, thoughts, and behavior, the ultimate functional output of the brain.

Neurons

Neurons have four major components: (1) cell body, (2) axons, (3) dendrites, and (4) synapses (Figure 2.1). The *cell body* contains the nucleus and receives inputs, providing the machinery for the generation of neurotransmitters and action potentials. An *action potential* occurs when a neuron's membrane is depolarized beyond its threshold. This depolarization is propagated along the axon. The *axon* is the "sending" part of the neuron, and it conducts these action potentials to the synapse to release neurotransmitters. The *synapse* is a specialized space or contact zone between neurons that allows interneuronal communication. One or more dendrites comprise the "receiving" part of the neuron, providing a massive receptive area for the neuronal surface (Figure 2.2).

Neurons act on other neurons to exert three major functions: inhibition, excitation, and

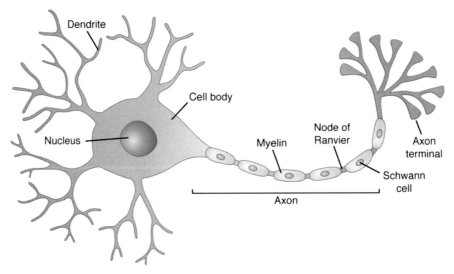

FIGURE 2.1 **Anatomy of a neuron.**

neuromodulation. Inhibition means that one neuron inhibits another neuron, often through the release of an inhibitory neurotransmitter at the synapse. Excitation means that one neuron activates another neuron through the release of an excitatory neurotransmitter at the synapse. Neuromodulation means that a neuron influences neurotransmission, often at a long distance.

Neurotransmission

The communication between neurons can be distilled into six major steps of neurotransmission relevant to the neuropharmacology of addiction (Figure 2.3).

Step 1: Neurotransmitter synthesis, involving the molecular mechanisms of peptide precursors and enzymes for further synthesis or cleavage.

Step 2: Neurotransmitter storage.

Step 3: Neurotransmitter release from the axon terminal into the synaptic cleft (or from a secreting dendrite some cases).

Step 4: Neurotransmitter inactivation caused by removal from the synaptic cleft through a reuptake process, or neurotransmitter breakdown by enzymes in the synapse or presynaptic terminal.

Step 5: Activation of the postsynaptic receptor, triggering a response of the postsynaptic cell.

Step 6: Subsequent signal transduction that responds to neurotransmitter receptor activation.

Drugs of abuse or drugs that counteract the effects of drugs of abuse can interact at any of these steps to dramatically or subtly alter chemical transmission to dysregulate or re-regulate, respectively, homeostatic function.

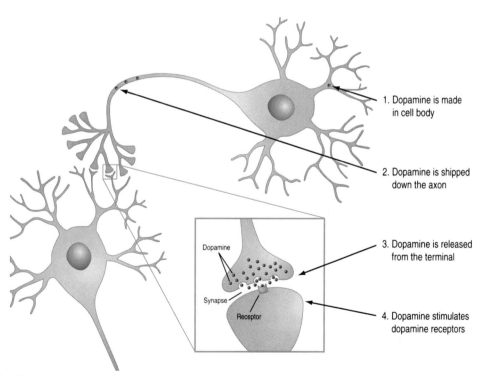

1. Dopamine is made in cell body

2. Dopamine is shipped down the axon

3. Dopamine is released from the terminal

4. Dopamine stimulates dopamine receptors

Dopamine

Synapse

Receptor

FIGURE 2.2 **Neurons, synapses, and neurotransmitters.** A typical example is shown for the neurotransmitter dopamine.

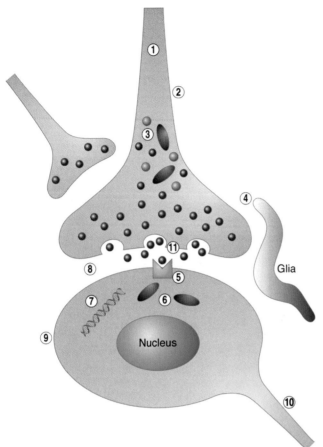

FIGURE 2.3 **Synaptic neurotransmission.** The figure shows a generalized process of synaptic transmission. (1) Various components of the neurotransmission machinery, such as enzymes, proteins, mRNA, and so on (depending on the neurotransmitter in question) are transported down the axon from the cell body. (2) The axonal membrane is electrically excited. (3) Organelles and enzymes in the nerve terminal synthesize, store, and release the neurotransmitter and activate the reuptake process. (4) Enzymes in the extracellular space and within the glia catabolize excess neurotransmitters released from nerve terminals. (5) The postsynaptic receptor triggers the response of the postsynaptic cell to the neurotransmitter. (6) Organelles within postsynaptic cells respond to the receptor trigger. (7) Interactions between genetic expression and postsynaptic nerve cells influence cytoplasmic organelles that respond to neurotransmitter action. (8) Certain steps are modifiable by events that occur at the synaptic contact zone. (9) The electrical portion of the nerve cell membrane integrates postsynaptic potentials in response to various neurotransmitters and produce an action potential. (10) The postsynaptic cell sends an action potential down its axon. (11) The neurotransmitter is released. The neurotransmitter that is released from the nerve terminal can be modulated by autoreceptors that respond to the neurotransmitter. [*Modified with permission from Iversen LL, Iversen SD, Bloom FE, Roth RH. Introduction to Neuropsychopharmacology. Oxford, New York, 2009, p. 26.*]

Glia

In addition to neurons, the central nervous system contains supporting cells. Supporting cells, generically called glia, can outnumber neurons by a factor of ten. Historically, *glia* were defined as the "nerve glue" that holds neurons together in the central nervous system. However, glia are now known to have key dynamic functions in the central nervous system, from myelin synthesis, to synapses, to serving as the innate brain defensive system against pathology. Glia consist of three types of supporting cells: oligodendrocytes, astrocytes, and microglia.

Oligodendrocytes synthesize myelin and provide an expedient way, via the myelin sheath, to significantly increase how fast an axon can conduct an action potential. Myelin is a long plasma membrane sheet that wraps around each axonal segment, leaving bare axons between myelin segments, known as the nodes of Ranvier (Figure 2.3). Myelin effectively forms insulation that allows the action potential to jump from node to node, known as salutatory conduction.

Astrocytes are star-shaped cells that have processes (branches) and both physical and biochemical support functions in the central nervous system. They physically isolate neurons and oligodendrocytes with long processes by making a cover over the nodes of Ranvier and covering the surface of capillaries, forming part of the blood–brain barrier. Astrocytes play a key role in the migration and guidance of neurons during neural circuit development. They control the formation, maturation, function, and removal of synapses. They also regulate neurotransmission and participate in reuptake processes, particularly for the excitatory neurotransmitter glutamate. Astrocytes produce growth factors and signals for activating cytokines, which can also regulate neurotransmission. They can be activated in a wide range of central nervous system disorders, ranging from neurodegenerative disorders and brain trauma to drug addiction (for further reading, see Clarke and Barres, 2013).

Microglia are immune-like cells in the central nervous system, comparable to macrophages in the immune system. A macrophage is a large cell that removes waste products, harmful microorganisms, and foreign material from the bloodstream. Immune cells are unlikely to enter the central nervous system because they cannot cross the blood–brain barrier making the brain an immunologically privileged site. However, microglia may be recruited in the brain to serve similar functions. Microglia in the central nervous system are activated by any form of central nervous system injury. They not only remove damaged cells in the brain but also remove synapses that are no longer functioning. When activated, microglia act as macrophages and, similarly to astrocytes, secrete growth factors and cytokines, both of which can modulate and regulate neurotransmission (for further reading, see Kettenmann et al., 2013).

PHARMACOLOGY FOR ADDICTION

What is a Drug, and What is Pharmacology?

The following terms need to be defined for pharmacological discussions of addiction. *Pharmacology* is the study of the interaction between

chemical reagents or drugs and living organisms. A *drug* is any chemical agent that affects an organism. Obviously, this definition can be murky in the domain of drugs of abuse, when one crosses into the realm of natural preparations that contain psychoactive or psychotropic drug entities. *Psychotropic* can be defined as an effect of a drug on the mind or behavior. For example, most drugs of abuse are derived from plant preparations. Many of them are alkaloids, such as nicotine in tobacco and caffeine in coffee and tea. An *alkaloid* is an organic compound that normally has basic chemical properties and contains mostly basic nitrogen atoms. So when does a compound transition from being a foodstuff to a drug? One metric is when it begins to have an identifiable psychotropic effect.

Other terms that are often used in the drug abuse field and should be defined in the context of this book are toxicology, pharmacotherapeutics, pharmacokinetics, and pharmacodynamics. *Toxicology* is the study of the harmful effects of drugs. *Pharmacotherapeutics* is the study of the diagnostic or therapeutic effects of drugs. *Pharmacokinetics* is the study of the factors that determine the amount of a given drug at a given site of action. *Pharmacodynamics* is the study of how a drug produces its biological effect.

Drug Nomenclature

Drugs generally have three names: a chemical name, a nonproprietary (generic) name, and a proprietary (trade) name. The chemical name describes the chemical structure. For example, 7-chloro-2-methylamino-5-phenyl-3-H-1,4-benzodiazapine-4-oxide is the chemical name for a benzodiazepine called chlordiazepoxide. Chlordiazepoxide is the nonproprietary or generic name, which is given to a drug when it has been demonstrated to have a therapeutic use. A proprietary or trade name is given by a drug company when the drug is patented. Two trade names for chlordiazepoxide are Librium and Mitran.

Drug Classification

Drugs can be classified three ways: behavioral classification, pharmacodynamic classification, and legal classification.

Behavioral classification includes five main categories: stimulants, opioids, sedative hypnotics, antipsychotics, antidepressants, and psychedelics (Table 2.1). Each of these categories is more or less self-explanatory.

- Stimulants include drugs that stimulate or produce arousal and behavioral activation. Examples of stimulants are cocaine, amphetamines, nicotine, and caffeine.
- Opioids are natural, semisynthetic, or synthetic drugs that bind to opioid receptors and produce analgesia. *Analgesia* can be defined as the reduction of pain or elevation of pain thresholds.
- Sedative hypnotics are drugs that sedate or decrease arousal, producing an anti-anxiety effect, hypnosis, or sleep. *Hypnosis* is defined as the induction of sleep. Two

examples of this class of drugs are alcohol and benzodiazepines.

- Antipsychotics are drugs that are used to treat psychosis and include the classic antipsychotics such as haloperidol (trade name: Haldol), and modern second generation drugs, such as olanzapine (trade name: Zyprexa).
- Antidepressants are drugs that are used to treat major depressive episodes and include selective serotonin reuptake inhibitors, such as fluoxetine (trade name: Prozac) and escitalopram (trade name: Lexapro), among others.
- Psychedelics are drugs that produce psychedelic experiences. *Psychedelic* can be defined as mind-altering. Another term that is often used to describe this drug class is hallucinogen, but the true meaning of the term hallucination is to experience something that is not there; therefore, the term *psychedelic* is preferred. Psychedelics include lysergic acid diethylamide (LSD) and psilocybin (derived from psychedelic mushrooms).

TABLE 2.1   Behavioral and Pharmacodynamic Classification of Psychotropic Drugs

Drug Class	Examples	Neurotransmitters
Stimulants	Caffeine Nicotine Cocaine Methamphetamine	Dopamine
Opiates	Morphine Heroin Meperidine (Demerol)	Enkephalins Endorphins
Sedative/Hypnotics	Alcohol Diazepam (Valium)	GABA
Antipsychotics	Haloperidol	Dopamine
Antidepressants	Fluoxetine (Prozac)	Norepinephrine Serotonin
Psychedelics/Hallucinogens	Lysergic acid diethylamide Psilocybin Marijuana	Serotonin Glutamate Endocannabinoids

A pharmacodynamic classification can utilize the same broad behavioral categories mentioned above and adopt them to describe the pharmacodynamic effects on brain neurotransmission (Table 2.1). For example, stimulants are indirect dopamine agonists. Opioids are direct opioid receptor agonists. Sedative hypnotics directly or indirectly facilitate γ-aminobutyric acid neurotransmission. Antipsychotics are currently dopamine D_2 receptor antagonists and serotonin 5-HT_2 receptor antagonists. Antidepressants are serotonin reuptake inhibitors, norepinephrine reuptake inhibitors, or a combination of serotonin/norepinephrine reuptake inhibitors. Psychedelics all facilitate serotonergic activity either directly or indirectly by increasing serotonin release.

Legal classification involves two categories: prescription vs. nonprescription and drug abuse. The modern era of the legal classification of drugs with abuse potential in the United States began in 1970 with the passage of the Controlled Substances Act. Five Schedules were created. The Department of Justice (Drug Enforcement Administration and Federal Bureau of Investigation) and Department of Health and Human Services (Food and Drug Administration) determine which drugs are on which schedule. The classification decisions are made on the basis of specific criteria for the potential of abuse, accepted medical use in the United States, and the potential for dependence. Drugs are classified on a continuum of increasing abuse potential, with or without a medical use.

Schedule I:	No officially recognized medical use, lack of accepted safety for use under medical supervision, high abuse potential, and cannot be legally prescribed in the United States. Examples: heroin, LSD, Δ^9-THC, and methylenedioxymethamphetamine (MDMA or Ecstasy).
Schedule II:	Officially recognized medical use and high abuse potential that may lead to severe psychological or physical dependence. Examples: methamphetamine, morphine.

Schedule III:	Officially recognized medical use and abuse potential that is less than Schedules I and II that can lead to moderate or low physical dependence or high psychological dependence. Examples: ketamine, drug products that contain less than 15 mg hydrocodone per unit (Vicodin).
Schedule IV:	Officially recognized medical use and low abuse potential compared with Schedule III. Examples: alprazolam (Xanax), diazepam (Valium).
Schedule V:	Officially recognized medical use and low abuse potential relative to Schedule IV. These drugs consist mainly of preparations that contain limited amounts of certain narcotics. Example: Robitussin AC cough syrup, which contains less than 200 mg codeine per 100 ml.

PHARMACOKINETICS

Absorption

Absorption can be defined as the movement of a drug into the blood stream, which is dramatically affected by the route of drug administration (Table 2.2). By definition, intravenous administration goes directly into the veins, giving instantaneous absorption. Each route of administration has advantages and disadvantages. The intravenous route is highly titratable, hence the amount of drug administered over time can be controlled very carefully. One disadvantage, however, is that there is no turning back. Once absorbed intravenously, there is no easy way to remove the drug from the bloodstream before it enters the brain. The oral route, by contrast, is highly variable and generally less preferred by those who use addictive drugs, but it is generally the safest route of administration. The time course of the effects of a drug is also highly affected by the route of administration (Figure 2.4). Particularly relevant to drugs of abuse is the general principle that faster absorption is associated with a higher likelihood of

TABLE 2.2   Common Routes of Drug Administration

Route	Advantages	Disadvantages
Intravenous	Valuable for emergency use Titratable Suitable for large volumes Suitable for irritating substances	No turning back Increased risk of adverse effects Must inject slowly
Subcutaneous	Suitable for some insoluble suspensions Suitable for implantation of solid pellets	Not suitable for large volumes Possible pain Possible tissue damage
Intramuscular	Suitable for moderate volumes Suitable for some irritating substances	Contraindicated when concomitant with anticoagulants Possible pain Possible tissue damage
Oral	Reversible Generally safe Convenient Economical	Requires patient cooperation Erratic absorption Possible incomplete absorption Possible instability

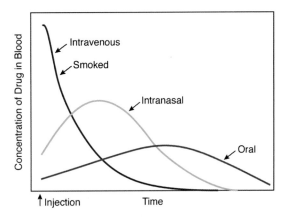

FIGURE 2.4 **Time course of blood levels of drug by different routes of administration.**

abuse. For example, amphetamines have high addiction potential when injected intravenously, but Adderall (a mixture of amphetamine isomers/salts) appears to have low addiction liability when used orally and appropriately for the treatment of attention-deficit/hyperactivity disorder.

The basis of the differences in absorption via different routes of administration depends on several factors. One obvious factor, however, is the number of physical membranes within the body that the drug needs to cross before it can be absorbed into the bloodstream (Figure 2.5). Drugs that enter the body through the gastrointestinal track, skin, or lungs must first cross an epithelial barrier and then the endothelial cells of capillary walls. Drugs that are administered subcutaneously or intramuscularly bypass the epithelial barrier but must also cross the endothelial cells of capillary walls. *Epithelial* cells line the cavities and structures of the body. *Endothelial* cells line the interior surface of blood vessels.

Drug Elimination

Drugs are eliminated from the body through metabolism in the liver, excretion from the kidneys, or a combination of both (usually metabolism followed by excretion). The classic drug that is largely metabolized is alcohol, and its elimination past a certain level is entirely metabolic and thus conforms to what is known as zero-order kinetics, in which the absolute amount of drug that is removed from the body over time is constant and

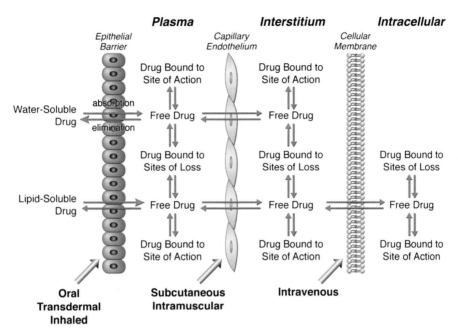

FIGURE 2.5 **Absorption of drugs through different routes of administration.** Drugs entering the body through the gastrointestinal tract (oral administration), skin (transdermal administration), or lungs (inhalation) must first cross the epithelial barrier before they can enter the interstitium (or interstitial fluid; the fluid that surrounds cells). Drugs administered subcutaneously or intramuscularly bypass the epithelial barrier and enter the interstitium directly and then must cross the capillary wall. Drugs administered intravenously further bypass the capillary wall and enter the blood stream directly. [*Modified with permission from Levine RR.* Pharmacology: Drug Actions and Reactions, *2nd edition. Little, Brown and Company, Boston, 1978.*]

conforms to the capacity of the liver to break down the drug. Thus, zero-order kinetics result from the liver's metabolism of drugs. For alcohol in a nontolerant social drinker, the average metabolism for a 70 kg male is approximately 0.01 gram percent (g%) per hour (for more information, see Chapter 6, Alcohol).

The excretion of a drug or drug metabolite follows first-order kinetics, in which a constant percentage of the drug in the blood stream is excreted over time. Such a concept reflects the drug's half-life. *Half-life* is defined as the time it takes to remove 50% of the drug from the blood stream. As an example, morphine administered intramuscularly at a dose of 10 mg in a 70 kg male produces a blood level of approximately 70 ng/ml. The half-life of morphine is approximately 2.5 h, so, as shown in Table 2.3, at the

7.5 h time point, the amount of morphine in the blood is reduced to 8.75 ng/ml. The half-life of some drugs can be changed by adjusting the pH of urine. For example, alkaloids, which constitute all major drugs of abuse with the exception of marijuana (see above), can have their half-life significantly shortened by acidifying the urine using ascorbic acid (vitamin C). This is used by physicians in an emergency room, who will intravenously administer ascorbic acid to a patient who presents with amphetamine-induced psychosis. The process by which this works is called *ion trapping*, in which there is a build-up of a high concentration of a drug across a cell membrane because of a difference in pH across the membrane. Therefore, a basic drug (one with a high pH) will accumulate in the acid (or low-pH) compartment (for example, acidic

TABLE 2.3   Drug Elimination

Half-life ($t_{1/2}$)	• The time it takes to remove 50% of the drug from the bloodstream • Independent from drug concentration • Constant rate

10 mg morphine, intramuscular injection

Time after injection	Concentration in blood
t = 0	70 ng/ml in blood
t = 2.5 h	35 ng/ml
t = 5 h	17.5 ng/ml
t = 7.5 h	8.75 ng/ml
$t_{1/2}$ = 2.5 h	

urine for amphetamine). In an acidic medium, the drug becomes more ionized (more polar/charged and less lipophilic) and thus is less likely to cross a lipid barrier or membrane.

Drug Receptors and Signal Transduction

A *receptor* is a cellular element of an organism with which a drug interacts to produce its effect. Most receptors are proteins, and most drugs bind to a specific binding site (although there are exceptions; for example, alcohol may interact with an ethanol-receptive element, perhaps in a water-containing pocket of receptors; see Chapter 6, Alcohol).

Drugs that bind to receptors and produce an effect are called *agonists*. Think of an agonist as a key and the receptor as a lock. The key is turned, producing an effect. An *antagonist* is a drug that binds to receptors and blocks the effect of an agonist. Think of an antagonist as a broken key that goes into a lock, cannot open the lock, and prevents another key from opening the lock. In the body, and particularly the brain, antagonists can produce effects on their own by blocking an endogenous agonist. For example, a dopamine receptor antagonist can

block the effects of a dopamine receptor agonist. On its own, however, the antagonist can produce motor initiation deficits by blocking the effects of endogenous dopamine. A drug that binds strongly to the binding site of the receptor with high affinity but is only partially effective (low efficacy) is termed a *partial agonist* (it partially activates the receptor).

Once a drug binds to a receptor, it must also trigger an effector domain in the receptor that activates various intracellular targets through intermediate components, collectively referred to as a *signal transduction cascade*. The brain has three major types of receptor binding/effector systems: enzymes, ligand-gated ion channels, and G-protein-coupled receptors. Enzymes and G-protein-coupled receptor systems have intermediate small molecules, called second messengers, which mediate a cascade of biochemical signals that ultimately change the function of cells or neurons in the brain. Ligand-gated ion channels bind some psychoactive agents, such as nicotine, that in turn can directly modulate neuronal excitation by opening or closing ion channels to let in excitatory sodium ions or inhibitory chloride ions. This leads to a fast response (within milliseconds). G-protein-coupled receptors, in contrast, use G proteins to transduce signals to multiple other intracellular proteins in the neuron that ultimately also affect excitability via calcium and potassium channels (Figure 2.6). For example, $G_{\alpha s}$ proteins *activate* adenylyl cyclase that in turn activates protein kinase A, which can inhibit potassium channels, facilitate excitatory glutamate neurotransmission, and increase neuronal excitability. $G_{\alpha i}$ proteins *inhibit* adenylyl cyclase and in turn inhibit protein kinase A and neuronal excitability. $G_{\alpha q}$ proteins activate a different enzyme, phospholipase C, causing the release of calcium from intracellular stores and increasing neuronal excitability. These G-protein responses are thought to occur over longer periods of time, from seconds to minutes.

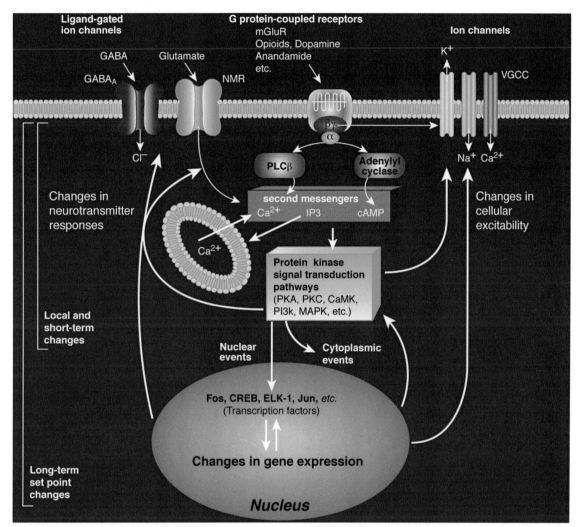

FIGURE 2.6 **Molecular mechanisms of neuroadaptation.** Shown are examples of ligand-gated ion channels such as the γ-aminobutyric acid-A (GABA$_A$) receptor and glutamate N-methyl-D-aspartate (NMDA) receptor (NMR) and G-protein-coupled receptors, such as opioid, dopamine, or cannabinoid CB$_1$ receptors, among others. These receptors modulate the levels of second messengers like cAMP and Ca^{2+}, which in turn regulate the activity of protein kinase transducers. *Cocaine and amphetamines*, as indirect sympathomimetics, stimulate the release of dopamine which acts at G-protein-coupled receptors, specifically D$_1$, D$_2$, D$_3$, D$_4$, and D$_5$. These G-protein receptors modulate via the α subunit the levels of second messengers like cyclic adenosine monophosphate (cAMP) and Ca^{2+}, which in turn regulate the activity of protein kinase transducers. Such protein kinases affect the functions of proteins located in the cytoplasm, plasma membrane, and nucleus. Among the membrane proteins affected are ligand-gated and voltage-gated ion channels (VGCC). G$_i$ and G$_o$ proteins also can regulate K$^+$ and Ca^{2+} channels directly through their βγ subunits. Protein kinase transduction pathways also affect the activities of transcription factors. Some of these factors, like cyclic adenosine monophosphate (cAMP) response element binding protein (CREB), are regulated post-translationally by phosphorylation; others, like Fos, are regulated transcriptionally; still others, like Jun, are regulated both post-translationally and/or transcriptionally. While membrane and cytoplasmic changes may be only local (e.g., dendritic domains or synaptic boutons), changes in the activity of transcription factors may result in long-term functional changes. These may include changes in the gene expression of proteins involved in signal transduction and/or neurotransmission, resulting in altered neuronal responses. For example, chronic exposure to psychostimulants has

◀ FIGURE 2.6 (cont'd)

been reported to increase the levels of protein kinase A (PKA) and adenylyl cyclase in the nucleus accumbens and decrease the levels of $G_{\alpha i}$. Chronic exposure to psychostimulants also alters the expression of transcription factors themselves. CREB expression, for instance, is depressed in the nucleus accumbens by chronic cocaine treatment. Chronic cocaine induces a transition from Fos induction to the induction of the much longer-lasting Fos-related antigens such as ΔFosB. *Opioids*, by acting on neurotransmitter systems, affect the phenotypic and functional properties of neurons through the general mechanisms outlined in the diagram. Chronic exposure to opioids has been reported to increase the levels of PKA and adenylyl cyclase in the nucleus accumbens and decrease the levels of $G_{\alpha i}$. Chronic exposure to opioids also alters the expression of transcription factors themselves. CREB expression, for instance, is depressed in the nucleus accumbens and increased in the locus coeruleus by chronic morphine treatment, whereas chronic opioid exposure activates Fos-related antigens such as ΔFosB. *Alcohol*, by acting on neurotransmitter systems, affects the phenotypic and functional properties of neurons through the general mechanisms outlined in the diagram. Alcohol, for instance, has been proposed to affect the $GABA_A$ response via protein kinase C (PKC) phosphorylation. G_i and G_o proteins also can regulate K^+ and Ca^{2+} channels directly through their $\beta\gamma$ subunits. Chronic exposure to alcohol has been reported to increase the levels of PKA and adenylyl cyclase in the nucleus accumbens and decrease the levels of $G_i\alpha$. Moreover, chronic ethanol induces differential changes in subunit composition in the $GABA_A$ and glutamate inotropic receptors and increases the expression of VGCCs. Chronic exposure to alcohol also alters the expression of transcription factors themselves. CREB expression, for instance, is increased in the nucleus accumbens and decreased in the amygdala by chronic alcohol treatment. Chronic alcohol induces a transition from Fos induction to the induction of the longer-lasting Fos-related antigens. *Nicotine* acts directly on ligand-gated ion channels. These receptors modulate the levels of Ca^{2+}, which in turn regulate the activity of protein kinase transducers. Chronic exposure to nicotine has been reported to increase the levels of PKA in the nucleus accumbens. Chronic exposure to nicotine also alters the expression of transcription factors themselves. CREB expression, for instance, is depressed in the amygdala and prefrontal cortex and increased in the nucleus accumbens and ventral tegmental area. Δ^9-*Tetrahydrocannabinol (THC)*, by acting on neurotransmitter systems, affects the phenotypic and functional properties of neurons through the general mechanisms outlined in the diagram. Cannabinoids act on the cannabinoid CB_1 G-protein-coupled receptor. The CB_1 receptor also is activated by endogenous cannabinoids such as anandamide. This receptor modulates (inhibits) the levels of second messengers like cAMP and Ca^{2+}, which in turn regulate the activity of protein kinase transducers. Chronic exposure to THC also alters the expression of transcription factors themselves. CaMK, Ca^{2+}/calmodulin-dependent protein kinase; ELK-1, E-26-like protein 1; PLCβ, phosphlipase C β; IP3, inositol triphosphate; MAPK, mitogen-activated protein kinase; PI3K, phosphoinositide 3-kinase; R, receptor. [*Modified with permission from Koob GF, Sanna PP, Bloom FE. Neuroscience of addiction.* Neuron, *1998, (21), 467–476.*]

Dose-Response Functions

The effects of drugs vary according to the dose administered. The relationship between a given dose and the effects that this specific dose generates is called the dose-effect function (or dose–response curve). In many areas of pharmacology, dose-effect functions are monotonic (the functions move in only one direction), such as the relationship between an opioid dose and the response generated, which is typically analgesia (Figure 2.7). As the dose increases, pain relief increases – up to a point. At a certain level, called the asymptote, additional doses of the drug are unable to produce any additional effects. Dose–effect functions, however, can also be non-monotonic, such as the classic inverted U-shaped curve associated with locomotor activation produced by psychostimulant drugs (Figure 2.8). In such a dose-response function,

the decreased effectiveness of cocaine/amphetamine in producing locomotor activity is attributable to an increase in stereotyped behavior.

Dose–effect functions describe two key characteristics of drug action: efficacy and potency. These two terms are often confused. *Efficacy* is the percentage of a maximum response. This can be seen on the Y-axis of the dose–response function in Figure 2.7. *Potency* is the dose required to produce a given effect relative to a standard. This can be seen on the X-axis of the dose-response function. Increases or decreases in effectiveness can be observed when comparing the levels reached by acetaminophen and morphine on the Y-axis in Figure 2.9. All three opioids shown in the figure are both more effective than acetaminophen (they produce a higher level of pain relief on the Y-axis). Further inspection of the figure also shows that the three opioids, although they have similar efficacy, have different potencies, reflected by parallel shifts of the dose to the right or left on the X-axis: codeine is less potent than morphine, and morphine is less potent than hydromorphone.

Therapeutic Ratio

The therapeutic ratio is an index of the safety of a drug. The way to calculate the therapeutic

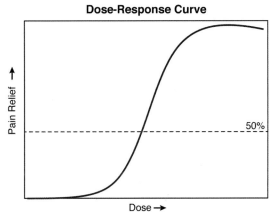

FIGURE 2.7 **A typical example of a drug's dose–response curve.** As the dose of the drug increases, its effect increases – up to a certain point.

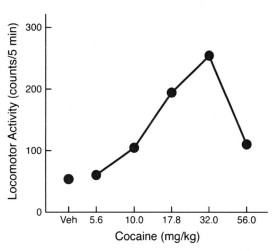

FIGURE 2.8 **A classic example of an inverted U-shaped dose–response curve.** Increasing doses of cocaine progressively increase locomotor activity – up to a point. When the dose gets high enough, locomotor activity starts to decrease. With cocaine, high doses cause stereotyped behavior. [*Modified with permission from Baladi MG, Koek W, Aumann M, Velasco F, France CP. Eating high fat chow enhances the locmotor-stimulating effects of cocaine in adolescent and adult female rats.* Psychopharmacology, *2012, (222), 447–457.*]

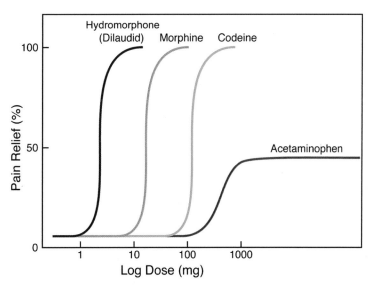

FIGURE 2.9 **Comparisons of efficacy and potency between different analgesics.** Notice that hydromorphone is more potent than morphine but has similar efficacy. Acetaminophen is both less potent and less effective than the opioid analgesics. [*Modified with permission from Levine RR.* Pharmacology: Drug Actions and Reactions, *2nd edition. Little, Brown and Company, Boston, 1978.*]

Therapeutic Ratios

$$\text{Therapeutic Ratio} = \frac{\text{Lethal Dose (LD}_{50})}{\text{Effective Dose (ED}_{50})}$$

Examples:

$$\text{Morphine} = \frac{80 \text{ mg (LD}_{50})}{10 \text{ mg (ED}_{50})} = 8$$

$$\text{Alcohol} = \frac{0.4 \text{ gram\% (LD}_{50})}{0.4 \text{ gram\% (ED}_{50})} = 1$$

FIGURE 2.10 **Example of how to calculate a drug's therapeutic ratio.**

ratio is to divide the lethal dose (LD$_{50}$) by the effective dose (ED$_{50}$) (Figure 2.10). The LD$_{50}$ is the dose that produces death in 50% of the population. The ED$_{50}$ is the dose that produces a desired therapeutic effect in 50% of the population. High therapeutic ratios indicate a substantial spread between the lethal dose and the dose required to produce the desired therapeutic effect. Therefore, higher therapeutic ratios usually reflect greater drug safety. For example, the LD$_{50}$ for morphine is 80 mg in a nontolerant person. The ED$_{50}$ for morphine to produce analgesia is 10 mg (intramuscularly). Therefore, the therapeutic ratio for morphine is 8, indicating the relative safety of using morphine to produce pain relief. By contrast, the therapeutic ratio for alcohol to produce anesthetic effects is 1. Alcohol's LD$_{50}$ is a blood level of approximately 0.4% in a nontolerant person. Alcohol's ED$_{50}$ to produce anesthesia is also 0.4%. Therefore, using alcohol to produce anesthesia for, say, tooth extraction in the 1800s would also have a good chance of killing the patient.

BASIC NEUROBIOLOGY OF ADDICTION

Dopamine

Two major dopamine systems project to the basal ganglia from cell bodies in the ventral part of the midbrain: the mesocorticolimbic dopamine system and the nigrostriatal dopamine system. The nigrostriatal dopamine system projects from the substantia nigra to corpus striatum. Degeneration of this system is the primary basis for many of the motor dysfunctions associated with Parkinson's disease. The activation of this system is also implicated in the focused repetitive behavior, called stereotyped behavior, that is associated with high doses of psychostimulants, such as cocaine and methamphetamine (Figure 2.11).

The mesocorticolimbic dopamine system projects from the ventral tegmental area to the nucleus accumbens, olfactory tubercle, amygdala, and frontal cortex. This system has been implicated in psychostimulant-induced locomotor activity, drug reward, and non-drug motivational attributes, such as incentive salience, conditioned reinforcement, and conditioned approach (for further reading, see Schultz, 2006).

Thus, dopamine neurons that project to the forebrain are associated with the initiation of behavior, reward, and motivational processes. Pharmacological manipulations that increase or decrease dopaminergic function provided early evidence of the role of the midbrain dopamine systems in reward. Pharmacological activation of dopamine synaptic activity, for example with the dopamine indirect agonist cocaine or amphetamine, produces behavioral activation, facilitated responding for many reinforcers, and decreased reward thresholds (that is, less stimulation is needed for a subject to perceive a stimulus as rewarding). Conversely, blockade of dopamine function decreases responding for both positive and negative reinforcers. Electrophysiological studies that measure the electrical activity of cells have shown that both unpredictable and predictable stimuli activate the firing of midbrain dopamine neurons. Some argue that mainly appetitive or rewarding events (like eating chocolate, having sex, or winning a card game) activated dopamine neurons in the mesocorticolimbic dopamine system. Such hedonic selectivity of the activation of dopamine neurons

Dopamine

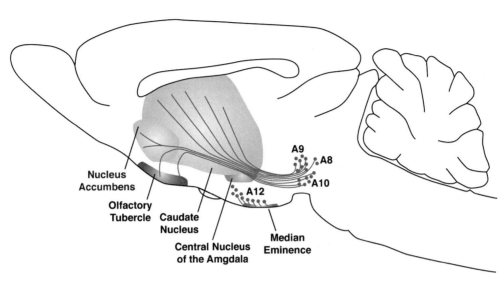

FIGURE 2.11 **Dopamine localization.** Schematic illustration of central dopamine pathways. Groups A8 and A9 give rise to nigrostriatal dopamine pathway. Group A10 gives rise to the mesolimbic dopamine pathway. Group A12 gives rise to the tubero-infundibular dopamine neurons. [*Modified from Fuxe K, Hokfelt T, Olson L, Ungerstedt U. Central monoaminergic pathways with emphasis on their relation to the so-called "extrapyramidal motor system."* Pharmacology and Therapeutics B, *1977, (3), 169–210.*]

provides intriguing insights into the conceptualization of what constitutes positive rewards or incentives. Midbrain dopamine neurons may be part of the process by which rewards motivate or guide behavior, referred to as incentive motivation or incentive salience. Positive incentives paired with previously neutral stimuli through activation of the mesocorticolimbic dopamine system facilitate species-specific approach responses or changes in direction toward important incentives via dopamine release. As discussed in the various drug-specific chapters in this book, such incentive salience provides a powerful mechanism by which associations are made between previously neutral stimuli and drugs of abuse that pharmacologically facilitate the release of mesocorticolimbic dopamine.

Five different dopamine receptors, D_1 through D_5, have been identified. Dopamine acts through these receptors to produce its functional effects. The dopamine receptors fall into two main categories: D_1-like (which are coupled to G_s proteins to *activate* adenylate cyclase; these include D_1 and D_5 receptors) and D_2-like (which are coupled to G_i proteins to *inhibit* adenylate cyclase; these include D_2, D_3, and D_4). Most pharmacological studies have been performed using agonists and antagonists of D_1, D_2, and D_3 receptors, mainly because agents that are selective for these receptors are available. D_1 and D_2 receptors are widely distributed throughout the mesocorticolimbic and nigrostriatal dopamine systems. D_3 receptors are localized to more specific subregions of the terminals of the mesocorticolimbic dopamine system in the rat, namely the shell subdivision of the nucleus accumbens and the Islands of Calleja.

Norepinephrine

Norepinephrine (also known as noradrenaline) is widely distributed in the central nervous system. It is involved in arousal, attention, stress, anxiety, and mood disorders. Cell bodies for norepinephrine in the brain originate in the dorsal pons and brainstem (Figure 2.12). The dorsal pons contains the locus coeruleus, which is the source of the dorsal noradrenergic pathway to the cortices and hippocampus. The brainstem projections converge in the ventral noradrenergic bundle to innervate or activate the basal forebrain and hypothalamus. Norepinephrine, particularly in the forebrain, is released in the brain during stressful events and plays an important role in the anxiety/stress-like responses associated with drug dependence. Noradrenergic projections from the locus coeruleus play a key role in maintaining attentional homeostasis (regulating arousal/attention setpoint). For example, both increases and decreases in the activity of norepinephrine in the locus coeruleus are associated with disruptions in working memory.

Norepinephrine binds to three distinct receptors: α_1, α_2, and β. The α receptor subtypes are coupled to the inositol phosphate second messenger system via G_q proteins, or they inhibit adenylate cyclase by coupling to the inhibitory G_i protein. The β receptor subtype activates adenylate cyclase by coupling to the G_s protein.

Opioid Peptides

Opioid peptides – β-endorphin, enkephalin, and dynorphin – are the endogenous ligands that naturally exist in the body and activate opioid receptors. Both *opiate* and *opioid* drugs bind to the same opioid receptor. An *opiate* is an alkaloid that resembles morphine and is derived from the opium poppy. An *opioid* is any drug (whether synthetic, semisynthetic, or endogenous) that binds to opioid receptors and has morphine-like effects. There are three types of opioid receptors: μ (mu), δ (delta), and κ (kappa).

Opioids have profound analgesic effects and rewarding properties. As such, they have both high medical use potential and high abuse potential. The analgesic effects of opioids are mediated by all three types of receptors. Their rewarding

Norepinephrine

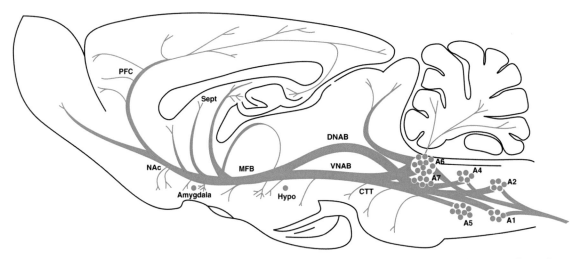

FIGURE 2.12 **Norepinephrine localization.** Origin and distribution of central noradrenergic pathways in the rat brain. PFC, prefrontal cortex; Sept, septum; NAc, nucleus accumbens; MFB, medial forebrain bundle; Hypo, hypothalamus; DNAB, dorsal noradrenergic ascending bundle; VNAB, ventral noradrenergic ascending bundle; CTT, central tegmental tract. *[Modified with permission from Robbins TW, Everitt BJ. Central norepinephrine neurons and behavior. In: Bloom FE, Kupfer DJ (eds.) Psychopharmacology: The Fourth Generation of Progress. New York, Raven Press, 1995, pp. 363–372.]*

effects and dependence and addiction liability, however, are all largely mediated by the μ receptor.

β-endorphin, the endogenous ligand for μ opioid receptors, is largely derived from proopiomelanocortin cells in the arcuate nucleus in the brain. It is distributed throughout the brainstem and basal forebrain and released from corticotropes in the anterior lobe of the pituitary.

Methionine and leucine enkephalins are endogenous ligands for δ opioid receptors. They are derived from the proenkephalin gene and have a widespread distribution in the basal forebrain, including the basal ganglia and midbrain, such as the periaqueductal gray.

Dynorphins can bind to all three opioid receptor subtypes but show a preference for κ receptors. They are derived from the prodynorphin precursor and contain the leucine (leu)-enkephalin sequence at the N-terminal portion of the molecule. Dynorphins are widely distributed in the central nervous system and play important roles in neuroendocrine regulation, pain regulation, motor activity, cardiovascular function, respiration, temperature regulation, feeding behavior, and stress responsivity. Dynorphin cell bodies and axon terminals are heavily localized to the central nucleus of the amygdala, bed nucleus of the stria terminalis, and nucleus accumbens shell (Figure 2.13). Activation of the dynorphin-κ receptor system produces actions that are similar to other opioids, such as analgesia, but the actions are often opposite to those of μ opioid receptors in the motivational domain. For example, μ agonists cause euphoria-like effects, and κ agonists produce dysphoric-like effects in animals and humans. Some evidence suggests that they also mediate negative emotional states. As a link between dopaminergic and opioidergic systems, dopamine D_1 receptor activation in the nucleus accumbens shell can phosphorylate (turn on) cyclic adenosine monophosphate response element binding protein (CREB) and subsequently alter gene expression, notably the transcription of protachykinin and prodynorphin. Such activation of dynorphin systems has been suggested to contribute

to the dysphoric-like syndrome associated with cocaine dependence and feedback to decrease dopamine release. Such enhanced dynorphin action may also drive corticotropin-releasing factor (a key neurotransmitter in the stress system) responses or be driven by activation of this stress hormone (see Chapter 4).

Corticotropin-Releasing Factor

Stress is a major factor in drug relapse, and corticotropin-releasing factor (CRF) is key to the body's stress response. A large, 41-amino-acid polypeptide with a wide distribution throughout the brain, CRF cell bodies are prominent in the paraventricular nucleus of the hypothalamus, basal forebrain (notably the extended amygdala), and brainstem (Figure 2.14). When CRF is administered directly into rodents, it mimics behavioral activation and the stress response, and CRF receptor antagonists generally have anti-stress effects.

Two major CRF receptors have been identified: CRF_1 and CRF_2. CRF_1 receptor activation is associated with activation of the hypothalamic–pituitary–adrenal (HPA) axis neuroendocrine response to stress and increased stress responsiveness at the behavioral and physiological (autonomic) extrahypothalamically (outside the HPA axis). The HPA axis is a term that describes the relationship between direct releasing factor/hormonal actions and feedback between the hypothalamus, pituitary gland, and adrenal gland. CRF_2 receptor activation is associated with decreased feeding behavior and decreased stress responsiveness, although there is some controversy in this area. Both CRF receptor subtypes belong to a subfamily of G-protein-coupled receptors. CRF itself has preferential affinity for CRF_1 rather than CRF_2 receptors. Other CRF-related neuropeptides include urocortins, and some of these preferentially bind CRF_2 receptors. The distribution of CRF_1 receptors in the brain is highly consistent across mammalian species in stress-responsive brain regions, including the neocortex, central

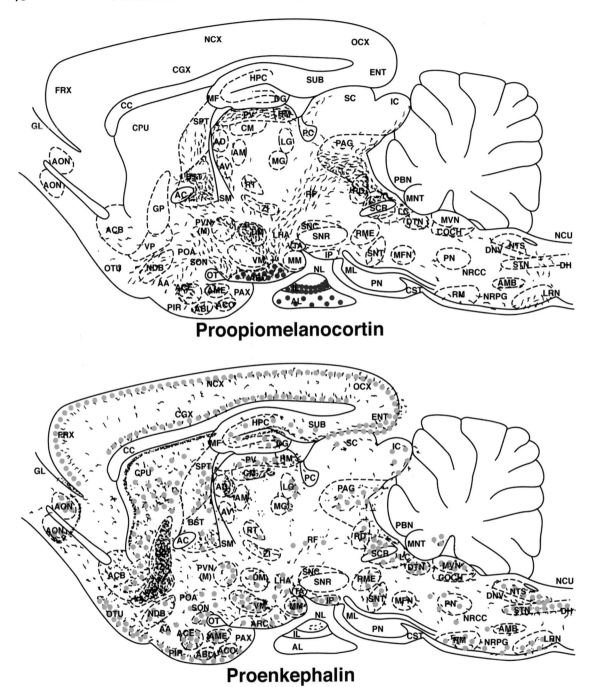

FIGURE 2.13 Dynorphin localization. Schematic representation of the distribution of prodynorphin-derived peptides in the rat's central nervous system determined by immunohistochemistry. Prodynorphin codes for several active opioid peptides containing the sequence of [Leu]enkephalin, including dynorphin A, dynorphin B, and α-neoendorphin. This precursor

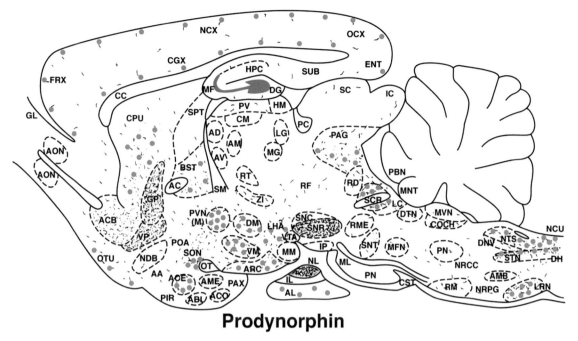

Prodynorphin

FIGURE 2.13 Cont'd

is distributed in neuronal systems found at all levels of the neuraxis. Like their proenkephalin counterparts, the prodynorphin neurons form both short- and long-tract projections often found in parallel with the proenkephalin systems. Neuronal peri-karya are shown as solid circles, and fiber-terminals are shown as short curved lines and dots. AA, anterior amygdala; ABL, basolateral nucleus of amygdala; AC, anterior commissure; ACB, nucleus accumbens; ACE, central nucleus of the amygdala; ACO, cortical nucleus of amygdala; AD, anterodorsal nucleus of thalamus; AL, anterior lobe of pituitary; AM, anteromedial nucleus of thalamus; AMB, nucleus ambiguus; AME, medial nucleus of the amygdala; AON, anterior olfactory nucleus; ARC, arcuate nucleus; AV, anteroventral nucleus of thalamus; BST, bed nucleus of the stria terminalis; CC, corpus callosum; CGX, cingulate cortex; CM, central-medial nucleus of thalamus; COCH, cochlear nuclear complex; CPU, caudate-putamen; CST, corticospinal tract; DH, dorsal horn of spinal cord; DG, dentate gyrus; DM, dorsomedial nucleus of hypothalamus; DNV, dorsal motor nucleus of vagus; DTN, dorsal tegmental nucleus; ENT, entorhinal cortex; FN, fastigial nucleus of cerebellum; FRX, frontal cortex; GL, glomerular layer of olfactory bulb; GP, globus pallidus; HM, medial habenular nucleus; HPC, hip-pocampus; IC, inferior colliculus; IL, intermediate lobe of pituitary; IP, interpeduncular nuclear complex; LC, nucleus locus coeruleus; LG, lateral geniculate nucleus; LHA, lateral hypothalamic area; LRN, lateral reticular nucleus; MF, mossy fibers of hippocampus; MFN, motor facial nucleus; MG, medial geniculate nucleus; ML, medial lemniscus; MM, medial mammil-lary nucleus; MNT, mesencephalic nucleus of trigeminal; MVN, medial vestibular nucleus; NCU, nucleus cuneatus; NCX, neocortex; NDB, nucleus of diagonal band; NL, neural lobe of pituitary; NRGC, nucleus reticularis gigantocellularis; NRPG, nucleus reticularis paragigantocellularis; NTS, nucleus tractus solitarius; OCX, occipital cortex; OT, optic tract; OTU, olfac-tory tubercle; PAG, periaqueductal gray; PAX, periamygdaloid cortex; PBN, parabrachial nucleus; PC, posterior commissure; PIR, piriform cortex; PN, pons; POA, preoptic area; PP, perforant path; PV, periventricular nucleus of thalamus; PVN(M), paraventricular nucleus (pars magnocellularis); PVN(P), paraventricular nucleus (pars parvocellularis); RD, nucleus raphe dorsalis; RE, nucleus reuniens of thalamus; RF, reticular formation; RM, nucleus raphe magnus; RME, nucleus raphe media-nus; SC, superior colliculus; SCP, superior cerebellar peduncle; SM, stria medullaris thalami; SNC, substantia nigra (pars compacta); SNR, substantia nigra (pars reticulata); SNT, sensory nucleus of trigeminal (main); SON, supraoptic nucleus; SPT, septal nuclei; STN, spinal nucleus of trigeminal; SUB, subiculum; VM, ventromedial nucleus of hypothalamus; VP, ventral pallidum; ZI, zona incerta. *[Modified with permission from Khachaturian H, Lewis ME, Schafer MKH, Watson SJ. Anatomy of the CNS opioid systems.* Trends in Neurosciences, *1985, (8), 111–119.]*

Corticotropin-Releasing Factor

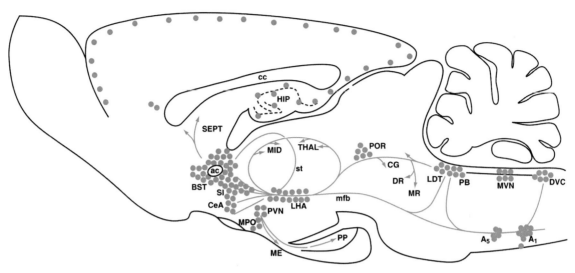

FIGURE 2.14 **Corticotropin-releasing factor localization.** The major CRF-stained cell groups (dots) and fiber systems in the rat brain. Most of the immunoreactive cells and fibers appear to be associated with systems that regulate the output of the pituitary and autonomic nervous system and with cortical interneurons. Most of the longer central fibers course either ventrally through the medial forebrain bundle and its caudal extension in the reticular formation, or dorsally through a periventricular system in the thalamus and brainstem central gray. The direction of fibers in these systems is unclear because they appear to interconnect regions that contain CRF-stained cell bodies. Three adjacent CRF-stained cell groups – laterodorsal tegmental nucleus, locus coeruleus, parabrachial nucleus – lie in the dorsal pons. It is uncertain which of these cell groups contributes to each of the pathways shown and which of them receives inputs from the same pathways. ac, anterior commissure; BST, bed nucleus of the stria terminalis; cc, corpus callosum; CeA, central nucleus of the amygdala; CG, central gray; DR, dorsal raphe; DVC, dorsal vagal complex; HIP; hippocampus; LDT, laterodorsal tegmental nucleus; LHA; lateral hypothalamic area; ME; median eminence; mfb, medial forebrain bundle; MID THAL, midline thalamic nuclei; MPO, medial preoptic area; MR, median raphe; MVN, medial vestibular nucleus; PB, parabrachial nucleus; POR, perioculomotor nucleus; PP, peripeduncular nucleus; PVN, paraventricular nucleus; SEPT, septal region; SI, substantia innominata; st, stria terminalis. *[Modified with permission from Swanson LW, Sawchenko PE, Rivier J, Vale W. Organization of ovine corticotropin-releasing factor immunoreactive cells and fibers in the rat brain: an immunohistochemical study. Neuroendocrinology, 1983, (36), 165–186.]*

division of the extended amygdala, medial septum, hippocampus, hypothalamus, thalamus, cerebellum, and autonomic midbrain and hindbrain nuclei. This receptor distribution, concordant with its natural ligand CRF, is consistent with the role for CRF_1 receptors outside the HPA axis in behavioral and physiological (autonomic) stress responses.

Vasopressin

Vasopressin has an hormonal function as an antidiuretic hormone that helps control water balance in the body. It is derived from the posterior pituitary within the HPA axis but also has extrahypothalamic actions in the central nervous system. Vasopressin is distributed widely in the brain outside of the HPA axis, with the highest concentrations in the suprachiasmatic and supraoptic nuclei and substantial levels in the septum and locus coeruleus. Vasopressin neurons innervate the extended amygdala and are derived from cell bodies in the medial bed nucleus of the stria terminalis. The distribution of vasopressin receptors is prominent in the rat's extended amygdala, with high concentrations

Vasopressin

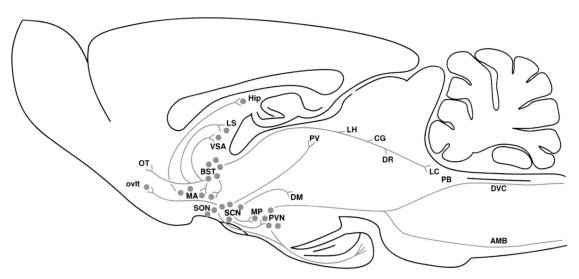

FIGURE 2.15 **Vasopressin localization.** Schematic of the most prominent vasopressin-immunoreactive projections. AMB, ambiguus nucleus; BST, bed nucleus of the stria terminalis; CG, midbrain central gray; DM, dorsomedial nucleus of the hypothalamus; DR, dorsal raphe nucleus; DVC, dorsal vagal complex; HIP, ventral hippocampus; LC, locus coeruleus; LH; lateral habenular nucleus; LS; lateral septum; MA, medial nucleus of the amygdala; MP; medial preoptic area; OT, olfactory tubercle; ovlt; organum vasculosum laminae terminalis; PB, parabrachial nucleus; PV, periventricular nucleus of the hypothalamus; PVN, paraventricular nucleus; SCN, suprachiasmatic nucleus; SON, supraoptic nucleus; VSA, ventral septal area. *[Modified with permission from de Vries GJ, Miller MA. Anatomy and function of extrahypothalamic vasopressin systems in the brain. In: Urban IJA, Burbach JPH, de Wied D (eds.)* Advances in Brain Vasopressin *(series title:* Progress in Brain Research, *vol 119). Elsevier, New York, 1998, pp. 3–20.]*

in the lateral and supracapsular bed nucleus of the stria terminalis, central nucleus of the amygdala, and nucleus accumbens shell. Vasopressin produces autonomic arousal-promoting effects in brain structures relevant to memory, including the hippocampus. Vasopressin V_{1b} receptor antagonists have been shown to produce anxiolytic-like and antidepressant-like effects in animal models, and such anxiolytic-like actions were shown to be localized to the amygdala (Figure 2.15).

Neuropeptide Y

Neuropeptide Y (NPY) is a 36-amino-acid polypeptide that is also widely distributed throughout the central nervous system, with particularly high concentrations in the hypothalamus, periaqueductal gray, and extended amygdala (Figure 2.16). Administration of NPY directly into the brain increases feeding behavior, reduces anxiety-like behavior, and augments the effects of sedative hypnotics. The amygdala is a possible site that mediates the anti-stress effects of NPY. Multiple NPY receptor subtypes have been identified, and the Y_1 and Y_2 receptors have been the most implicated in stress actions. The Y_1 receptor has a wide distribution in the rat brain. It is found most abundantly in the cortex, olfactory tubercle, hippocampus, hypothalamus, and thalamus. The distribution of Y_2 receptors is similar to that of the Y_1 receptors, although Y_2 receptors are less abundant in the cortex and thalamus and more abundant in the hippocampus.

Neuropeptide Y

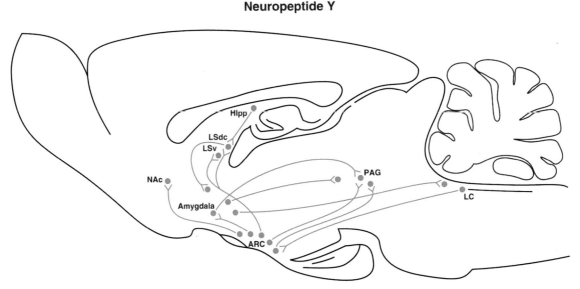

FIGURE 2.16 **Neuropeptide Y localization.** Pathways hypothesized to be involved in NPY effects related to stress and emotionality. ARC, arcuate nucleus; Hipp, hippocampus; LC, locus coeruleus; LSdc, lateral septum-dorsocaudal; LSv, lateral septum-ventral; NAc, nucleus accumbens; PAG, periaqueductal gray matter. *[Modified with permission from Heilig M. The NPY system in stress, anxiety and depression.* Neuropeptides, *2004, (38), 213–224.]*

Nociceptin

Nociceptin (also known as orphanin FQ) is a 17-amino-acid polypeptide that is structurally related to the opioid peptide dynorphin A. It is the endogenous ligand for the nociceptin opioid (NOP) receptor (formerly referred to as opioid receptor-like-1). Nociceptin does not bind to μ, δ, or κ opioid receptors, and no known exogenous or endogenous opioids bind to the NOP receptor. The neuroanatomical distribution of nociceptin and its receptor are distinct from other opioid peptides. The highest density of nociceptin and the NOP receptor is in the cortex, amygdala, bed nucleus of the stria terminalis, medial prefrontal cortex, ventral tegmental area, lateral hypothalamus, nucleus accumbens, and many brainstem areas, including the locus coeruleus and raphe (Figure 2.17).

NOP receptor agonists and antagonists have numerous functional effects that are related to anxiety-like and stress-like states. Nociceptin blocks stress-induced analgesia triggered by the release of endogenous opioids. Nociceptin generally attenuates adaptive behaviors to stress, such as opioid and non-opioid stress-induced analgesia and stress-induced anorexia. Nociceptin and small-molecule synthetic nociceptin analogs have a broad anxiolytic-like profile in animals and also reverse stress-induced anorexia. Nociceptin may play a role in the addiction process that is independent of any classic opioid action. Nociceptin and synthetic NOP receptor agonists decrease the acute rewarding effects of drugs of abuse in the conditioned place preference paradigm. They also block alcohol consumption in a genetically selected line of rats that is known to be hypersensitive to stressors and decrease reinstatement of drug seeking behavior.

Nociceptin/Orphanin FQ

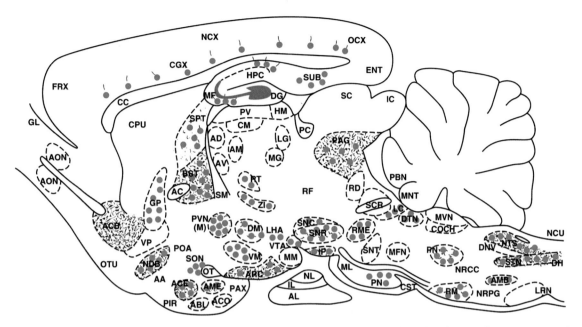

FIGURE 2.17 **Nociceptin/orphanin FQ localization.** Schematic representation of the distribution of nociceptin peptide in the rat central nervous system determined by immunohistochemistry and *in situ* hybridization. Neuronal perikarya are shown as solid circles, and fiber-terminals are shown as short curved lines and dots. AA, anterior amygdala; ABL, basolateral nucleus of amygdala; AC, anterior commissure; ACB, nucleus accumbens; ACE, central nucleus of the amygdala; ACO, cortical nucleus of amygdala; AD, anterodorsal nucleus of thalamus; AL, anterior lobe of pituitary; AM, anteromedial nucleus of thalamus; AMB, nucleus ambiguus; AME, medial nucleus of the amygdala; AON, anterior olfactory nucleus; ARC, arcuate nucleus; AV, anteroventral nucleus of thalamus; BST, bed nucleus of the stria terminalis; CC, corpus callosum; CGX, cingulate cortex; CM, central-medial nucleus of thalamus; COCH, cochlear nuclear complex; CPU, caudate-putamen; CST, corticospinal tract; DH, dorsal horn of spinal cord; DG, dentate gyrus; DM, dorsomedial nucleus of hypothalamus; DNV, dorsal motor nucleus of vagus; DTN, dorsal tegmental nucleus; ENT, entorhinal cortex; FN, fastigial nucleus of cerebellum; FRX, frontal cortex; GL, glomerular layer of olfactory bulb; GP, globus pallidus; HM, medial habenular nucleus; HPC, hippocampus; IC, inferior colliculus; IL, intermediate lobe of pituitary; IP, interpeduncular nuclear complex; LC, nucleus locus coeruleus; LG, lateral geniculate nucleus; LHA, lateral hypothalamic area; LRN, lateral reticular nucleus; MF, mossy fibers of hippocampus; MFN, motor facial nucleus; MG, medial geniculate nucleus; ML, medial lemniscus; MM, medial mammillary nucleus; MNT, mesencephalic nucleus of trigeminal; MVN, medial vestibular nucleus; NCU, nucleus cuneatus; NCX, neocortex; NDB, nucleus of diagonal band; NL, neural lobe of pituitary; NRGC, nucleus reticularis gigantocellularis; NRPG, nucleus reticularis paragigantocellularis; NTS, nucleus tractus solitarius; OCX, occipital cortex; OT, optic tract; OTU, olfactory tubercle; PAG, periaqueductal gray; PAX, periamygdaloid cortex; PBN, parabrachial nucleus; PC, posterior commissure; PIR, piriform cortex; PN, pons; POA, preoptic area; PP, perforant path; PV, periventricular nucleus of thalamus; PVN(M), paraventricular nucleus (pars magnocellularis); PVN(P), paraventricular nucleus (pars parvocellularis); RD, nucleus raphe dorsalis; RE, nucleus reuniens of thalamus; RF, reticular formation; RM, nucleus raphe magnus; RME, nucleus raphe medianus; SC, superior colliculus; SCP, superior cerebellar peduncle; SM, stria medullaris thalami; SNC, substantia nigra (pars compacta); SNR, substantia nigra (pars reticulata); SNT, sensory nucleus of trigeminal (main); SON, supraoptic nucleus; SPT, septal nuclei; STN, spinal nucleus of trigeminal; SUB, subiculum; VM, ventromedial nucleus of hypothalamus; VP, ventral pallidum; ZI, zona incerta. *[Taken with permission from Koob GF. A role for brain stress systems in addiction.* Neuron, *2008, (59), 11–34.]*

BRAIN STRUCTURES AND FUNCTIONS RELEVANT TO THE THREE STAGES OF THE ADDICTION CYCLE

As described in Chapter 1, a three-stage framework can be used to explore the behavioral, neurobiological, and treatment perspectives of addiction: *binge/intoxication, withdrawal/ negative affect*, and *preoccupation/anticipation*. One can also utilize this framework to understand the basic neuroanatomy and neurocircuitry of addiction.

Binge/Intoxication Stage – Basal Ganglia

The *binge/intoxication* stage heavily involves the basal ganglia. The basal ganglia are considered a key part of the extrapyramidal motor system and are historically associated with a number of key functions, including voluntary motor control, procedural learning related to routine behaviors or habits, and action selection. The basal ganglia include the following structures: striatum, globus pallidus, substantia nigra, and subthalamic nucleus (Figure 2.18). The striatum can be further divided into the ventral striatum and dorsal striatum. The ventral striatum includes the nucleus accumbens, olfactory tubercle, and ventral pallidum. This is a subarea of the basal ganglia that has gained recognition for its involvement in motivation and reward function. The ventral striatum is now considered a major integrative center for converting motivation to action. In the domain of addiction, it mediates the rewarding effects of drugs of abuse. The basal ganglia receive neurochemical inputs (or afferents) from the prefrontal cortex and midbrain dopamine system. They then send neurochemical signals (or efferents) from the globus pallidus to the thalamus, which then relays motor and sensory signals to the cerebral cortex. The functions of the basal ganglia involve a series of cortical–striatal–pallidal–thalamic–cortical loops that encode habits related to compulsive behavior (Figure 2.19).

Positive reinforcement with drugs of abuse occurs when presentation of a drug increases the probability of a response to obtain the drug and usually refers to producing a positive hedonic state. Animal models of the positive reinforcing or rewarding effects of drugs in the absence of withdrawal or deprivation are extensive and well validated. These models include intravenous drug self-administration, conditioned place preference, and decreased brain stimulation reward thresholds (see Chapter 3, Animal Models).

The acute reinforcing effects of drugs of abuse are mediated by brain structures connected by the medial forebrain bundle reward system, with a focus on the ventral tegmental area, nucleus accumbens, and amygdala. Much evidence supports the hypothesis that the mesocorticolimbic dopamine system, projecting from the ventral tegmental area to the nucleus accumbens, is dramatically activated by psychostimulant drugs during limited-access self-administration. This system is critical for mediating the rewarding effects of cocaine, amphetamines, and nicotine. However, although acute administration of other drugs of abuse activates the dopamine systems, opioids and alcohol have both dopamine-dependent and -independent rewarding effects (Figure 2.20). μ opioid receptors in both the nucleus accumbens and ventral tegmental area mediate the reinforcing effects of opioid drugs. Opioid peptides in the ventral striatum and amygdala mediate the acute reinforcing effects of alcohol, largely observed experimentally through the effects of opioid antagonists and in knockout mice. γ-Aminobutyric acid (GABA) systems are activated pre- and postsynaptically in the extended amygdala by alcohol at intoxicating doses, and GABA receptor antagonists block alcohol self-administration. A specific nicotinic receptor, the $\alpha_4\beta_2$ subtype, either in the ventral tegmental area or nucleus accumbens, mediates the reinforcing effects of nicotine

Neurobiology of Addiction: Binge/Intoxication Stage

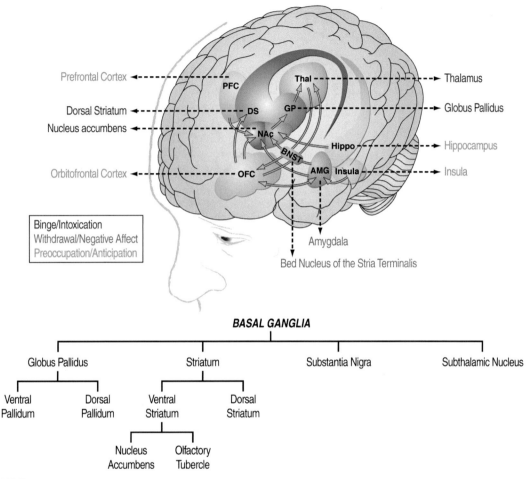

FIGURE 2.18 **Brain regions recruited during the *binge/intoxication* stage of the addiction cycle.** *[Modified with permission from Koob GF, Volkow ND. Neurocircuitry of addiction. Neuropsychopharmacology Reviews, 2010, (35), 217–238 (erratum: 35: 1051).]*

via actions on the mesocorticolimbic dopamine system. The cannabinoid CB_1 receptor, involving the activation of dopamine and opioid peptides in the ventral tegmental area and nucleus accumbens, mediates the reinforcing actions of marijuana.

Drugs of abuse have a profound effect on the response to previously neutral stimuli to which the drugs become paired; a phenomenon called conditional reinforcement and now linked with

the concept of "incentive salience." Psychostimulants caused rats to show compulsive-like lever pressing in response to a cue that was previously paired with a water reward (for further reading of this seminal finding, see Robbins, 1976).

In a subsequent series of studies that recorded the electrical activity of ventral tegmental area dopamine neurons in primates during repeated presentation of rewards and presentation of stimuli associated with

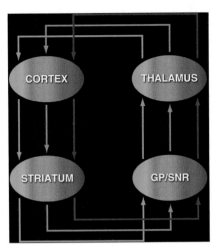

FIGURE 2.19 **Functional topography of cortico-basal ganglia-thalamocortical circuits.** Each color represents a different function. Each functional region of the cortex projects to a specific region of the striatum, represented by the same color. The striatum projects to a specific region of the globus pallidus/substantia nigra pars reticulata, also represented by the same color. The globus pallidus/substantia nigra pars reticulata projects to a specific thalamic region and back to the cortical region of origin. *[Taken with permission from Haber S, McFarland NR. The place of the thalamus in frontal cortical-basal ganglia circuits.* Neuroscientist, 2001, (7), 315–324.]

reward, dopamine cells fired at the first exposure to the novel reward, but repeated exposure caused the neurons to stop firing during reward consumption and instead fire when they were exposed to stimuli that were *predictive* of the reward (for further reading, see Schultz et al., 1997). Through the process of conditioning, previously neutral stimuli are linked to either a natural or drug reinforcer and acquire the ability to increase dopamine levels in the nucleus accumbens in anticipation of the reward, thus engendering strong motivation to seek the drug, termed incentive salience.

As noted previously, all drugs of abuse can initially elicit increased physiological dopamine release in the nucleus accumbens. This drug-induced dopamine signaling can eventually trigger neuroadaptations in other basal ganglia brain circuits that are related to habit formation. Key synaptic changes involve glutamate-modulated N-methyl-D-aspartate (NMDA) receptors and α-amino-3-hydroxy-5-methyl-4-isoxazolepropionic acid (AMPA) receptors in glutamatergic projections from the prefrontal cortex and amygdala to the ventral tegmental area and nucleus accumbens (for further reading, see Kalivas, 2009; Lüscher and Malenka, 2011; Wolf and Ferrario, 2010). The power of initial dopamine release (and activation of opioid peptide systems) upon initial drug taking begins the neuroadaptations that lead to tolerance and withdrawal and triggers the ability of drug-associated cues to increase dopamine levels in the dorsal striatum, a region that is involved in habit formation (for further reading, see Belin et al., 2009) and the strengthening of those habits as addiction progresses. The recruitment of these circuits is significant for the progression through the addiction cycle because such conditioned responses help explain the intense desire for the drug (craving) and its compulsive use when subjects with addiction are exposed to drug cues. Conditioned responses within the incentive salience process can drive dopamine signaling to maintain the motivation to take the drug even when the direct pharmacological effects of the drug lessen.

Withdrawal/Negative Affect Stage – Extended Amygdala

The *withdrawal/negative affect* stage involves key elements of the extended amygdala. The extended amygdala consists primarily of three structures: the central nucleus of the amygdala, bed nucleus of the stria terminalis, and a transition zone in the nucleus accumbens shell (for those interested in learning more about the anatomy of this structure, see Alheid et al., 1995). The extended amygdala can also be divided into two major divisions: central division and medial division. These two divisions have important anatomical structural differences and dissociable afferent and efferent connections.

The central division of the extended amygdala includes the central nucleus of the amygdala, central sublenticular extended amygdala, lateral bed nucleus of the stria terminalis, and a transition area in the medial and caudal portions of the nucleus accumbens (Figure 2.21). These structures in the central division have similar morphology (structure), immunohistochemistry (proteins associated with neurotransmission), and connectivity, and they receive afferent connections from limbic cortices, the hippocampus, the basolateral amygdala, the

**Converging Acute Actions of Drugs of Abuse on the
Ventral Tegmental Area and Nucleus Accumbens**

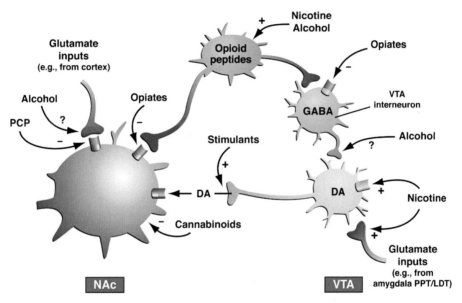

FIGURE 2.20 **Simplified schematic of converging acute actions of drugs of abuse on the ventral tegmental area (VTA) and nucleus accumbens (NAc).** Drugs of abuse, despite diverse initial actions, produce some common effects on the VTA and NAc. Stimulants directly increase dopaminergic transmission in the NAc. Opiates do the same indirectly: they inhibit γ-aminobutyric acid (GABA) interneurons in the VTA, which disinhibits VTA dopamine neurons. Opiates also directly act on opioid receptors on NAc neurons, and opioid receptors, like dopamine (DA) D_2 receptors, signal via G_i proteins. Hence, the two mechanisms converge within some NAc neurons. The actions of the other drugs remain more conjectural. Nicotine seems to activate VTA dopamine neurons directly by stimulating nicotinic cholinergic receptors on those neurons and indirectly by stimulating its receptors on glutamatergic nerve terminals that innervate dopamine cells. Alcohol, by promoting $GABA_A$ receptor function, may inhibit GABAergic terminals in the VTA and hence disinhibit VTA dopamine neurons. It may similarly inhibit glutamatergic terminals that innervate NAc neurons. Many additional mechanisms (not shown) are proposed for alcohol. Cannabinoid mechanisms seem complex, and they involve the activation of cannabinoid CB_1 receptors (which, like D_2 and opioid receptors, are G_i-linked) on glutamatergic and GABAergic nerve terminals in the NAc and on NAc neurons themselves. Phencyclidine (PCP) may act by inhibiting postsynaptic NMDA glutamate receptors in the NAc. Finally, there is some evidence that nicotine and alcohol may activate endogenous opioid pathways and that these and other drugs of abuse (such as opiates) may activate endogenous cannabinoid pathways (not shown). PPT/LDT, peduncular pontine tegmentum/lateral dorsal tegmentum. *[Modified with permission from Nestler EJ. Is there a common molecular pathway for addiction?* Nature Neuroscience, *2005, (8), 1445–1449.]*

midbrain, and the lateral hypothalamus. The efferent connections from this complex include the posterior medial (sublenticular) ventral pallidum, ventral tegmental area, various brainstem projections, and a considerable projection to the lateral hypothalamus. The extended amygdala includes major components of the brain stress systems associated with the negative reinforcement of dependence. The central division has also been found to receive cortical information and regulate the hypothalamic–pituitary–adrenal stress axis.

The medial division of the extended amygdala consists of the medial bed nucleus of the stria terminalis, medial nucleus of the amygdala, and medial sublenticular extended amygdala. It appears to be more involved in

sympathetic (fight-or-flight) and physiological responses and receives olfactory information. Most motivational experimental manipulations that modify the reinforcing effects of drugs of abuse through both positive and negative reinforcement appear to do so by impacting the central division : central nucleus of the amygdala and lateral bed nucleus of the stria terminalis.

Negative reinforcement occurs when the removal of an aversive event increases the probability of a response. In the case of addiction, negative reinforcement involves the removal of a negative emotional state associated with withdrawal, such as dysphoria, anxiety, irritability, sleep disturbances, and hyperkatifeia. Such negative emotional

Neurobiology of Addiction: Withdrawal/Negative Affect Stage

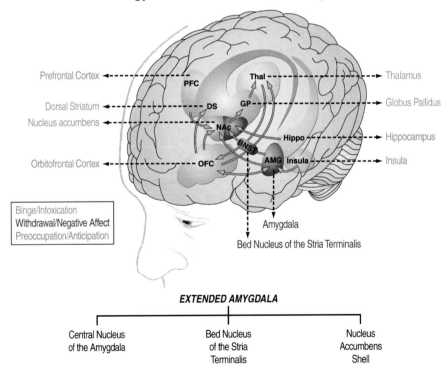

FIGURE 2.21 **Brain regions recruited during the** *withdrawal/negative affect* **stage of the addiction cycle.** *[Modified with permission from Koob GF, Volkow ND. Neurocircuitry of addiction.* Neuropsychopharmacology Reviews, 2010, (35), 217–238 *(erratum: 35: 1051).]*

states are thought to derive from two sources: within-system changes and between-system changes.

- *Within-system neuroadaptations in the reward system.* During the development of dependence, the brain systems in the ventral striatum that are important for the acute reinforcing effects of drugs of abuse, such as dopamine and opioid peptides, become compromised and begin to contribute to a negative reinforcement mechanism, in which the drug is administered to restore the decreased function of the reward systems. Within-system changes within medium spiny neurons in the nucleus accumbens during acute withdrawal include decreased long-term potentiation, increased trafficking of AMPA receptors to the surface of neurons, increased adenylate cyclase activity, and increased CREB phosphorylation. Some of these changes may precede or drive between-system neuroadaptations. Neurochemical evidence of within-system neuroadaptations includes the observation that chronic administration of all drugs of abuse decreases the function of the mesocorticolimbic dopamine system. Decreases in neuronal firing rate in the mesocorticolimbic dopamine system and decreases in serotonergic neurotransmission in the nucleus accumbens occur during drug withdrawal. Decreases in the firing of dopamine neurons in the ventral tegmental area have also been observed during withdrawal from opioids, nicotine, and ethanol. Imaging studies in drug-addicted humans have also consistently shown long-lasting decreases in the number of dopamine D_2 receptors in drug abusers compared with controls. Additionally, drug abusers have reduced dopamine release in response to a pharmacological challenge with drugs. Decreases in the number of dopamine D_2 receptors, coupled with the decrease in

dopaminergic activity in cocaine, nicotine, and alcohol abusers, results in decreased sensitivity of reward (incentive salience) circuits to stimulation by natural reinforcers. These findings suggest an overall reduction of the sensitivity of the dopamine component of reward circuitry to natural reinforcers and other drugs in drug-addicted individuals (Figure 2.22).

- *Between-system neuroadaptations in the extended amygdala.* The neuroanatomical substrates for many of the motivational effects of drug dependence may also involve between-system neuroadaptations that occur in the ventral striatum and extended amygdala, which includes neurotransmitters associated with the brain stress systems involved in the negative reinforcement of dependence. Several neurotransmitters localized to the extended amygdala, such as CRF, norepinephrine, and dynorphin, are activated during states of stress and anxiety and during drug withdrawal (Figure 2.22). Antagonists of these neurochemical systems selectively block drug self-administration in dependent animals, suggesting a key role for these neurotransmitters in the ventral striatum and extended amygdala in the negative reinforcement associated with drug dependence.

To summarize the roles of positive and negative reinforcement in addiction, the brain reward (incentive salience) system is implicated in both the positive reinforcement produced by drugs of abuse and the negative reinforcement produced by dependence, mediated by dopamine in the ventral striatum. Neuropharmacological studies in animal models of addiction have provided evidence of the dysregulation of specific neurochemical mechanisms in specific positive reinforcement (reward) systems in the ventral striatum (dopamine, opioid peptides, and GABA). Importantly, however, brain stress systems (CRF, dynorphin, and norepinephrine)

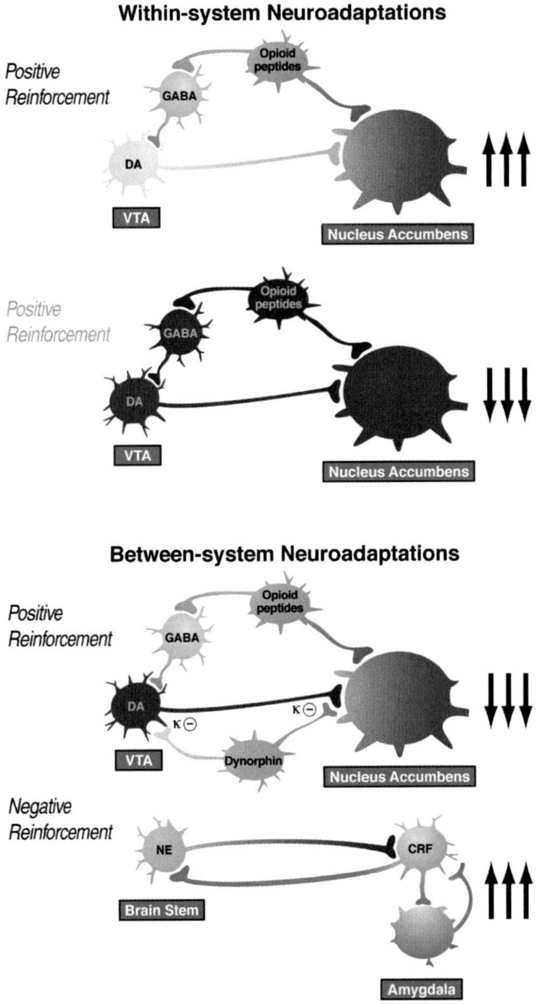

FIGURE 2.22 **Diagram of the hypothetical "within-system" and "between-system" changes that lead to the "dark side" of addiction.** (Top) Circuitry for drug reward with major contributions from mesolimbic dopamine and opioid peptides that converge on the nucleus accumbens. During the *binge/intoxication* stage of the addiction cycle, the reward circuitry is excessively engaged. (Middle) Such excessive activation of the reward system triggers "within-system" neurobiological adaptations during the *withdrawal/negative affect* stage, including activation of cyclic adenosine monophosphate (cAMP) and cAMP response element binding protein (CREB), downregulation of dopamine D$_2$ receptors, and decreased firing of ventral tegmental area (VTA) dopaminergic neurons. (Bottom) As dependence progresses and the *withdrawal/negative affect* stage is repeated, two major "between-system" neuroadaptations occur. One is activation of dynorphin feedback that further decreases dopaminergic activity. The other is recruitment of extrahypothalamic norepinephrine (NE)-corticotropin-releasing factor (CRF) systems in the extended amygdala. Facilitation of the brain stress system in the prefrontal cortex is hypothesized to exacerbate the between-system neuroadaptations while contributing to the persistence of the dark side into the *preoccupation/anticipation* stage of the addiction cycle. *[Taken with permission from Koob GF. Negative reinforcement in drug addiction: the darkness within.* Current Opinion in Neurobiology, *2013, (23), 559–563.]*

are also recruited in the extended amygdala to contribute to the negative motivational state associated with drug abstinence, which in turn drives an additional source of negative reinforcement in drug addiction.

Preoccupation/Anticipation Stage – Prefrontal Cortex

The *preoccupation/anticipation* ("craving") stage involves key elements of the prefrontal cortex. The global function of the prefrontal cortex is to mediate executive function. *Executive function* can be conceptualized as the ability to organize thoughts and activities, prioritize tasks, manage time, and make decisions. To accomplish such complex tasks in the context of the neurobiology of addiction, the prefrontal cortex can be divided into two opposing systems: the Go system and the Stop system. The Go system engages habit systems, possibly even subconsciously and automatically. The Stop system inhibits such systems. The result of the interactions between these two systems produces the well-known impulsivity associated with the addiction process, both during the initiation of drug intake and relapse.

The Go system involves the anterior cingulate cortex and dorsolateral prefrontal cortex. The anterior cingulate cortex facilitates the maintenance and selection of responses, particularly under high attentional demands (like comprehending the information contained in this book), planning (for the midterm exam), self-initiation (getting yourself to class), and self-monitoring of goal-directed behaviors. The functions of the dorsolateral prefrontal cortex involve working memory, planning, and strategy.

The Stop system largely involves the ventrolateral prefrontal cortex and orbitofrontal cortex. The functions of the ventrolateral prefrontal cortex involve response inhibition, sustained attention, memory retrieval, rule generation, and shifting. The functions of the

orbitofrontal cortex, including the ventromedial prefrontal cortex, include the assignment of value (valuation) and integration of reward and punishment (Figure 2.23). The anterior cingulate cortex and dorsolateral prefrontal cortex in humans correspond to the anterior cingulate cortex and prelimbic cortex in rats, and the ventromedial prefrontal cortex and orbitofrontal cortex in humans correspond to the infralimbic cortex and orbitofrontal cortex in rats (Figure 2.24).

The *preoccupation/anticipation* stage of the addiction cycle is a key element of relapse in humans, defining addiction as a chronic relapsing disorder. Although often linked to the construct of craving, the concept of craving *per se* has been difficult to measure in human clinical studies and often does not correlate with relapse. Nevertheless, the stage of the addiction cycle at which an individual reinstates drug seeking behavior after abstinence remains a challenging focus of neurobiological studies and medication development.

Animal models of craving can be divided into two domains:

i) Drug seeking induced by the drug or stimuli paired with drug taking (reward craving), and
ii) Drug seeking induced by an acute stressor or state of stress (relief craving; Table 2.4).

Drug-induced reinstatement appears to be localized to a medial prefrontal cortex/ventral striatum circuit mediated by the neurotransmitter glutamate. Cue-induced reinstatement appears to involve the basolateral amygdala, with a possible feed-forward mechanism that goes through the same prefrontal cortex system involved in drug-induced reinstatement. Neurotransmitter systems involved in drug-induced reinstatement include a glutamate projection from the frontal cortex to nucleus accumbens that is modulated by dopamine in the frontal cortex. Cue-induced reinstatement also involves a glutamate projection from the basolateral amygdala and ventral

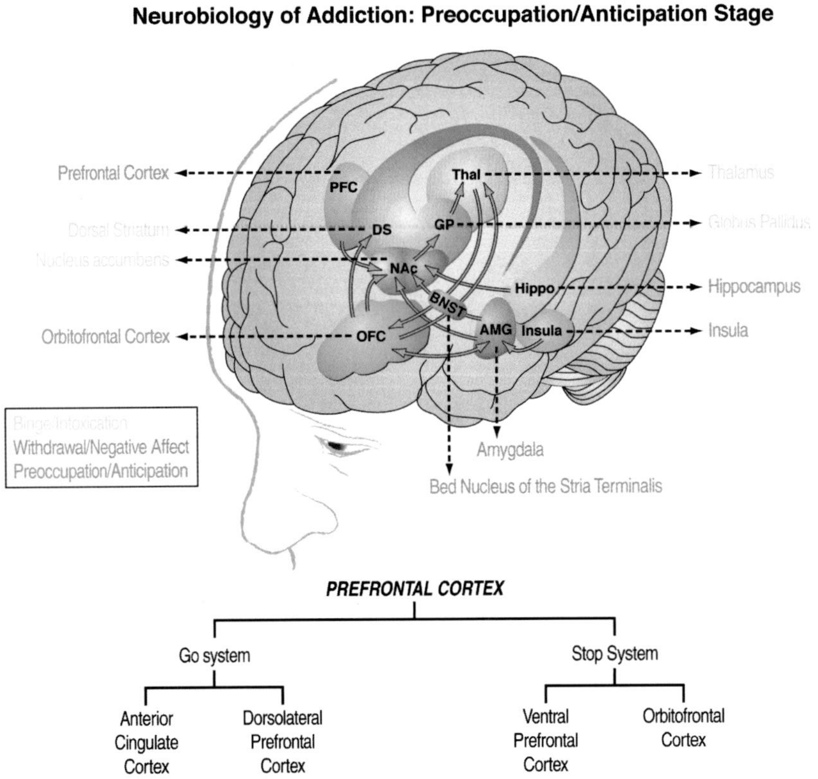

Neurobiology of Addiction: Preoccupation/Anticipation Stage

FIGURE 2.23   **Brain regions recruited during the *preoccupation/anticipation* stage of the addiction cycle.** *[Modified with permission from Koob GF, Volkow ND. Neurocircuitry of addiction.* Neuropsychopharmacology Reviews, 2010, (35), 217–238 *(erratum: 35: 1051).]*

subiculum to the nucleus accumbens. Stress-induced reinstatement depends on activation of both CRF and norepinephrine in the extended amygdala. Protracted abstinence, largely described in alcohol dependence models, involves both an overactive glutamatergic Go system and sensitized CRF systems. Brain CRF stress systems remain hyperactive during protracted abstinence, and this hyperactivity has motivational significance for excessive alcohol drinking.

Executive control over incentive salience is essential to maintain goal-directed behavior and the flexibility of stimulus-response associations. The prefrontal cortex sends glutamatergic projections directly to mesocortical dopamine neurons in the ventral tegmental area, exerting excitatory control on dopamine in the prefrontal cortex. Thus, the ventral part of the prefrontal cortex (the Stop system) can inhibit incentive salience and suppress conditioned behavior when a salient cue is present. It follows that lesions of the prefrontal cortex can induce impulsivity. Withdrawal from alcohol is associated with increased glutamate release in the nucleus accumbens and other brain areas. However, cue-induced reinstatement of psychostimulant-seeking behavior dramatically increases dorsal prefrontal cortex activity (Go system) and glutamate release in the nucleus accumbens. The increased activity of the prefrontal–glutamatergic system during

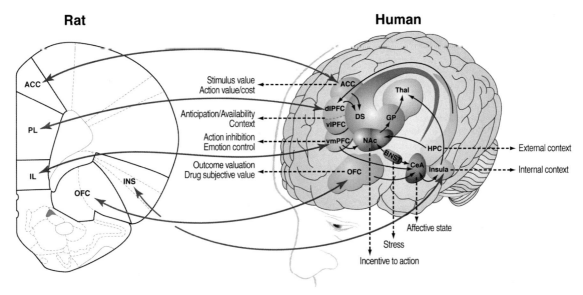

FIGURE 2.24   **Correspondence between rat and human brain regions that are relevant to the addiction process.** Rats are commonly studied to unveil the neurobiological mechanisms of addiction because they have a well-characterized central nervous system whose neurochemical and molecular pathways in subcortical areas correspond reasonably well to those in humans. ACC, anterior cingulate cortex; PL, prelimbic cortex; IL, infralimbic cortex; OFC, orbitofrontal cortex; INS, insula; dlPFC, dorsolateral prefrontal cortex; vlPFC, ventrolateral prefrontal cortex; DS, dorsal striatum; Thal, thalamus; GP, globus pallidus; NAC, nucleus accumbens; BNST, bed nucleus of the stria terminalis; CeA, central nucleus of the amygdala; HPC, hippocampus. *[Modified with permission from George O, Koob GF. Control of craving by the prefrontal cortex. Proceedings of the National Academy of Sciences USA, 2013, (110), 4165–4166.]*

relapse may elicit a dramatic glutamatergic response that may in turn mediate craving-like responses during the *preoccupation/anticipation* stage.

Behavioral procedures have been developed to reinstate drug self-administration using previously neutral stimuli that are paired with alcohol self-administration or that predict alcohol self-administration. Cue-induced reinstatement can by blocked by opioid receptor antagonists, dopamine D_1 and D_2 receptor antagonists, and glutamate receptor antagonists. Stress exposure can also reinstate responding for drugs in rats that are extinguished from drug-seeking behavior. Such stress-induced reinstatement can be blocked by CRF antagonists, dynorphin antagonists, and norepinephrine antagonists.

Human imaging studies reveal similar circuit dysregulation during the *preoccupation/* *anticipation* stage to that demonstrated in animal models. Decreased frontal cortex activity parallels deficits in executive function in neuropsychologically challenging tasks. Individuals with alcoholism exhibit impairments in the maintenance of spatial information, disruption of decision making, and impairments in behavioral inhibition. Such frontal cortex-derived executive function disorders have been linked to the ineffectiveness of some behavioral treatments in individuals with alcoholism. Thus, individual differences in the prefrontal cortical control of incentive salience may also explain individual differences in the vulnerability to addiction. Excessive attribution of incentive salience to drug-related cues and residual hypersensitivity of the brain stress systems may perpetuate excessive drug intake, compulsive behavior, and relapse.

TABLE 2.4   Drug Craving

Drug craving	"Drug craving is the desire for the previously experienced effects of a psychoactive substance. This desire can become compelling and can increase in the presence of both internal and external cues, particularly with perceived substance availability. It is characterized by an increased likelihood of drug-seeking behavior and, in humans, drug-related thoughts." (United Nations International Drug Control Programme. *Informal Expert Group Meeting on the Craving Mechanism* (report no. V92–54439T). United Nations International Drug Control Programme and World Health Organization, Geneva, 1992.)
Reward Craving	• Induced by stimuli that have been paired with drug self-administration such as environmental cues. • Termed conditioned positive reinforcement in experimental psychology. • Animal model: Cue-induced reinstatement where a cue previously paired with access to a drug reinstates responding for a lever that has been extinguished.
Relief Craving	• State of protracted abstinence in drug-dependent individuals weeks after acute withdrawal. • Conceptualized as a state change characterized by anxiety and dysphoria. • Animal model: Residual hypersensitivity to states of stress and environmental stressors that lead to relapse to drug-seeking behavior.

NEUROADAPTATIONAL SUMMARY

Drug addiction involves a three-stage cycle – *binge/intoxication, withdrawal/negative affect,* and *preoccupation/anticipation* – that worsens over time and involves allostatic changes in the brain reward and stress systems. Two primary sources of reinforcement, positive and negative reinforcement, have been hypothesized to play a role in this allostatic process (see Chapter 1).

The construct of negative reinforcement is defined as drug taking that alleviates a negative emotional state. The negative emotional state that drives such negative reinforcement is hypothesized to derive from dysregulation of key neurochemical elements involved in the brain reward and stress systems within the ventral striatum, extended amygdala, and frontal cortex. Specific neurochemical elements in these structures include decreases in reward system function (within-system opponent processes), recruitment of the classic stress axis mediated by CRF in the frontal cortex and extended amygdala, and recruitment of aversive dynorphin-κ opioid systems in the frontal cortex, ventral striatum, and extended amygdala (both between-system opponent processes). Acute withdrawal from all major drugs of abuse increases reward thresholds, decreases mesocorticolimbic dopamine activity, increases anxiety-like responses, increases extracellular levels of CRF in the central nucleus of the amygdala, and increases dynorphin in the ventral striatum. CRF receptor antagonists block anxiety-like responses associated with withdrawal. They also block increases in reward thresholds produced by withdrawal from drugs of abuse and blunt compulsive-like drug taking during extended access.

Excessive activation of dopamine receptors in the nucleus accumbens via the release of mesocorticolimbic dopamine or opioid peptide activation of opioid receptors also activates the dynorphin-κ opioid system, which in turn can decrease dopaminergic activity in the mesocorticolimbic dopamine system. Blockade of the κ opioid system can also block the dysphoric-like effects associated with withdrawal from drugs of abuse and block the development of compulsive-like responding during extended access to drugs of abuse, suggesting another powerful brain stress system that contributes to compulsive drug seeking. Thus, the brain reward systems become compromised, and the brain stress systems become activated by acute excessive drug intake. These changes become sensitized during repeated withdrawal, continue into protracted abstinence, and contribute to the development and persistence of addiction. The loss of reward function and recruitment of brain stress systems provide a powerful neurochemical basis for the negative emotional states that are responsible for the negative reinforcement that drives the compulsivity of addiction. Excessive drug taking also activates CRF in the medial prefrontal cortex, paralleled by deficits in executive function that may facilitate the transition to compulsive-like responding. Dysregulation of the prefrontal cortex can impair executive function and drive impulsivity and help perpetuate disinhibition of the brain stress systems. The combination of the facilitation of incentive salience for drugs, reward dysfunction, stress sensitization, and impaired executive function captures most of the addiction phenotype.

Suggested Reading

Alheid, G.F., De Olmos, J.S., Beltramino, C.A., 1995. Amygdala and extended amygdala. In: Paxinos, G. (Ed.), The Rat Nervos System, second ed. Academic Press, San Diego, pp. 495–578.

Belin, D., Jonkman, S., Dickinson, A., Robbins, T.W., Everitt, B.J., 2009. Parallel and interactive learning processes within the basal ganglia: relevance for the understanding of addiction. Behav. Brain. Res. 199, 89–102.

Clarke, L.E., Barres, B.A., 2013. Emerging roles of astrocytes in neural circuit development. Nat. Rev. Neurosci. 14, 311–321. [erratum: 2013, 14: 451].

Kalivas, P.W., 2009. The glutamate homeostasis hypothesis of addiction. Nat. Rev. Neurosci. 10, 561–572.

Kettenmann, H., Kirchhoff, F., Verkhratsky, A., 2013. Microglia: new roles for the synaptic stripper. Neuron 77, 10–18.

Lüscher, C., Malenka, R.C., 2011. Drug-evoked synaptic plasticity in addiction: from molecular changes to circuit remodeling. Neuron 69, 650–663.

Robbins, T.W., 1976. Relationship between reward-enhancing and stereotypical effects of psychomotor stimulant drugs. Nature 264, 57–59.

Schultz, W., Dayan, P., Montague, P.R., 1997. A neural substrate of prediction and reward. Science 275, 1593–1599.

Schultz, W., 2006. Behavioral theories and the neurophysiology of reward. Annu. Rev. Psychol. 57, 87–115.

Wolf, M.E., Ferrario, C.R., 2010. AMPA receptor plasticity in the nucleus accumbens after repeated exposure to cocaine. Neurosci. Biobehav. Rev. 35, 185–211.

Animal Models of Addiction

The definition of drug addiction to be used in this book draws on several different meanings of drug addiction (see What is Addiction? Chapter 1):

1) Compulsion to seek and take the drug,
2) Loss of control in limiting intake, and
3) Emergence of a negative emotional state (e.g., dysphoria, anxiety, irritability) when access to the drug is prevented.

Much of the recent progress in understanding the mechanisms of addiction has derived from the study of animal models of addiction that use specific drugs, such as opiates, cocaine, and alcohol. No single animal model of addiction fully emulates the human condition, but various models permit researchers to investigate specific elements of the addiction process. Some models evaluate psychological constructs, such as positive and negative reinforcement. Other models evaluate different stages of the addiction cycle, and still others evaluate actual symptoms of addiction from a psychiatric perspective. For the purposes of this chapter, animal models will be categorized based on the three stages of the addiction cycle and the actual psychiatric symptoms of addiction.

Drug addiction can be heuristically characterized as a cycle that includes three stages: (1) *preoccupation/anticipation*, (2) *binge/intoxication*, and (3) *withdrawal/negative affect*. A primary focus of animal studies has been on the central nervous system mechanisms and synaptic sites where drugs of abuse initially act to produce their positive reinforcing effects, but newer, more refined animal models can assess the negative reinforcing effects of dependence and how the central nervous system adapts to drug use.

The constructs of *reinforcement* and *motivation* are crucial parts of all animal models of addiction. The process by which a stimulus increases the probability of a response is termed *reinforcement*. A *reinforcer*, which can be a drug, is any event that increases the probability of a response. This definition can also apply to the definition of *reward*, and the two words are often

used interchangeably. However, *reward* often connotes some additional emotional value, such as pleasure. Multiple powerful sources of reinforcement have been identified during the course of drug addiction research. Positive reinforcement is defined as the presentation of an event that increases the probability of a response. An example is drug seeking in a nondependent individual. Negative reinforcement occurs when the removal of an aversive event increases the probability of a response. One example is a person who self-administers a drug to provide relief from the aversive aspects of drug abstinence or withdrawal.

These sources of reinforcement provide the motivation to compulsively use drugs, with a concomitant loss of control over intake (Wikler, 1973). *Motivation* has several definitions. Donald Hebb defined it as "stimulation that arouses activity of a particular kind" (Hebb, 1949). C.P. Richter stated that "spontaneous activity arises from certain underlying physiological origins and such 'internal' drives are reflected in the amount of general activity" (Richter, 1927). A behavioristic view put forth by Kling and Riggs is that motivation is "the property of energizing of behavior that is proportional to the amount and quality of the reinforcer" (Kling and Riggs, 1971). Dalbir Bindra defined it as a "rough label for the relatively persisting states that make an animal initiate and maintain actions leading to particular outcomes or goals" and went further by defining it from a more neurobehavioral perspective: "[a] set of neural processes that promote actions in relation to a particular class of environmental objects" (Bindra, 1976).

As noted above, the primary pharmacological effect of a drug can produce a direct effect through either positive or negative reinforcement. The secondary pharmacological effects of a drug also can have motivating properties. For example, conditioned positive reinforcement involves the pairing of a previously neutral stimulus, perhaps a particular room or a favorite bar, with the acute positive reinforcing effects of a drug. Conditioned negative reinforcement involves the pairing of a previously neutral stimulus with the aversive stimulus effects of withdrawal or abstinence (Table 3.1).

One approach to the development of animal models that has gained wide acceptance in the research community is that they should have construct validity or predictive validity, in which the model mimics specific signs or symptoms associated with a particular psychopathological condition. Animal models of a complete syndrome of a human psychiatric disorder are unlikely to be possible either conceptually or practically. Certain areas of the human condition are obviously difficult to model in animals, like kleptomania, child abuse, etc. From a practical standpoint, psychiatric disorders are based on a classification of diseases that is complex and constantly evolving. Such disorders often have multiple subtypes and diverse etiologies, and many of them are in fact constellations of many different disorders. Any animal model that attempts to reproduce entire syndromes of the human condition would require multiple endpoints, making the practical study of the underlying mechanisms very difficult.

Under such a framework of mimicking only very precise signs or symptoms of a psychopathological condition, specific "observables" (symptoms that one can observe) that have been identified in addiction provide a focus for animal studies. The reliance of animal models on a given observable also eliminates a fundamental problem associated with animal models of human psychopathology – the frustration of attempting to provide complete validation of an entire syndrome. More definitive information related to a specific domain of addiction can be generated, thus increasing the confidence of cross-species validity. This framework also leads to a more pragmatic approach to the study of the neurobiological mechanisms of the behavior in question.

In the present chapter, these observables are organized under the framework of the *binge/intoxication*, *withdrawal/negative affect*, and *preoccupation/anticipation* (craving) stages of the addiction cycle. Further on in the chapter, however, these observables are linked to the actual criteria for addiction in the *Diagnostic and Statistical Manual of Mental Disorders*, 4th edition (DSM IV), and human clinical laboratory models of addiction. The particular behavioral parameter being assessed in an animal model may or may not be a particular symptom of the disorder, but it still must be defined objectively and observed reliably. The behavior being analyzed may actually be found in both pathological and nonpathological states but still have predictive validity. A good example of such a situation is the widespread, and sometimes misguided, use of drug reinforcement or reward as a definitive animal model of addiction. Drug reinforcement does *not* necessarily lead to addiction. Take, for instance, a social drinker who does not develop alcoholism. Nonetheless, drug self-administration by animals has significant predictive validity for the *binge/intoxication* stage of addiction, and one may confidently state that drug addiction indeed cannot happen without drug reinforcement.

TABLE 3.1 Relationship of Addiction Components and Behavioral Constructs

Addictive Component	Behavioral Construct
Pleasure	Positive reinforcement
Self-medication	Negative reinforcement
Habit	Conditioned positive reinforcement
Habit	Conditioned negative reinforcement

VALIDATION OF ANIMAL MODELS OF DRUG ADDICTION

Animal models are critical for understanding the neuropharmacological mechanisms involved in the development of addiction. As mentioned above, no animal model fully emulates the complete addiction process, but several models do reflect many elements of the syndrome. An animal model can be viewed as an experimental protocol that is used to study a given phenomenon found in humans.

Construct validity refers to the interpretability, "meaningfulness," or explanatory power of a model and incorporates most other measures of validity, in which multiple measures or dimensions are associated with conditions known to affect the construct. This is the most relevant conceptualization of validity for animal models of addiction (Ebel, 1961). An alternative conceptualization of construct validity is the requirement that the model must be functionally equivalent, defined as "assessing how controlling variables influence outcome in the model and the target disorders" (Katz and Higgins, 2003). The most efficient process for evaluating functional equivalence is through common experimental manipulations that should have similar effects in the animal model and the target condition. This process is very similar to the construct *predictive validity* (see below).

Face validity is often the starting point in animal models in which animal syndromes are produced that resemble those found in humans to study specific parts of the human syndrome (McKinney, 1988). For example, rats that intravenously self-administer drugs of abuse show patterns of responding that are identical to those of humans.

Reliability refers to the stability of the model and the consistency with which the dependent variable can be measured. Reliability is said to be achieved when small within- and between-subject variability is found after repeated measurements of the variable, and the phenomenon is readily reproduced under similar circumstances (Geyer and Markou, 2002).

Predictive validity refers to the model's ability to lead to accurate predictions about the human phenomenon based on the animal's response within the model. This type of validity is used most often in animal models of psychiatric disorders to refer to the ability of the model to identify pharmacological agents with potential therapeutic value in humans. However, when predictive validity is more broadly extended to understanding the physiological mechanisms of action of psychiatric disorders, it can incorporate other types of validity – etiological, convergent, concurrent, or discriminant – that are also considered important for the model.

The present chapter describes various animal models that have been shown to be reliable, and in many cases to have construct validity for the various stages of the addiction process, including *binge/intoxication, withdrawal/negative affect,* and *preoccupation/anticipation.*

ANIMAL MODELS OF THE *BINGE/ INTOXICATION* STAGE OF THE ADDICTION CYCLE

Intravenous Drug Self-Administration

Both animals and humans will readily self-administer drugs in the nondependent state. Drugs of abuse have powerful positive reinforcing properties. Animals will perform many different tasks to obtain drugs, even when not dependent. Drugs that have positive reinforcing effects, measured by direct self-administration, lowering of brain stimulation reward thresholds, and conditioned place preference in rodents and primates, correspond very well with the drugs that have high abuse potential in humans, including alcohol, cocaine, and heroin, among many others (Table 3.2).

The animal model of intravenous drug self-administration is a powerful tool for exploring the neurobiology of positive reinforcement. Intravenous cocaine and heroin self-administration in rodents produces a characteristic and predictable pattern of behavior that lends itself to pharmacological and neuropharmacological study. Rats on a simple schedule of continuous reinforcement, such as a fixed-ratio 1 schedule

TABLE 3.2   Animal Models of the *Binge/Intoxication* Stage of the Addiction Cycle

Intravenous and oral drug self-administration

Brain stimulation reward

Conditioned place preference

Drug discrimination

Genetic animal models of high drinking

Drug taking in the presence of aversive consequences

(in which one press of a lever or one nosepoke in a hole results in one drug delivery), will develop a highly stable pattern of drug self-administration in a limited-access situation (Caine et al., 1993; Figure 3.1). If the dose is decreased, then the animals increase their rate of self-administration. Conversely, if the dose is increased, then the animals decrease their rate of self-administration. Thus, experimental manipulations that increase the self-administration rate on this fixed-ratio schedule, such as administering a drug that counteracts the effects the drug of abuse, mimic a decrease in the unit dose and may be interpreted as decreasing the reinforcing potency of the drug under study.

As predicted by this dose-response model, low to moderate doses of dopamine receptor antagonists *increase* cocaine self-administration maintained on a fixed-ratio schedule in a manner that is similar to decreasing the dose of cocaine, suggesting that dopamine receptor antagonism by a dopamine receptor antagonist reduces the reinforcing potency of cocaine. Conversely, dopamine receptor agonists *decrease* cocaine self-administration in a manner similar to increasing the dose of cocaine, suggesting that the combined effects of dopamine receptor agonists and cocaine on self-administration can be additive, perhaps because of their common activation of the same neural substrates.

The use of different schedules of reinforcement (differential delivery of the reinforcer based on time or effort, in which the reinforcer is the discrete delivery of a drug) in intravenous self-administration models can provide an important control for nonspecific effects (that is, effects that are different from the primary endpoints under study, such as increases in exploratory activity and locomotion) and motivational effects, such as a loss of reinforcement efficacy. Such schedules can include progressive-ratio, second-order, and multiple schedules of reinforcement.

To model a measure of reinforcer efficacy for a self-administered drug, researchers can use a progressive-ratio schedule of reinforcement, in which the response requirement (like the number of times the animal has to press a lever) to receive a reinforcer (drug infusion) increases. This type of schedule will determine the *breakpoint* at which an animal will no longer respond to receive the drug. This schedule effectively determines the relative reinforcing strength of different reinforcers, including drugs. The dose-response model discussed above has shown that increasing the unit dose of a self-administered drug will increase an animal's breakpoint on a progressive-ratio schedule. Dopamine receptor antagonists have been shown to decrease the breakpoint for cocaine self-administration (Figure 3.2). To bring such an animal model back to the perspective of the human condition, performance on a progressive-ratio schedule can be linked to the following DSM-5 criterion for addiction: "a great deal of time spent in activities necessary to obtain the substance."

Oral Drug Self-Administration

Oral self-administration almost exclusively involves alcohol because of the obvious face validity. Such animal models include two-bottle choice responding and operant self-administration. Historically, home-cage drinking and preference have been used to characterize genetic differences in drug preference, most often with alcohol, and to explore the effects of pharmacological treatments on drug intake and preference.

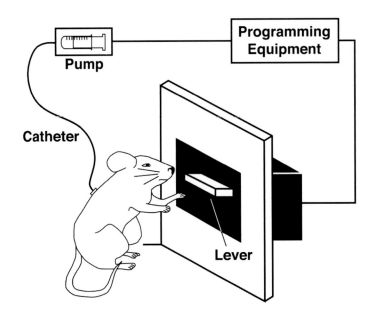

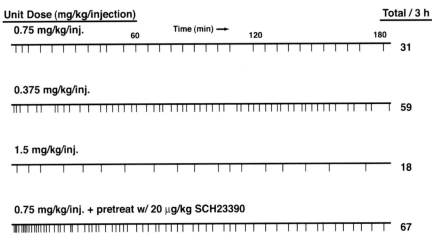

FIGURE 3.1   (*Top*) Drawing describing the procedure for intravenous self-administration in the rat. (*Bottom*) Event record and dose-response relationship relating dose of cocaine to the number of infusions. Rats implanted with intravenous catheters and trained to self-administer cocaine with limited access (3 h/day) will show stable and regular drug intake over each daily session. No obvious tolerance or dependence develops. Rats are generally maintained on a low-requirement, fixed-ratio (FR) schedule for intravenous infusion of the drug, such as an FR1 or FR5. In an FR1 schedule, one lever press is required to deliver one intravenous infusion of cocaine. In an FR5 schedule, five lever presses are required to deliver one infusion of cocaine. A special aspect of using an FR schedule is that the rats appear to regulate the amount of drug that they self-administer. Lowering the dose from the training level of 0.75 mg/kg/injection increases the number of self-administered infusions and *vice versa*. [*Taken with permission from Caine SB, Lintz R, Koob GF. Intravenous drug self-administration techniques in animals. In: Sahgal A (ed) Behavioral Neuroscience: A Practical Approach, vol 2. IRL Press, Oxford, 1993, pp. 117–143.*]

(A)

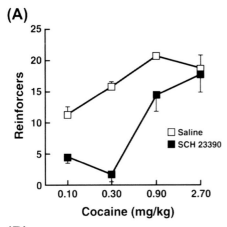

(B)

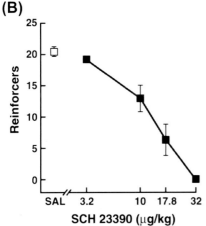

FIGURE 3.2 **Effect of SCH 23390 pretreatment in rats on the number of reinforcers obtained under a progressive-ratio schedule of reinforcement.** (A) Each point represents the average number of reinforcers obtained in a session with saline or SCH 23390 (10 μg/kg, s.c.) pretreatment. (B) Each point represents the average number of reinforcers obtained in a session with subcutaneous pretreatment with saline or SCH 23390. Saline or SCH 23390 was tested against the training dose of cocaine (0.90 mg/kg). *[Taken with permission from Depoortere RY, Li DH, Lane JD, Emmett-Oglesby MW. Parameters of self-administration of cocaine in rats under a progressive-ratio schedule.* Pharmacology Biochemistry and Behavior, *1993, (45), 539–548.]*

In a two-bottle choice procedure, a choice is offered between two bottles: one that contains a drug solution and one that contains alternative solutions (often water). Researchers will then simply measure the weight of each bottle after the experimental session and determine the proportion of drug intake relative to total intake, yielding the preference ratio. For two-bottle choice testing for alcohol in mice and rats, the animals are housed one per cage. The researcher places two bottles in the cage: one that contains alcohol and one that contains water. Most commonly, the animals are allowed free choice between these bottles for successive 24h periods, with simultaneous free access to food.

Two variations of the two-bottle choice procedure can result in binge-like drinking in rodents (see Chapter 1, What is Addiction? for the definition of a *binge*). In the intermittent-access model, originally developed by Wise (1973) and revisited by Simms et al. (2008), rats are given intermittent access to alcohol in a two-bottle choice procedure for 24h on Mondays, Wednesdays, and Fridays; on the intervening days, the rats have no access to alcohol (only water). Rats in the intermittent-access model progressively escalate their alcohol intake over the course of 2–3weeks, reaching blood alcohol levels that are equivalent to human binge drinking (50–100mg%).

A new variant of binge-like drinking in mice is called drinking-in-the-dark, in which mice drink intoxicating amounts of alcohol with limited 2–4h access, beginning 3h after lights out, a time when rodents normally initiate eating and drinking behavior (Rhodes et al., 2005). The mice are initially allowed to drink a 20% alcohol solution under this schedule for three consecutive days. On the fourth day, they are given 4h access, also 3h after lights out. Under such experimental conditions, the mice drink at levels of 80mg% or above.

For operant alcohol self-administration, animals can be trained to lever press for alcohol using a variety of techniques, but first the researchers much overcome the challenge of getting the animals to drink alcohol, which typically has an aversive taste. To do this, the animals are initially given an alcohol solution that contains a specific amount of a sweetener, usually saccharin. This is called a sweetened solution fading procedure. As the animals learn to lever press for alcohol, the amount of sweetener can be gradually faded out, to the point that the animals respond for concentrations up to about 40% (80 proof). Using such a procedure, animals can be trained to perform the operant task on both fixed-ratio and progressive-ratio schedules of reinforcement, obtaining significant blood alcohol levels in a 30 min session (Figure 3.3). The operant oral self-administration of alcohol has also been validated as a measure of the reinforcing effects of alcohol in primates. The advantages of the operant approach are that the effort to obtain the substance can be separated from the consummatory response (e.g., drinking), and intake can easily be charted over time.

Intracranial Self-Stimulation

Researchers have discovered other ways to assess the rewarding or reinforcing effects of various drugs of abuse. One widely used method is called brain stimulation reward (or intracranial self-stimulation [ICSS]). Animals will perform a

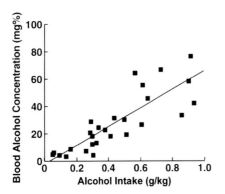

FIGURE 3.3 **Different degrees of alcohol exposure in individual rats that lever-press to obtain a 10% alcohol solution in a free choice operant task, following training with the saccharin fade-out procedure.** *The data were derived from Rassnick S, Pulvirenti L, Koob GF. SDZ 205,152, a novel dopamine receptor agonist, reduces oral ethanol self-administration in rats. Alcohol, 1993, (10), 127–132.*

variety of tasks to self-administer short electrical pulses (approximately 250 ms) directly into many areas of the brain (Olds and Milner, 1954). The brain site that supports the highest rates of self-stimulation is the medial forebrain bundle, which courses bidirectionally from the midbrain to basal forebrain. Several seminal studies found that ICSS directly activates many of the same neuronal circuits that are activated by conventional reinforcers, such as food, water, sex, and drugs, leading many to hypothesize that ICSS studies can reveal the brain systems involved in motivated behavior. The acute administration of drugs of abuse *decreases* ICSS thresholds, in which less electrical stimulation is needed for the animal to perceive the stimulation as rewarding. Conversely, withdrawal from drugs of abuse *increases* reward thresholds, meaning that more stimulation is needed to perceive the stimulation as rewarding. There is good correspondence between the ability of drugs to decrease ICSS thresholds and their abuse potential (Kornetsky and Esposito, 1979; Kornetsky and Bain, 1990). Two ICSS procedures that have been used extensively to measure the changes in reward threshold are the rate-frequency curve shift procedure (Campbell et al., 1985) and the discrete-trial, current-intensity procedure (Kornetsky and Esposito, 1979; Markou and Koob, 1992; Figures 3.4–3.6).

Conditioned Place Preference

Conditioned place preference, or place conditioning, is a non-operant procedure that can also assess the reinforcing effects of drugs using classical or Pavlovian conditioning. In a simple version of the place preference paradigm, animals experience two distinct neutral environments that are paired with distinct drug or nondrug states (Figure 3.7). The animal is then given the choice to enter and explore either environment, and the time spent in the drug-paired environment is considered an index of the reinforcing value of the drug. Animals exhibit a conditioned

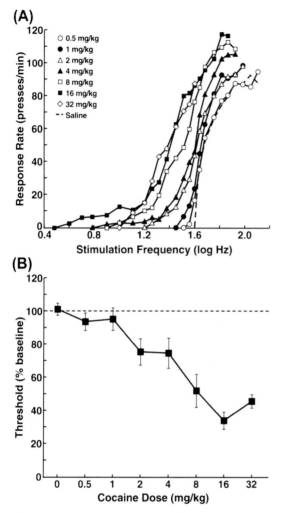

FIGURE 3.4 (A) Lever pressing in rats during the first 15 min after a cocaine injection as a function of the frequency of electrical stimulation of the lateral hypothalamus and cocaine dosage. (B) Self-stimulation frequency threshold (expressed as a percentage of baseline) as a function of cocaine dosage. The data are expressed as the means from the first threshold determination in the first hour after the injection. Each reference (baseline) value is the mean from the two threshold determinations taken just before the respective drug test. *[Taken with permission from Bauco P, Wise RA. Synergistic effects of cocaine with lateral hypothalamic brain stimulation reward: lack of tolerance or sensitization.* Journal of Pharmacology and Experimental Therapeutics, *1997, (283), 1160–1167.]*

preference for an environment associated with drugs that function as positive reinforcers (that is, they spend more time in a drug-paired environment than in a placebo-paired environment). They also avoid environments that are paired with aversive states, like drug withdrawal – a paradigm called conditioned place aversion (but more on that in the *withdrawal/negative affect* section below).

Drug Discrimination

Drug discrimination procedures can identify the relative reinforcing effects of drugs, thus indicating the relative abuse potential of these drugs (Holtzman, 1990). In this procedure, an animal is trained to emit a particular response (like pressing the right lever) for a food reinforcer in a drug-induced state and then to emit a different response (like pressing the left lever) for the same food reinforcer in a placebo-induced or nondrug state. The interoceptive cue state produced by the drug controls the behavior as a discriminative stimulus or cue that informs the animal to make the appropriate response to gain reinforcement. So if a rat is trained to respond on the left lever while intoxicated with D-amphetamine and the right lever when given vehicle injections while not intoxicated, then on the test day the rat will be given methamphetamine and allowed to choose. The rat will choose the D-amphetamine lever. In such a test, the rat "reports" its internal drug-like state caused by methamphetamine. The choice of the response that follows administration of an unknown test compound can provide valuable information about the similarity of that drug's interoceptive cue properties to those of the training drug.

Genetic Animal Models of High Alcohol Drinking

Many genetically selected lines of rats have been bred that have high and low drinking

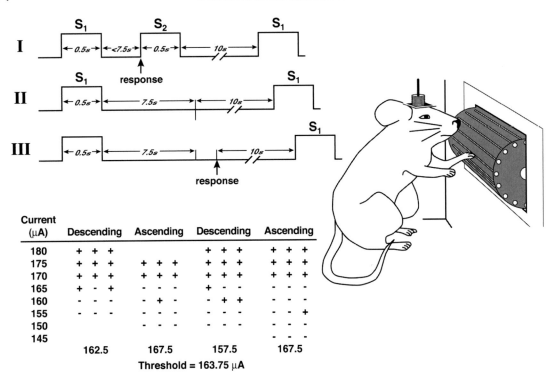

FIGURE 3.5   Intracranial self-stimulation threshold procedure. A rat is trained to turn a wheel (usually a quarter turn) to receive rewarding electrical stimulation directly in the brain. Panels I, II, and III illustrate the timing of events during three hypothetical discrete trials. Panel I shows a trial during which the rat responded within the 7.5 s following the delivery of the noncontingent stimulus (positive response). Panel II shows a trial during which the animal did not respond (negative response). Panel III shows a trial during which the animal responded during the intertrial interval (negative response). For demonstration purposes, the intertrial interval was set at 10 s. In reality, however, the interresponse interval has an average duration of 10 s, ranging from 7.5 to 12.5 s. The table at the bottom shows a hypothetical session and demonstrates how thresholds are defined for the four individual series. The threshold of the session is the mean of the four series' thresholds. *[Taken with permission from Markou A, Koob GF. Construct validity of a self-stimulation threshold paradigm: effects of reward and performance manipulations.* Physiology and Behavior, *1992, (51), 111–119.]*

preferences. Some of these genetic lines include University of Chile A and B rats, Alko alcohol and non-alcohol rats, University of Indiana alcohol-preferring and non-preferring rats, University of Indiana high-alcohol-drinking and low-alcohol-drinking rats, and Sardinian alcohol-preferring and non-preferring rats. The alcohol-preferring animals can voluntarily consume 6.5 g/kg alcohol per day when given a free choice between alcohol and water, attaining blood alcohol levels in the 50–200 mg% range.

Drug Taking in the Presence of Aversive Consequences

Drug taking or drug-seeking behavior that is impervious to environmental adversity or punishment captures elements of the compulsive nature of drug addiction associated with the *binge/intoxication* stage of the addiction cycle. From the perspective of the DSM-IV, such drug seeking fits well with the criterion of continued substance use despite knowledge of having a persistent physical or psychological problem.

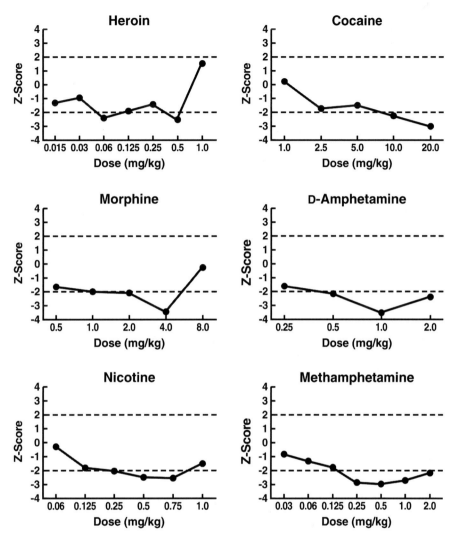

FIGURE 3.6   **Changes in intracranial self-stimulation reward thresholds (Z-scores) in rats for various doses of heroin, morphine, nicotine, cocaine, D-amphetamine, and methamphetamine.** A Z-score is based on the pre- and post-drug changes in threshold, and a Z-score of ±2.0 indicates the 95% confidence limit based on the mean and standard deviation for all saline days. *[Taken with permission from Hubner CB, Kornetsky C. Heroin, 6-acetylmorphine and morphine effects on threshold for rewarding and aversive brain stimulation.* Journal of Pharmacology and Experimental Therapeutics, *1992, (260), 562–567 (heroin, morphine); Huston-Lyons D, Kornetsky C. Effects of nicotine on the threshold for rewarding brain stimulation in rats.* Pharmacology Biochemistry and Behavior, *1992, (41), 755–759 (nicotine); Izenwasser S, Kornetsky C. Brain stimulation reward: a method for assessing the neurochemical bases of drug-induced euphoria. In: Watson RR (ed.)* Drugs of Abuse and Neurobiology. *CRC Press, Boca Raton FL, 1992, pp. 1–21 (cocaine); Kornetsky C. Brain stimulation reward: a model for the neuronal bases for drug-induced euphoria. In: Brown RM, Friedman DP, Nimit Y (eds.)* Neuroscience Methods in Drug Abuse Research *(series title: NIDA Research Monograph, vol. 62). National Institute on Drug Abuse, Rockville MD, 1985, pp. 30–50 (D-amphetamine); Sarkar M, Kornetsky C. Methamphetamine's action on brain-stimulation reward threshold and stereotypy.* Experimental and Clinical Psychopharmacology, *1995, (3), 112–117 (methamphetamine).]*

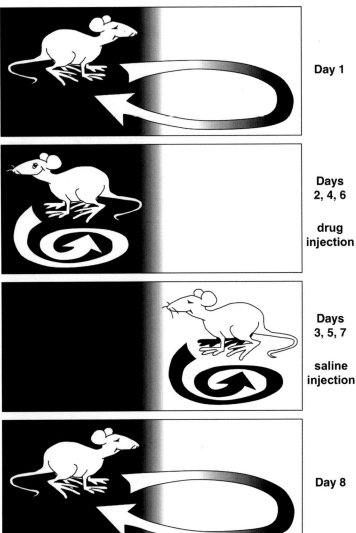

Day 1

Days
2, 4, 6

drug
injection

Days
3, 5, 7

saline
injection

Day 8

FIGURE 3.7 **The place conditioning procedure in the rat.** Animals experience two distinct neutral environments (here, black and white shaded) paired spatially and temporally with distinct unconditioned stimuli (here, drug on days 2, 4, and 6 and saline on days 3, 5, and 7). On day 8, the rat is given the opportunity to enter either environment in a drug-free state, and the time spent in each environment is used as an index of the reinforcing value of each unconditioned stimulus. These time values are often compared with baseline preference for each environment (here, measured on day 1). *[Taken with permission from Swerdlow NR, Gilbert D, Koob GF. Conditioned drug effects on spatial preference: critical evaluation. In: Boulton AA, Baker GB, Greenshaw AJ (eds.) Psychopharmacology (series title: Neuromethods, vol. 13). Humana Press, Clifton NJ, 1989, pp. 399–446.]*

The presentation of an aversive stimulus, like a mild footshock, suppresses cocaine-seeking behavior in rats that have limited access (e.g., less than 3h access to the drug per day). The aversive stimulus also suppresses sucrose seeking (a conventional reinforcer). This situation changes, however, when the animals are given extended access for, say, 6h. The animals' sucrose-seeking behavior continues to be suppressed by the aversive stimulus, but the rats' cocaine-seeking behavior does not diminish when confronted with the same aversive conditioned stimulus. For example, dependent rats display more persistent alcohol consumption than nondependent rats as increasing amounts of the bitter-tasting, aversive substance quinine is added to the solution (that is, dependent rats continue to consume alcohol

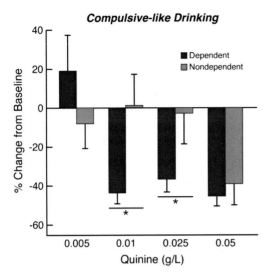

FIGURE 3.8　**Compulsive-like drinking (i.e., persistent alcohol drinking despite the aversive bitter taste of quinine added to the alcohol solution) in dependent alcohol vapor-exposed rats during acute alcohol withdrawal.** The data represent the percentage change from baseline (i.e., lever presses for alcohol alone before quinine adulteration). *[Taken with permission from Vendruscolo LF, Barbier E, Schlosburg JE, Misra KK, Whitfield T Jr., Logrip ML, Rivier CL, Repunte-Canonigo V, Zorrilla EP, Sanna PP, Heilig M, Koob GF. Corticosteroid-dependent plasticity mediates compulsive alcohol drinking in rats.* Journal of Neuroscience, 2012, (32), 7563–7571.]

despite the aversive bitter taste of quinine). This is considered a measure of compulsive-like alcohol intake (Figure 3.8).

Summary of Animal Models of the *Binge/Intoxication* Stage

The experimental paradigms outlined above have proven reliability and predictive validity in their ability to understand the neurobiological basis of the acute reinforcing effects of drugs of abuse and compulsive drug seeking associated with the *binge/intoxication* stage of the addiction cycle. However, one could reasonably argue that drug addiction also involves counteradaptive mechanisms that go far beyond solely the acute reinforcing effects. Nonetheless, understanding the neurobiological mechanisms of the positive

reinforcing effects of drugs of abuse can provide a framework for understanding specific changes in a drug's motivational effects as addiction develops. One strength of the models outlined above is that any of the operant measures can be used in within-subjects designs, meaning that the same animals can be subjected to different manipulations, thus limiting the number of animals required for research. Once an animal is trained to, say, press a lever, full dose-effect functions can be generated for different drugs, and the animal can be tested for weeks or even months. Once an animal is tested with a particular experimental drug, additional pharmacological manipulations can be done with standard reference compounds, using the same animals, to validate the effects. A rich literature on the experimental analysis of behavior is available to explore the actions of various drugs, which can be used to develop additional experimental protocols that attempt to alter drug reinforcement by modifying the history and contingencies of reinforcement.

The advantage of the ICSS paradigm as a model of the effects of drugs on motivation and reward is that the threshold provided by ICSS is easily quantifiable. Such threshold estimations are very stable over long periods of time, up to several months (Stellar and Stellar, 1985). Another considerable advantage of the ICSS technique is its high reliability of predicting the abuse liability of drugs. A false-positive result has never been obtained with the discrete trials threshold procedure.

Place conditioning has several advantages as a model for evaluating drugs of abuse: it is highly sensitive to even very low doses of drugs; it can be used to study both the positive and negative reinforcing effects of drugs; and it tests drug reward under drug-free conditions. It also allows for the precise control of interactions between environmental cues and drug administration.

Animal models associated with responding in the face of punishment and the progressive-ratio

schedule have both face and construct validity. Numerous studies in humans have found
that people who meet the criteria for substance
dependence will work hard to obtain drugs
and show increased motivation for drug
taking. As addiction develops, an individual's
behavioral repertoire narrows toward drug
seeking and taking. Progressive-ratio studies in humans have found similar patterns
of responding to those in the animal models.
Clearly, responding in the face of punishment
and progressive-ratio responding in rodents
show individual differences that are reminis-
cent of the individual differences found in the
human population. From the perspective of
construct validity, responding in the face of
punishment and progressive-ratio paradigms
predict a key role for midbrain dopamine systems in the reinforcing effects of cocaine. Second-order schedules of reinforcement with a
well-established cocaine "habit" have revealed
a key role for dorsal striatal mechanisms in the
increased motivation to work for cocaine.

ANIMAL MODELS OF THE WITHDRAWAL/NEGATIVE AFFECT STAGE OF THE ADDICTION CYCLE

Drug withdrawal from chronic drug administration is usually characterized by responses
and effects that are opposite to the acute initial actions of the drug. The physical signs of
withdrawal are often drug-specific. Many of
the overt physical signs associated with withdrawal from drugs (for example, alcohol and
opiates) can be easily observed and quantified,
providing specific markers for the study of the
neurobiological mechanisms of dependence.
Standard rating scales have been developed
for opiate, nicotine, and alcohol withdrawal
(Gellert and Holtzman, 1978; Malin et al., 1992;
Macey et al., 1996).

However, the motivational measures of withdrawal have more validity in understanding

the counteradaptive neurobiological mechanisms that drive addiction. Such motivational
measures have proved to be extremely sensitive
to drug withdrawal and are powerful tools for
exploring the neurobiological bases of the motivational aspects of drug dependence.

Animal models of the motivational effects
of drug withdrawal include operant schedules, conditioned place aversion, ICSS, the
elevated plus maze, and drug discrimination,
which include some of the same motivational
measures of drug seeking used to characterize
the *binge/intoxication* stage (Table 3.3). Each of
these models can address different theoretical constructs associated with a given motivational aspect of withdrawal. Some might
reflect general malaise, and others might
reflect specific components of the withdrawal
syndrome.

Intracranial Self-Stimulation

Withdrawal from the chronic administration of virtually all major drugs of abuse ele-
vates ICSS thresholds (i.e., decreases reward;
Figure 3.9).

Notice that we use the word "elevate" to
describe the increase in reward threshold. This
has become a convention in the field. Conversely, the word "lower" is used to describe a
decrease in threshold.

TABLE 3.3   Animal Models of the *Withdrawal/Negative Affect* Stage of the Addiction Cycle

Intracranial self-stimulation

Conditioned place aversion

Disrupted operant schedules

Drug discrination

Measures of anxiety-like responses

Drug self-administration with extended access

Drug self-administration in dependent animals

Conditioned Place Aversion, Disrupted Operant Responding, and Drug Discrimination

The aversive stimulus effects of withdrawal can be measured using a variant of the conditioned place conditioning procedure, termed conditioned place aversion. When studying opioid dependence, one method is to precipitate or induce withdrawal by administering a competitive opioid receptor antagonist, such as naloxone (Hand et al., 1988). Although naloxone itself can produce a conditioned place aversion in nondependent rats, the dose required to produce such a place aversion decreases significantly in dependent rats. Place aversions have also been observed with precipitated nicotine withdrawal and acute *spontaneous* alcohol withdrawal, in which the animal is simply no longer allowed access to alcohol. The response-disruptive effects of drug withdrawal in operant schedules have also been associated with an "amotivational" state of withdrawal, in which an animal is less motivated or willing to perform the task (Figure 3.10).

Drug discrimination has also been used to characterize both specific and nonspecific aspects of withdrawal. For alcohol withdrawal, for example, animals have been trained to discriminate between saline and the anxiogenic (anxiety-inducing) drug pentylenetetrazol (Gauvin and Holloway, 1991). Generalization to a convulsant-like cue during alcohol withdrawal suggested that the withdrawal syndrome has an anxiogenic-like component. Opiate-dependent animals have been trained to discriminate an opioid receptor antagonist from saline. This generalization to an opioid antagonist provided a general nonspecific measure of the intensity of opiate withdrawal and its time course.

Measures of Anxiety-Like Responses

A common response to acute withdrawal and protracted abstinence from all major drugs of abuse is the manifestation of anxiety-like responses, such as fear, panic, irritability, hypervigilance, sweating, increased heart rate, increased blood pressure, and distractibility. The dependent variable can be a *passive* response to a novel or aversive stimulus, such as an open field or the elevated plus maze. In such paradigms, the animal is simply placed on or in the apparatus, and its behavior is watched and recorded. Another kind of dependent variable is an *active* response to an aversive stimulus, such as in the defensive burying test. Withdrawal from repeated administration of cocaine, opioids, ethanol, and cannabinoids produces anxiogenic-like responses in both the elevated plus maze and defensive burying test (Box 3.1).

In the defensive burying test, a rat or mouse is placed in a box with woodchip bedding material. Protruding into the box is an electrified metal probe. Rodents have a natural defense reaction to unfamiliar and potentially dangerous objects. When the animal incidentally touches the probe, it receives a mild shock. The rat or mouse then vigorously pushes the bedding material to cover the probe (presumably in an effort to prevent itself from touching the probe). Researchers will watch this active response and record how long it takes the animal to start burying the probe (latency), the total time spent burying, the total number of burying acts, and the height of the bedding material deposited over the probe. All of these measures have been validated to reflect emotionality in this test (Andrews and Broekkamp, 1993).

The elevated plus maze is an ethologically based exploratory model of anxiety that measures how animals, typically rats and mice, respond to a novel approach/avoidance situation by measuring their relative exploration of two distinct environments. The elevated plus maze is elevated about 2 feet (60 cm) from the floor. It is shaped as a plus sign, consisting of a bright and exposed runway and a dark and walled runway

3. ANIMAL MODELS OF ADDICTION

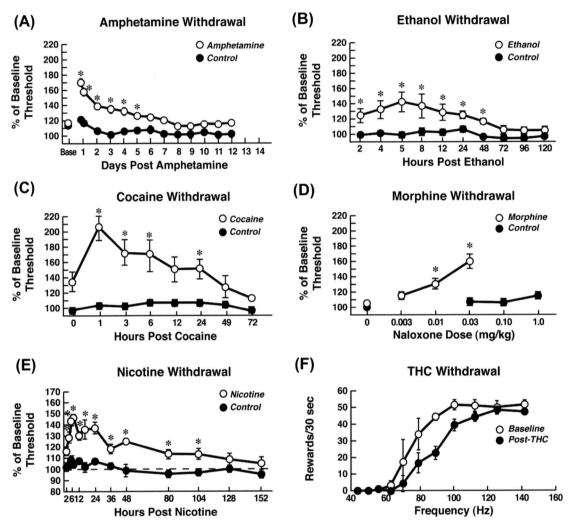

FIGURE 3.9   (A) Mean intracranial self-stimulation (ICSS) reward thresholds in rats during amphetamine withdrawal (10 mg/kg/day for 6 days). The data are expressed as a percentage of the mean of the last five baseline values prior to drug treatment. *$p < 0.05$, significant differences from the saline control group.
(B) Mean ICSS thresholds in rats during ethanol withdrawal (blood alcohol levels reached 197.29 mg%). Elevations in thresholds were time-dependent. *$p < 0.05$, significant differences from the control group.
(C) Mean ICSS thresholds in rats during cocaine withdrawal 24 h following the cessation of cocaine self-administration. *$p < 0.05$, significant differences from the control group.
(D) Mean ICSS thresholds in rats during naloxone-precipitated morphine withdrawal. The minimum dose of naloxone that elevated ICSS thresholds in the morphine group was 0.01 mg/kg. *$p < 0.05$, significant differences from the control group.
(E) Mean ICSS thresholds in rats during spontaneous nicotine withdrawal following surgical removal of osmotic minipumps that delivered nicotine hydrogen tartrate (9 mg/kg/day) or saline. *$p < 0.05$, significant differences from the control group.
(F) Mean ICSS thresholds in rats during withdrawal from an acute 1.0 mg/kg dose of Δ^9-tetrahydrocannabinol (THC). Withdrawal significantly shifted the reward function to the right (indicating diminished reward).
Note that because different equipment systems and threshold procedures were used in the collection of the above data, direct comparisons among the magnitude of effects induced by these drugs cannot be made.

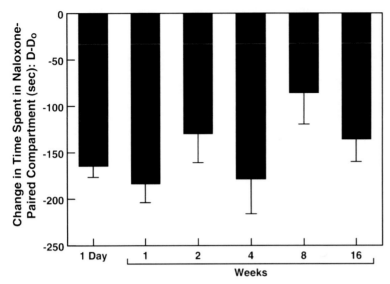

FIGURE 3.10 **Place conditioning with naloxone (15 μg/kg, s.c.) in morphine-dependent rats.** D_0 indicates the time spent in the naloxone-paired compartment before conditioning. The rats were then evaluated 1 day and 1, 2, 4, 8, and 16 weeks later. The data are expressed as the mean ± SEM time spent in the naloxone compartment after conditioning minus the time spent in the naloxone compartment before conditioning. [*Data from Stinus L, Caille S, Koob GF. Opiate withdrawal-induced place aversion lasts for up to 16 weeks. Psychopharmacology, 2000, (149), 115–120.*]

that intersect in the middle. The animal is usually placed at the intersection, facing an open arm. It is then freely allowed to seek the relative safety of one of the closed arms or venture out onto the open arms. An "anxious" animal will spend less time in the open arms and visit the open arms a lower percentage of time relative to the total number of visits it makes to both the open and closed arms. A rodent's behavior on the elevated plus maze is very sensitive to stress, drug withdrawal, and treatments that produce disinhibition, such as sedative/hypnotic drugs or alcohol.

Drug Self-Administration with Extended Access and Drug Self-Administration in Dependent Animals

A progressive increase in the frequency and intensity of drug use is one of the major behavioral phenomena that characterize the development of addiction. Such an escalation has face validity with a number of DSM-IV criteria for addiction, including "Need for markedly increased amounts of substance to achieve intoxication or desired effect," "Important

[Panel A. Taken with permission from Paterson NE, Myers C, Markou A. Effects of repeated withdrawal from continuous amphetamine administration on brain reward function in rats. Psychopharmacology, 2000, (152) 440–446.]

[Panel B. Taken with permission from Schulteis G, Markou A, Cole M, Koob G. Decreased brain reward produced by ethanol withdrawal. Proceedings of the National Academy of Sciences USA, 1995, (92) 5880–5884.]

[Panel C. Taken with permission from Markou A, Koob GF. Post-cocaine anhedonia: an animal model of cocaine withdrawal. Neuropsychopharmacology, 1991, (4) 17–26.]

[Panel D. Taken with permission from Schulteis G, Markou A, Gold LH, Stinus L, Koob GF. Relative sensitivity to naloxone of multiple indices of opiate withdrawal: a quantitative dose-response analysis. Journal of Pharmacology and Experimental Therapeutics, 1994, (271) 1391–1398.]

[Panel E. Data adapted with permission from Epping-Jordan MP, Watkins SS, Koob GF, Markou A. Dramatic decreases in brain reward function during nicotine withdrawal. Nature, 1998, (393) 76–79.]

[Panel F. Taken with permission from Gardner EL, Vorel SR. Cannabinoid transmission and reward-related events. Neurobiology of Disease, 1998, (5) 502–533.]

BOX 3.1

DESCRIBING ANXIETY IN ANIMAL MODELS

Notice in this chapter and throughout the book, we often use the word "-like" to describe behaviors in animals, such as "anxiety-like behavior." The word anxiety or other such terms are used by people to describe their own subjective internal states; what they themselves are thinking or feeling. When studying animals, however, we cannot ask the rat to report what it is experiencing. Its behavioral or physiological state can be observed by researchers, and such states can bear a striking resemblance to the states observed in people (face validity). Nevertheless, scientists and researchers are discouraged from using anthropomorphisms to describe human-like characteristics in nonhuman organisms. Therefore, we say that such states are like those in humans. We cannot say with absolute certainty that the rat feels "anxious," but its outward manifestation is objectively close enough to the human condition that we can say it is presenting "anxiety-like" behavior.

social, occupational, or recreational activities given up or reduced because of substance use," "A great deal of time spent in activities necessary to obtain substance, to use substance, or recover from its effects," and "Substance in larger amounts or over a longer period than the person intended."

A framework with which to model the transition from drug use to drug addiction can be found in relatively recently developed animal models of prolonged access to drug self-administration and drug self-administration in dependent animals during withdrawal (Figure 3.11). Before the extended-access model was developed, rodents were typically given access to the drug for less than 3h per day, which produced stable and reliable responding for the drug over time. In contrast, in the extended-access model with cocaine, drug access was increased to 6h per day, which produced dramatic increases in self-administration compared with animals that had the usual 1h access. This escalation in responding has now been observed with extended access to all major drugs of abuse, including methamphetamine, heroin, nicotine, and alcohol. A similar phenomenon of increased

intake is observed when rats are tested repeatedly after the induction of alcohol dependence. They show reliable increases in self-administration after a period of withdrawal, in which the amount of intake can increase 3–4 fold and the animals maintain blood alcohol levels of 100–150 mg% when allowed to self-administer alcohol during withdrawal. In each of these models of extended access, the animals show increased responding on a progressive-ratio schedule when tested during withdrawal, suggesting an increase in reward value or efficacy of the drug when they are dependent.

Summary of Animal Models of the *Withdrawal/Negative Affect* Stage

Motivational measures of drug withdrawal have significant face validity for the motivational measures of drug withdrawal in humans. Dysphoria, hypohedonia, loss of motivation, anxiety, and irritability can all be reflected in the animal models described above. ICSS threshold procedures also have high predictive validity for changes in the reward value of the drug. The disruption of operant responding during drug abstinence reflects general malaise. Drug discrimination allows a powerful and sensitive comparison to other drug states. Conditioned place aversion reflects an aversive unconditioned stimulus. The escalation of intake of all drugs of abuse is also associated with an increased breakpoint on a progressive-ratio schedule, indicating that animals will work harder to obtain the drug – possibly reflecting either enhanced motivation to seek the drug or the enhanced reward value of the drug, or both.

As more and more data are generated that establish the neurobiological bases of negative emotional states in animals that correspond to such negative emotional states in humans, these measures will gain construct validity (Koob and Volkow, 2010). The use of multiple dependent variables in studies of the motivational effects of withdrawal reveal numerous overlapping neurobiological substrates, laying a framework for identifying the counteradaptive mechanisms that drive addiction. The reinforcing value of drugs may change as an individual becomes dependent. The neurobiological basis for such changes is only beginning to be investigated. Thus, drug dependence can produce an aversive or negative motivational state, manifested by changes in numerous behavioral measures, such as response disruption, changes in reward thresholds, and conditioned place aversions.

ANIMAL MODELS OF THE PREOCCUPATION/ANTICIPATION STAGE OF THE ADDICTION CYCLE

A defining characteristic of addiction is its chronic, relapsing nature. Animal models of relapse fall into three general conditioning constructs: (1) drug-induced reinstatement, (2) cue-induced reinstatement, and (3) stress-induced reinstatement (Table 3.4). The general conceptual framework for this conditioning conceptualization is that cues, both internal and external, can become associated with the positive and negative reinforcing actions of drugs and abstinence through classical conditioning, which can then elicit drug use.

Drug-Induced Reinstatement

The persistence of drug seeking behavior in the absence of response-contingent drug availability can be measured using extinction procedures, but extinction is also a key element of most animal models of relapse. When noncontingent drug injections are administered after extinction, they increase responding at the lever that previously delivered the drug. Such responding is called drug-induced reinstatement (Stewart and de Wit, 1987; Figure 3.12).

Cue-Induced Reinstatement

Environmental cues paired with drug self-administration can also reliably and robustly reinstate responding after extinction. In this procedure, animals are trained to self-administer drugs of abuse using an operant response procedure, usually lever pressing. A cue, such as a tone or light, precedes the drug delivery. When the animal acquires stable responding, it is then subjected to extinction, in which further lever presses do not deliver any drugs or cues. After responding is extinguished, reinstatement sessions are conducted. The cue by itself is presented, and the animal is allowed to press the lever (Figure 3.13). The cue then elicits vigorous lever pressing. This procedure is widely used to explore the neurobiological substrates of relapse (Shaham et al., 2003). Place conditioning can also be used as a model of cue-induced reinstatement. A place preference is induced by a drug, followed by extinction sessions. Conditioned place preference can then be induced again by a cue presentation.

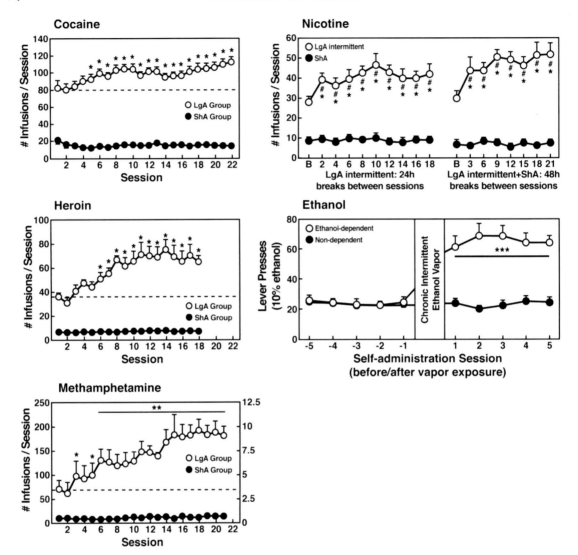

FIGURE 3.11 **Escalation of drug intake with extended access.** (Cocaine) Effect of drug availability on cocaine intake. In long-access (LgA) rats with 6h access ($n = 12$) but not short-access (ShA) rats with 1 h access ($n = 12$), the mean total cocaine intake began to increase significantly from session 5 ($p < 0.05$; sessions 5 to 22 compared with session 1) and continued to increase thereafter ($p < 0.05$; session 5 compared with sessions 8–10, 12, 13, and 17–22).

(Heroin) Effect of drug availability on total intravenous heroin self-infusions. During the escalation phase, the rats had access to heroin (40 μg per infusion) for 1h (ShA rats, $n = 5$–6) or 11 h per session (LgA rats, $n = 5$–6). Regular 1-h (ShA rats) or 11-h (LgA rats) sessions of heroin self-administration were performed for 6 days per week. The dotted line indicates the mean ± SEM number of heroin self-infusions in LgA rats during the first 11-h session. *$p < 0.05$, different from the first session.

(Methamphetamine) Effect of extended access to intravenous methamphetamine on self-administration as a function of daily sessions in rats trained to self-administer 0.05, 0.1, and 0.2 mg/kg/infusion of intravenous methamphetamine during the 6h session. ShA, 1h session (each unit dose, $n = 6$). LgA, 6h session (0.05 mg/kg/infusion, $n = 4$; 0.1 mg/kg/infusion, $n = 6$; 0.2 mg/kg/infusion, $n = 5$). *$p < 0.05$, **$p < 0.01$, compared with day 1.

(Nicotine) Nicotine intake in rats that self-administered nicotine under a fixed-ratio (FR) 1 schedule in either 21h (long-access [LgA]) or 1h (short-access [ShA]) sessions. LgA rats increased their nicotine intake on an intermittent schedule with 24–48h breaks between sessions, whereas LgA rats on a daily schedule did not. The left shows the total number of nicotine infusions per session when the intermittent schedule included 24h breaks between sessions. The right shows the total number of

Context-Induced Reinstatement

Drug-associated stimuli that signal the response-contingent availability of intravenous drug also reliably elicit drug seeking behavior in experimental animals, and responding for these stimuli is highly resistant to extinction (See et al., 1999). Subsequent re-exposure to the drug discriminative stimulus after extinction but not re-exposure to a nonreward discriminative stimulus produces strong recovery of responding at the previously active lever in the absence of any further drug availability. Cues associated with the availability of oral alcohol self-administration can also reinstate responding in the absence of the primary reinforcer (Katner et al., 1999; Ciccocippo et al., 2001; Crombag et al., 2002, 2008).

TABLE 3.4   Animal Models of the *Preoccupation/Anticipation* Stage of the Addiction Cycle

Resistance to extinction associated with drug self-administration

Drug-induced reinstatement

Cue-induced reinstatement

Context-induced reinstatement ("renewal")

Cue-induced reinstatement without extinction ("relapse")

Stress-induced reinstatement

Second-order schedules of reinforcement

Protracted abstinence

Conditioned withdrawal

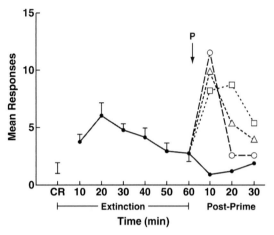

FIGURE 3.12   **Mean number of responses in rats per 10 min during self-administration (continuous reinforcement, CR), during extinction, and after cocaine priming injections of 2.0, 1.0, and 0.5 mg/kg or after a "dummy trial" (0.0 mg/kg).** "P" indicates the point at which the priming injection was given. The mean values during extinction are based on eight determinations for each of five rats; the means after the priming infusions are based on two determinations per rat for each of five rats. Closed circles, 0.0 mg/kg; open circles, 0.5 mg/kg; triangles, 1.0 mg/kg; squares, 2.0 mg/kg. *[Taken with permission from de Wit H, Stewart J. Reinstatement of cocaine-reinforced responding in the rat.* Psychopharmacology, *1981, (75), 134–143.]*

nicotine infusions per session when the intermittent schedule included 48 h breaks between sessions. [#]$p < 0.05$, compared with baseline; [*]$p < 0.05$, compared with daily self-administration group ($n = 10$ per group).

(Ethanol) Ethanol self-administration in ethanol-dependent and nondependent animals. The induction of ethanol dependence and correlation of limited ethanol self-administration before and excessive drinking after dependence induction following chronic intermittent ethanol vapor exposure is shown. [***]$p < 0.001$, significant group × test session interaction. With all drugs, escalation is defined as a significant increase in drug intake within-subjects in extended-access groups, with no significant changes within-subjects in limited-access groups.

[Cocaine: Taken with permission from Ahmed SH, Koob GF. Transition from moderate to excessive drug intake: change in hedonic set point. Science, *1998, (282), 298–300.]*

[Heroin. Taken with permission from Ahmed SH, Walker JR, Koob GF. Persistent increase in the motivation to take heroin in rats with a history of drug escalation. Neuropsychopharmacology, *2000, (22), 413–421.]*

[Methamphetamine. Taken with permission from Kitamura O, Wee S, Specio SE, Koob GF, Pulvirenti L. Escalation of methamphetamine self-administration in rats: a dose-effect function. Psychopharmacology, *2006, (186), 48–53.]*

[Nicotine. Taken with permission from Cohen A, Koob GF, George O. Robust escalation of nicotine intake with extended access to nicotine self-administration and intermittent periods of abstinence. Neuropsychopharmacology, *2012, (37), 2153–2160.]*

[Ethanol. Taken with permission from Edwards S, Guerrero M, Ghoneim OM, Roberts E, Koob GF. Evidence that vasopressin V_{1b} receptors mediate the transition to excessive drinking in ethanol-dependent rats. Addiction Biology, *2011, (17), 76–85.]*

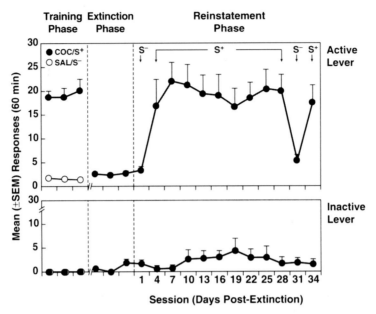

FIGURE 3.13   **Lever-press responses at an active (A) and inactive (B) lever in rats during self-administration training, extinction, and reinstatement sessions.** Training Phase: Cocaine-reinforced (●) and saline/nonreinforced (○) responses during the final 3 days of the self-administration phase in rats trained to associate discriminative stimuli with the availability of intravenous cocaine (S+) or saline (S−). Rats were designated for tests of resistance to the extinction of cocaine-seeking behavior induced by the cocaine S+ during the Reinstatement Phase. Extinction Phase: Extinction responses at criterion (<4 responses/session over three consecutive days). The number of days required to reach the criterion was 15.3 ± 3.9. Reinstatement Phase: Responses in the presence of the S+ and S−. Exposure to the S+ elicited significant recovery of responding in the absence of further drug availability, whereas responding in the presence of the S− remained at extinction levels. *[Taken with permission from Weiss F, Martin-Fardon R, Ciccocioppo R, Kerr TM, Smith DL, Ben-Shahar O. Enduring resistance to extinction of cocaine-seeking behavior induced by drug-related cues.* Neuropsychopharmacology, 2001, (25), 361–372.]

Cue-Induced Reinstatement without Extinction

Another model of drug seeking that has been termed a "relapse" model is one in which animals undergo cue-induced exposure following forced abstinence from chronic drug self-administration without extinction outside the testing cage (Yahyavi-Firouz-Abadi and See, 2009). This paradigm is based on the well-established "incubation effect," in which cocaine seeking induced by re-exposure to drug-associated cues progressively increases over the first two months of withdrawal from cocaine (Lu et al., 2004). Cues paired with drugs produce a robust increase in cocaine

seeking after abstinence without extinction. This paradigm has more face validity for the human condition, because individuals with drug addiction rarely experience explicit extinction of drug seeking related to drug-paired cues.

Stress-Induced Reinstatement and Conditioned Withdrawal

In human studies, stressful situations are the most likely triggers of relapse. Animal models of stress-induced reinstatement also show that stressors elicit strong recovery of extinguished drug-seeking behavior in the absence of any further drug availability (Erb et al., 1996).

Acute intermittent footshock reinstates cocaine-seeking behavior after prolonged extinction, and this effect is as strong as a priming injection of cocaine. Such effects are observed even after a 4–6 week drug-free period and appear to be specific to drugs because food-seeking behavior is not reinstated. Stressors other than shock can effectively reinstate drug seeking, including food deprivation, restraint stress, tail pinch stress, swim stress, conditioned fear, social defeat stress, and administration of the α_2-adrenergic receptor antagonist yohimbine (which activates the sympathetic nervous system).

The motivational aspects of withdrawal can also be conditioned, and conditioned withdrawal has been repeatedly observed in both opiate-dependent animals and humans. Cues paired with withdrawal can elicit a withdrawal-like response in numerous animal paradigms, ranging from the suppression of operant responding to conditioned place aversions (Shippenberg and Koob, 2002).

Second-Order Schedules of Reinforcement

Second-order schedules of reinforcement involve training animals to work for a previously neutral stimulus that ultimately predicts drug availability. These schedules maintain high rates of responding (e.g., up to thousands of responses per session in monkeys) and can motivate the animal to emit extended sequences of behavior before any drug is administered. Such extended schedules minimize potentially disruptive, nonspecific, acute drug and treatment effects on response rates. High response rates are maintained even for doses that decrease rates of responding on a regular fixed-ratio schedule, indicating that performance on the second-order schedule is unaffected by the acute effects of the drug that would otherwise disrupt operant responding. The maintenance of performance under second-order schedules with drug-paired stimuli appears to be analogous to the maintenance and reinstatement of drug seeking behavior in humans who are also presented with drug-paired stimuli.

Protracted Abstinence

Relapse to drugs of abuse commonly occurs even after the physical and motivational signs of withdrawal have subsided, from days to weeks to months to even years later. This suggests that the neurochemical changes that occur during the *development* of dependence can persist far beyond the overt signs of acute withdrawal end. Animal work has shown that prior dependence lowers an individual's "dependence threshold." For example, previously ethanol-dependent animals made dependent again display even more severe withdrawal symptoms than when they received alcohol for the first time (Branchey et al., 1971; Baker and Cannon, 1979; Becker and Hale, 1989; Becker, 1994). Alcohol experience and the development of dependence in particular can lead to long-lasting motivational alterations in responsiveness to alcohol.

Increases in alcohol self-administration that persist long past acute withdrawal and detoxification can be observed in rats that have been made dependent (Roberts et al., 2000). The persistent alterations in ethanol self-administration and residual sensitivity to stressors have been arbitrarily defined as a state of "protracted abstinence" (or prolonged abstinence). Protracted abstinence in the rat begins after the acute physical signs of withdrawal have disappeared, with elevations in ethanol intake over baseline and increased stress responsivity persisting 2–8 weeks after withdrawal from chronic ethanol.

A robust and reliable feature of animal models of alcohol drinking is an increase in consumption after a period of deprivation. This is called the "alcohol deprivation effect" and has been observed in mice, rats, monkeys, and human drinkers.

Summary of Animal Models of the *Preoccupation/Anticipation* Stage

Each of the models of this stage of the addiction cycle has face validity with the human condition, and all provide frameworks for understanding the neurobiological bases of various aspects of craving. The DSM-IV criteria that apply to the craving stage and loss of control over drug intake include "any unsuccessful effort or persistent desire to cut down or control substance use."

Second-order schedules of reinforcement can assess the motivational value of a drug in the absence of the drug's acute effects that could otherwise influence performance or processes that can interfere with motivational function. Reinstatement models have demonstrated face validity, but their predictive validity remains to be established, with little evidence of predictive validity from studies of pharmacological treatments for drug relapse. Very few clinical trials have tested medications that effectively prevent reinstatement, and very few anti-relapse medications that have been tested in animal models of reinstatement have had success in human laboratory studies or clinical trials. However, drug re-exposure or priming, stressors, and cues paired with drugs all produce reinstatement in animal models and promote relapse in humans, providing some support for the functional equivalence and construct validity of these modes.

A challenge for future studies will be to develop cross-species endophenotypes, from animals to humans, which will allow further construct validity and functional equivalence in studies of genetic and environmental vulnerability and the neurobiological mechanisms therein.

ANIMAL MODELS OF VULNERABILITY TO ADDICTION

Acquisition of Drug Seeking

Models of the vulnerability to addiction have historically involved acquisition studies, in which subjects that are naive to a particular drug learn a simple operant response to obtain an intravenous delivery of the drug in a limited-access situation. Individual differences in the response to psychostimulants and other drugs of abuse in general have been widely demonstrated in humans and laboratory animals. Although the importance of individual differences in humans is well accepted in clinical practice, it has generally been neglected in animal studies. One of most sensitive models for testing the vulnerability to drugs of abuse is to provide naive animals with very low doses of drugs in an acquisition paradigm, such that only the more sensitive individuals develop self-administration. The differences are hypothesized to reflect the differential reactivity of specific neurotransmitters (Figure 3.14). Such types of differential responses have been shown for cocaine, amphetamine, and heroin. The difference between animals within a group can be further exaggerated by dividing the group in half or by the median (i.e., 50%–50%) or to maximize the phenotypic differences by comparing the lowest and highest interquartiles. Such models lead to at least two avenues of research:

i) Investigating the biological and brain parameters that differentiate behavioral phenotypes, and
ii) Characterizing the vulnerable vs. resistant phenotypes, so that the knowledge or the measure of a behavioral characteristic predicts the type of response to the drug.

These models have face validity because vulnerable subjects have a higher chance of developing addiction-like behavior, independent of the quantity of drug available (which appears to occur in the real, human world).

Vulnerability to Addiction

Another approach to investigating individual differences in the vulnerability to addiction has been to characterize individual animals in terms

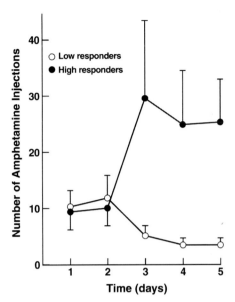

FIGURE 3.14 **Acquisition of amphetamine self-administration of rats in high-responder and low-responder groups after repeated intraperitoneal administration of saline.** After saline treatment, the groups ($n = 10$ per group) differed in their acquisition of self-administration both in terms of total amphetamine administered over the five days and in terms of the number of injections over the different days. *[Taken with permission from Piazza PV, Deminiere JM, Le Moal M, Simon H. Factors that predict individual vulnerability to amphetamine self-administration. Science, 1989, (245), 1511–1513.]*

of their propensity to show responses that relate to the DSM-IV (now DSM-5) criteria for addiction. Three domains have been identified from the DSM-5 criteria that can be linked to animals models:

i) Difficulty stopping or limiting drug use (items 3–4 in the DSM-IV),
ii) High motivation to seek and use the drug (items 5–6 in the DSM-IV), and
iii) Maintenance of drug use despite negative consequences (item 7 in the DSM-IV).

Using these three diagnostic domains, studies of intravenous cocaine self-administration in Sprague-Dawley rats have shown that the severity of cocaine use can be assessed in three

animal models that represent these diagnostic domains:

i) Drug seeking during periods when drug is not available,
ii) Breakpoints on a progressive-ratio schedule of reinforcement, and
iii) Persistence of self-administration despite punishment.

Using such criteria, a certain percentage of animals can be ranked according to addiction-like behavior, and an "addiction score" can be computed, from 0 (no addiction-like behavior) to 3 (high addiction-like behavior; Deroche-Gamonet et al., 2004; Belin et al., 2008). Animals with a score of 3 escalate drug intake more rapidly and to a much larger extent than animals with lower scores. They also show greater responses to contextual and drug-associated cues and exhibit much more reinstatement. This model is reliable and based on the link to DSM-IV and DSM-5 criteria. It also has some significant predictive validity.

SUMMARY OF ANIMAL MODELS OF ADDICTION

Most of the animal models discussed in this chapter have predictive validity for certain components of the addiction cycle and generate reliable effects in animals. For the positive reinforcing effects of drugs, drug self-administration, ICSS, and conditioned place preference each have predictive validity. Drug discrimination has predictive validity indirectly through generalization to the training drug. Animal models of withdrawal focus on the motivational components of withdrawal rather than overt somatic signs. Animal models of conditioned drug effects can predict the potential for conditioned drug effects in humans. Animal models of vulnerability in rats show promise for identifying factors that promote individual differences in the initial sensitivity to the rewarding effects of drugs and individual differences in developing compulsive-like responding for drugs with extended access. Achieving predictive validity is more problematic for constructs such as craving because of the nebulous conceptualizations and various definitions of craving in humans. Virtually all of the measures described herein for animal models of addiction have demonstrated reliability, consistency, stability of the measures, small within-subject and between-subject variability, and reproducibility of the phenomena.

Much remains to be explored about the face validity and predictive validity of unconditioned positive and negative motivational states, particularly the conditioned positive and negative motivational states associated with drug use and withdrawal. However, the gaps in our knowledge may lie more in the human clinical laboratory domain than in the animal models themselves (Koob, 2009). Determining the specific changes in the central nervous system associated with these models will provide further insights into both drug dependence and psychopathologies associated with anxiety and affective disorders. Animal models of addiction provide the foundation to begin such studies.

Suggested Reading

Andrews, J.S., Broekkamp, C.L.E., 1993. Procedures to identify anxiolytic or anxiogenic agents. In: Sahgal, A. (Ed.), Behavioral Neuroscience: A Practical Approach, vol. 2. IRL Press, Oxford, pp. 37–54.

Baker, T.B., Cannon, D.S., 1979. Potentiation of ethanol withdrawal by prior dependence. Psychopharmacology 60, 105–110.

Becker, H.C., 1994. Positive relationship between the number of prior ethanol withdrawal episodes and the severity of subsequent withdrawal seizures. Psychopharmacology 116, 26–32.

Becker, H.C., Hale, R.L., 1989. Ethanol-induced locomotor stimulation in C57BL/6 mice following RO15-4513 administration. Psychopharmacology 99, 333–336.

Belin, D., Mar, A.C., Dalley, J.W., Robbins, T.W., Everitt, B.J., 2008. High impulsivity predicts the switch to compulsive cocaine-taking. Science 320, 1352–1355.

Bindra, D., 1976. A Theory of Intelligent Behavior. Wiley, New York.

Branchey, M., Rauscher, G., Kissin, B., 1971. Modifications in the response to alcohol following the establishment of physical dependence. Psychopharmacologia 22, 314–322.

Caine, S.B., Lintz, R., Koob, G.F., 1993. Intravenous drug self-administration techniques in animals. In: Sahgal, A. (Ed.), Behavioral Neuroscience: A Practical Approach, vol. 2. IRL Press, Oxford, pp. 117–143.

Ciccocioppo, R., Angeletti, S., Weiss, F., 2001. Long-lasting resistance to extinction of response reinstatement induced by ethanol-related stimuli: role of genetic ethanol preference. Alcohol. Clin. Exp. Res. 25, 1414–1419.

Crombag, H.S., Bossert, J.M., Koya, E., Shaham, Y., 2002. Context-induced relapse to drug seeking: a review. Philos. Trans. R. Soc. London B Biol. Sci. 363, 3233–3243.

Deroche-Gamonet, V., Belin, D., Piazza, P.V., 2004. Evidence for addiction-like behavior in the rat. Science 305, 1014–1017.

Ebel, R.M., 1961. Must all tests be valid? Am. Psychol. 16, 640–647.

Erb, S., Shaham, Y., Stewart, J., 1996. Stress reinstates cocaine-seeking behavior after prolonged extinction and a drug-free period. Psychopharmacology 128, 408–412.

Gauvin, D.V., Holloway, F.A., 1991. Cue dimensionality in the three-choice pentylenetetrazole–saline–chlordiazepoxide discrimination task. Behav. Pharmacol. 2, 417–428.

Gellert, V.F., Holtzman, S.G., 1978. Development and maintenance of morphine tolerance and dependence in the rat by scheduled access to morphine drinking solutions. J. Pharmacol. Exp. Ther. 205, 536–546.

Geyer, M.A., Markou, A., 2002. The role of preclinical models in the development of psychotropic drugs. In: Davis, K.L., Charney, D., Coyle, J.T., Nemeroff, C. (Eds.), Neuropsychopharmacology: The Fifth Generation of Progress. Lippincott Williams and Wilkins, New York, pp. 445–455.

Hand, T.H., Koob, G.F., Stinus, L., Le Moal, M., 1988. Aversive properties of opiate receptor blockade: evidence for exclusively central mediation in naive and morphine-dependent rats. Brain. Res. 474, 364–368.

Hebb, D.O., 1949. Organization of Behavior: A Neuropsychological Theory. Wiley, New York.

Holtzman, S.G., 1990. Discriminative stimulus effects of drugs: relationship to potential for abuse. In: Adler, M.W., Cowan, A. (Eds.), Testing and Evaluation of Drugs of Abuse. series title: Modern Methods in Pharmacology, vol. 6. Wiley, New York, pp. 193–210.

Katner, S.N., Magalong, J.G., Weiss, F., 1999. Reinstatement of alcohol-seeking behavior by drug-associated discriminative stimuli after prolonged extinction in the rat. Neuropsychopharmacolcogy 20, 471–479.

Katz, J.L., Higgins, S.T., 2003. The validity of the reinstatement model of craving and relapse to drug use. Psychopharmacology 168, 21–30. [erratum: 168: 244].

Kling, J.W., Riggs, L.A., 1971. Woodworth and Schlosberg's Experimental Psychology, third ed. Holt, Rinehart and Winston, New York.

Koob, G.F., Volkow, N.D., 2010. Neurocircuitry of addiction. Neuropsychopharmacol. Rev. 35, 217–238. [erratum: (35) 1051].

Koob, G.F., 2009. New dimensions in human laboratory models of addiction. Addict. Biol. 14, 1–8.

Kornetsky, C., Bain, G., 1990. Brain-stimulation reward: a model for drug-induced euphoria. In: Adler, M.W., Cowan, A. (Eds.), Testing and Evaluation of Drugs of Abuse. series title: Modern Methods in Pharmacology, vol. 6. Wiley-Liss, New York, pp. 211–231.

Kornetsky, C., Esposito, R.U., 1979. Euphorigenic drugs: effects on the reward pathways of the brain. Fed. Proc. 38, 2473–2476.

Lu, L., Grimm, J.W., Hope, B.T., Shaham, Y., 2004. Incubation of cocaine craving after withdrawal: a review of preclinical data. Neuropharmacology 47 (suppl. 1), 214–226.

Macey, D.J., Schulteis, G., Heinrichs, S.C., Koob, G.F., 1996. Time-dependent quantifiable withdrawal from ethanol in the rat: effect of method of dependence induction. Alcohol 13, 163–170.

Malin, D.H., Lake, J.R., Newlin-Maultsby, P., Roberts, L.K., Lanier, J.G., Carter, V.A., Cunningham, J.S., Wilson, O.B., 1992. Rodent model of nicotine abstinence syndrome. Pharmacol. Biochem. Behav. 43, 779–784.

Markou, A., Koob, G.F., 1992. Construct validity of a self-stimulation threshold paradigm: effects of reward and performance manipulations. Physiol. Behav. 51, 111–119.

McKinney, W.T., 1988. Models of Mental Disorders: A New Comparative Psychiatry. Plenum, New York.

Olds, J., Milner, P., 1954. Positive reinforcement produced by electrical stimulation of septal area and other regions of rat brain. J. Comp. Physiol. Psychol. 47, 419–427.

Rhodes, J.S., Best, K., Belknap, J.K., Finn, D.A., Crabbe, J.C., 2005. Evaluation of a simple model of ethanol drinking to intoxication in C57BL/6J mice. Physiol. Behav. 84, 53–63.

Richter, C.P., 1927. Animal behavior and internal drives. Q. Rev. Biol. 2, 307–343.

Roberts, A.J., Heyser, C.J., Cole, M., Griffin, P., Koob, G.F., 2000. Excessive ethanol drinking following a history of dependence: animal model of allostasis. Neuropsychopharmacology 22, 581–594.

See, R.E., Grimm, J.W., Kruzich, P.J., Rustay, N., 1999. The importance of a compound stimulus in conditioned drug seeking behavior following one week of extinction from self-administered cocaine in rats. Drug. Alcohol. Depend. 57, 41–49.

Shaham, Y., Shalev, U., Lu, L., de Wit, H., Stewart, J., 2003. The reinstatement model of drug relapse: history, methodology and major findings. Psychopharmacology 168, 3–20.

Shippenberg, T.S., Koob, G.F., 2002. Recent advances in animal models of drug addiction and alcoholism. In: Davis, K.L., Charney, D., Coyle, J.T., Nemeroff, C. (Eds.), Neuropsychopharmacology: The Fifth Generation of Progress. Lippincott Williams and Wilkins, Philadelphia, pp. 1381–1397.

Simms, J.A., Steensland, P., Medina, B., Abernathy, K.E., Chandler, L.J., Wise, R., Bartlett, S.E., 2008. Intermittent access to 20% ethanol induces high ethanol consumption in Long-Evans and Wistar rats. Alcohol. Clin. Exp. Res. 32, 1816–1823.

Stellar, J.R., Stellar, E., 1985. The Neurobiology of Motivation and Reward. Springer-Verlag, New York.

Stewart, J., de Wit, H., 1987. Reinstatement of drug taking behavior as a method of assessing incentive motivational properties of drugs. In: Bozarth, M.A. (Ed.), Methods of Assessing the Reinforcing Properties of Abused Drugs. Springer-Verlag, New York, pp. 211–227.

Wikler, A., 1973. Dynamics of drug dependence: implications of a conditioning theory for research and treatment. Arch. Gen. Psychiatry. 28, 611–616.

Wise, R.A., 1973. Voluntary ethanol intake in rats following exposure to ethanol on various schedules. Psychopharmacologia 29, 203–210.

Yahyavi-Firouz-Abadi, N., See, R.E., 2009. Anti-relapse medications: preclinical models for drug addiction treatment. Pharmacol. Ther. 124, 235–247.

Psychostimulants

DEFINITIONS

Psychostimulant drugs, such as cocaine, D-amphetamine, and methamphetamine, have medical uses but also considerable abuse potential (Figure 4.1). Direct and indirect sympathomimetics, such as cocaine and amphetamine, and nonsympathomimetics are two major classes of psychostimulants (Table 4.1, Box 4.1). This chapter focuses solely on indirect sympathomimetics. All indirect sympathomimetic compounds are chemically similar and share a common structure – a benzene ring with an ethylamine side chain. Amphetamine differs from its parent compound, β-phenethylamine, by the addition of a methyl group, whereas methamphetamine has two additional methyl groups (Box 4.2).

Psychomotor stimulants are drugs that produce behavioral activation, usually accompanied by increased arousal, alertness, and motor activity. Historically, eras of increased stimulant addiction in the general population have been linked to the increased availability and distorted or misinformed perceptions of the abuse potential of these drugs. This chapter describes psychostimulant use, abuse, and addiction, and delves into the physiological, behavioral, and neuroscientific mechanisms by which the psychostimulant effects occur.

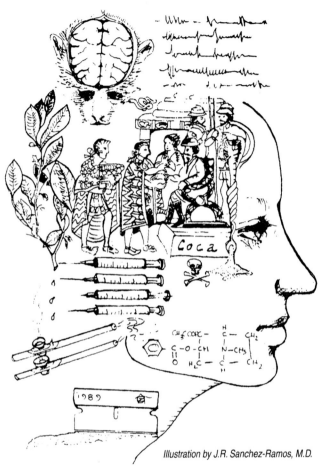

Illustration by J.R. Sanchez-Ramos, M.D.

FIGURE 4.1 **From nonhumans to humans, cocaine and related psychostimulants have numerous effects on the brain and behavior.** [From: Sanchez-Ramos JR, Neurological complications of cocaine abuse include seizure and strokes, The Psychiatric Times, 1990, February, pp. 20, 22. © 2013. UBM Medica. 103986:8135P.]

TABLE 4.1   Psychomotor Stimulant Drugs

Direct Sympathomimetics	Indirect Sympathomimetics	Nonsympathomimetics
Isoproterenol	Amphetamine	Caffeine
Epinephrine	Methamphetamine	Nicotine
Norepinephrine	Cocaine	Scopolamine
Phenylephrine	Methylphenidate	Strychnine
Phenylpropanolamine	Phenmetrazine	Pentylenetetrazol
Apomorphine	Pipradrol	Modafinil
	Tyramine	
	Pemoline	

BOX 4.1

WHAT IS AN INDIRECT SYMPATHOMIMETIC?

A drug that indirectly mimics "sympathin," which was the original term for norepinephrine (also known as noradrenaline). Norepinephrine is well known to be a primary mediator of the sympathetic nervous system ("fight or flight" response), which is a part of the autonomic nervous system. An indirect sympathomimetic is a drug that increases the availability of norepinephrine in the synapse by promoting neurotransmitter release, blocking neurotransmitter reuptake, or blocking transmitter metabolism. Note that the hormones norepinephrine (a.k.a., noradrenaline) and epinephrine (a.k.a., adrenaline) do not cross the blood-brain barrier. Therefore, any release in the brain is caused by the indirect sympathomimetics, which themselves cross the blood-brain barrier.

BOX 4.2

SYNOPSIS OF THE NEUROPHARMACOLOGICAL TARGETS FOR PSYCHOSTIMULANTS

Cocaine, amphetamines, and methamphetamine are indirect sympathomimetics that increase the availability of monoamine neurotransmitters at the synapse, such as dopamine, norepinephrine, and serotonin. All three drugs bind to the dopamine, norepinephrine, and serotonin reuptake transporters to block the reuptake of monoamines. Amphetamines and methamphetamine also bind to the vesicular transporter and enhance the release of monoamines into the synapse. The enhanced availability of monoamines at the synapse are transduced by five different dopamine receptors, two different families of norepinephrine receptors, and seven different families of serotonin receptors throughout different regions of the brain. The psychostimulant effects of indirect sympathomimetic psychostimulants are largely mediated by the release of dopamine which acts on dopamine receptors in the terminal areas of the mesocorticolimbic dopamine system and nigrostriatal dopamine system in the frontal cortex–nucleus accumbens-amygdala and corpus striatum, respectively. The addiction potential of psychostimulants largely derives from powerful within-system neuroadaptations (signal transduction mechanisms) and between-system neuroadaptations (neurocircuitry changes) in the brain motivational and stress systems.

HISTORY OF PSYCHOSTIMULANT USE

Cocaine derives from the coca plant *Erythroxylon coca* and has a long history as a stimulant (Figure 4.2, Box 4.3). Coca chewing originated in Peru at least as early as 3000 BC. Initially, its use was restricted to royalty but eventually came to the general population following the Spanish conquest to sustain the performance of laborers in the Peruvian silver mines. Cocaine has been used for centuries in tonics and other

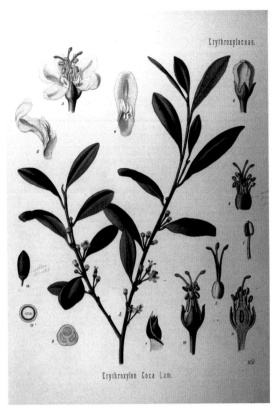

FIGURE 4.2 **Erythroxylon coca.** *[From: Bentley R, Trimen H. Medicinal plants: being descriptions with original figures of the principal plants employed in medicine and an account of the characters, properties and uses of their parts and products of medicinal value. Churchill, London, 1880.]*

preparations to allay fatigue, sustain performance, and treat a wide range of ailments. Cocaine once was a component of Coca Cola®. In 1886, the druggist John Styth Pemberton patented a medicine that contained two natural stimulants, cocaine and caffeine, to formulate the syrup base for Coca Cola®. He blended a whole-leaf extract of coca with an extract from the African Kola nut which contains caffeine. Coca Cola® was initially manufactured and marketed as an "intellectual beverage" and "brain tonic," and until 1903, Coca Cola® contained approximately 60 mg of cocaine per 8 ounce (237 ml) serving. In 1903, soon after the

dangers of cocaine were widely publicized, the manufacturer of Coca Cola® removed cocaine from its formulation, although an extract of the coca leaf is still found in the preparation today. However, the only stimulant now found in a typical can of Coke is ~34 mg caffeine.

The therapeutic effects of cocaine were propounded not only by manufacturers of Coca Cola®. In the late 19th century, Dr. Sigmund Freud also advocated the use of cocaine for the treatment of a variety of disorders, including psychiatric disorders and drug addiction. In fact, Freud used cocaine himself but quickly lost his enthusiasm after witnessing his first cocaine-induced psychosis in a colleague (more on cocaine psychoses will be discussed later in this chapter; see Box 4.4 for a modern example).

Cocaine and other indirect sympathomimetics have been involved in more than one episode of widespread drug abuse, both in the United States and worldwide (Table 4.2, Figure 4.3). Presumably because cocaine was used in numerous tonics and "healthful" preparations, extensive cultivation of cocaine occurred in South America, resulting in extensive exportation to the United States and Europe. With widespread supply, demand followed, and in the United States the first restriction of coca products occurred with the 1914 Harrison Narcotics Act, sponsored by Representative Francis Burton Harrison (Democrat, New York):

"An Act to provide for the registration of, with collectors of internal revenue, and to impose a special tax on all persons who produce, import, manufacture, compound, deal in, dispense, sell, distribute, or give away opium or coca leaves, their salts, derivatives, or preparations, and for other purposes...That it shall be unlawful for any person to sell, barter, exchange, or give away any of the aforesaid drugs except in pursuance of a written order of the person to whom such article is sold, bartered, exchanged, or given, on a form to be issued in blank for that purpose by the Commissioner of Internal Revenue...[but shall not apply to] the dispensing or distribution of any of the aforesaid drugs to a patient by a physician, dentist, or veterinary surgeon registered under this Act in the course of his professional practice [or] the sale, dispensing, or

BOX 4.3

COCAINE IS DERIVED FROM WHAT SOURCE?

Cocaine is derived from the leaves of the coca plant (*Erythroxylon coca*). Cocaine is an alkaloid found in the leaves of the plant and was first isolated in 1855 by Friedrich Gaedcke of Germany, who originally termed it "erythroxyline." An improved purification process was published in 1860 by Albert Niemann, who renamed the alkaloid "cocaine." Nearly 40 years later, in 1898, Richard Willstatter was the first to synthesize the cocaine molecule, beginning with tropinone, and define its chemical structure. Illicit cocaine production involves the extraction of crude coca paste from the coca leaf, purification of coca paste to coke base, and conversion of the base to cocaine hydrochloride. Cocaine hydrochloride can also be synthesized (that is, the process does not begin with a crude extract),

in which 2-carbomethoxytropinone is first produced, followed by conversion to methyl ecgonine, and finally benzoylation to cocaine. Licit or pharmaceutical-grade cocaine hydrochloride production generally follows this synthesis procedure but incorporates several more steps that yield cocaine hydrochloride with a purity greater than 99.5% (in contrast to illicit cocaine, which is ~80–97% pure).

Gaedcke F. Ueber das erythroxylin, dargestellt aus den blättern des in Südamerika cultivirten strauches erythroxylon coca. Archiv der Pharmazie, 1855, (132), 141–150.

Albert Niemann. Ueber eine neue organische base in den cocablättern. Archiv der Pharmazie, 1860, (153), 129–256.

Casale JF. A practical total synthesis of cocaine's enantiomers. Forensic Science International, 1987, (33), 275.

distributing of any of the aforesaid drugs by a dealer to a consumer under and in pursuance of a written prescription issued by a physician, dentist, or veterinary surgeon registered under this Act ... That any person who violates or fails to comply with any of the requirements of this Act shall, on conviction, be fined not more than $2,000 or be imprisoned not more than five years, or both, in the discretion of the court."

This legislation, however, may have unwittingly mislabeled cocaine-containing preparations as narcotics (Box 4.5), but the law, for the first time, penalized the possession, sale, and use of cocaine.

In the 1960s, cocaine use rose together with the monetary profits from illegal trafficking. In the 1970s, cocaine was most commonly administered intranasally in a powder form (as cocaine hydrochloride). The perception among users was that such a preparation was safe and non-addictive. In fact, the 1980 edition of the

Comprehensive Textbook of Psychiatry stated: "... used no more than two to three times a week, cocaine creates no serious problems. In daily and fairly large amounts, it can produce minor psychological disturbances. Chronic cocaine abuse does not appear as a medical problem." (Kaplan HI, Freedman AM, Sadock BJ (eds.) *Comprehensive Textbook of Psychiatry: Volume 2*, 3rd edition. Williams and Wilkins, Baltimore, 1980, pp. 1614–1629).

Cocaine hydrochloride itself cannot be smoked because it is quickly destroyed at high temperatures, and methods were developed to produce a smokeable preparation, in which the base of cocaine is separated from the salt. Termed "freebase" cocaine, such a preparation is very pure and originally appeared in the late 1970s and remained popular through the mid-1980s. Freebase vaporizes at 260°C. When heated, the crystals release vaporized cocaine

BOX 4.4

CASE REPORT

A 29-year-old white married unemployed man came to the outpatient clinic of the hospital with the complaints of marked anxiety and the fear that he was "going insane." His past history included several arrests and convictions for burglary and aggravated battery, as well as a psychiatric hospitalization a few years ago, when he was diagnosed as having "drug addiction" and a "sociopathic personality." He admitted using a variety of drugs (heroin, codeine, paregoric) for many years until about a year ago, when he stopped using these drugs and began instead to use Desoxyn (methamphetamine hydrochloride) alone. He related that once or twice a week he would dissolve about 15 tablets of Desoxyn (5 mg strength) into boiled water and then inject the solution intravenously in 2–4 divided doses over a 24 hour period. Following the last injection, he would stay up all night reading books on biology, medicine, and psychology, meditating, or looking at things through a microscope, which he bought a few months ago in order to find out more about the "secrets of Nature."

On examination, he was oriented, coherent and relevant. Almost throughout the interview he kept pulling the hair on the top of his head in a stereotyped manner. Asked why he was doing this, he replied that this was a "tic" he acquired a few months ago. His thought disorder became apparent, as he further explained that a few

months ago he came to believe that "twisted" hair in his head may cause cancer of the brain and schizophrenia, and he had to "untwist" it to prevent the occurrence of these illnesses. He was extremely concerned about it, since his father had died of a brain tumor a few years earlier. His preoccupation with "hair" was pervasive.

He pointed out that hair and sperm under the microscope look like worms; therefore [sic] they are worms, that the testes are bags of worms, and that the intestines and the brain and the whole human body are just big worms. Ideas of grandiosity and persecution were also present. He called attention to the fact that he was born on July 17, that Caesar's first name was Julius and that since the Romans celebrated the founding of Rome on the 17th of each month, it was more than likely that Julius Caesar was born on July 17. Since the patient was also Roman (Italian), he reasoned that he was Julius Caesar reincarnated. He expressed the belief that "police agents are everywhere"; he worried about [sic] "what they are doing to our food" and pointed out that the milk is not only pasteurized, but also *homogenized*, which means that "they poison our *genes* with milk." It is of interest that he denied ever having hallucinations.

Siomopoulos V. Thought disorder in amphetamine psychosis: a case report. Psychosomatics, 1976, (17), 42–44.

that can be inhaled. In one process, called freebase extraction, the hydrochloride salt is mixed with buffered ammonia, the alkaloidal (freebase) cocaine is extracted from the solution using ether, and the ether is evaporated to yield cocaine crystals. In another process, cocaine hydrochloride is combined with baking

soda (sodium bicarbonate), and the mixture is heated until it forms a solid. This smokeable form of cocaine became available as small, readily smokeable "rocks" and was called "crack" cocaine because the crystals make a crackling sound when heated. Since the mid-1980s, this has been the preferred method of

TABLE 4.2 History of Cocaine Use and Misuse

3000 B.C.	Cocaine is believed to have originated in the subtropical valleys of the eastern slopes of the Andes or Amazonian subtropical valleys. The earliest archeological evidence from Peru dates coca chewing to 3000 B.C.
1493–1527	Coca chewing was restricted to Incan royalty and religious figures. Coca leaves were used as offerings and were used in cultural and religious ceremonies.
1536	Coca chewing came to the masses following the Spanish conquest. Coca leaves were used by Indian slave laborers in the silver mines to keep themselves alert and working.
1859	Albert Niemann analyzes a sample of Peruvian coca in the lab of Fredrich Wöhler to determine active compound and isolates cocaine.
1868–1869	Coca is touted by Angelo Mariani who developed a coca based wine Vin Mariani. The wine contained no more than 300 mg of cocaine, was very popular, and was marketed as a tonic wine and cure-all.
1884	Karl Koller publishes work on using cocaine as an anesthetic during eye surgery.
	Sigmund Freud publishes *On Coca*. Recommends cocaine use for a variety of illnesses, notably for alcoholism and morphine addiction.
1886	Albert Erlenmeyer publishes a paper denouncing cocaine use as treatment for opioid addiction. Blames Freud for releasing "the third scourge of mankind."
1887	Freud publishes *Craving for and Fear of Cocaine*. He admits that cocaine should not be used to treat morphine addiction after his friend Ernst von Fleischl-Marxow experiences severe toxic symptoms of heavy cocaine use.
1885	Pemberton, a patent-medicine maker from Atlanta, produced a wine called *Cocaine – Ideal Nerve and Tonic Stimulant*. Because of overriding Prohibition restrictions, he launched a nonalcoholic extract of coca leaves and caffeine-rich African Kola nuts in a sweet, carbonated syrup he called *Coca Cola*.
1892	Coca Cola Company is founded. Coca Cola is touted as a medicinal drink.
1902	Due to negative public sentiment, Coca Cola "decocainizes" its preparation, replacing cocaine with caffeine.
1910	President Howard Taft presents a State Department report on drug use to Congress. Cocaine officially becomes "Public Enemy #1."
	"The illicit sales…and the habitual use of it temporarily raises the power of a criminal to a point where in resisting arrest there is no hesitation to murder. It is more appalling in its effects than any other habit-forming drug used in the United States."
1914	The Harrison Narcotic Act is passed which tightly regulates the distribution and sale of drugs. Because of public anti-cocaine sentiment the Harrison Act was largely supported and was rather successful.
1970	Cocaine use increases following a backlash against amphetamine use. Stimulant users rediscover cocaine as a "safe" recreational drug. Most use is social-recreational among friends or acquaintances.
	Controlled Substances Act passes in United States Congress. Cocaine is made a Schedule II drug by the Drug Enforcement Administration (abusable drugs with officially sanctioned medical uses).
1974	"Freebasing" develops in southern California.
1975	A White Paper issued by the United States government indicated that cocaine is "not physically addictive" and "usually does not result in serious social consequences such as crime, hospital emergency room admission, or death."
1980	Approximately 20% of those aged 15–25 admit to using cocaine. Drug abuse treatment facilities and hospitals report dramatic increases in cocaine freebase admission.

From: Siegel RK. Cocaine smoking. Journal of Psychoactive Drugs, 1982, (14), 271–359.

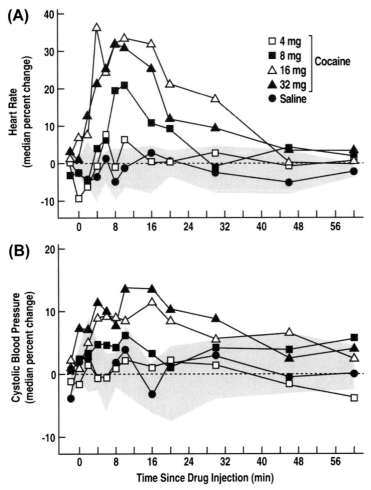

(A)

(B)

FIGURE 4.3 (A) Median percentage change in heart rate in humans for 1 h after an intravenous injection of saline or 4–32 mg cocaine. The percentage change was calculated for each dose of cocaine with reference to its own 30 min pre-drug baseline. The saline function represents data collected on day 8 of the experimental series. The shaded region indicates the semi-interquartile range of those data. (B) Median percent change in systolic blood pressure after an intravenous injection of saline or 4–32 mg cocaine. The percent change was calculated for each dose of cocaine from the pre-drug baseline measured during the 30 min prior to the injection of that dose. The saline function represents the data collected on day 8 of the experimental series. The shaded area indicates the semi-interquartile range for those data. *These figures show the relative effectiveness and potency of cocaine in producing increases in heart rate and blood pressure.* [From Fischman MW, Schuster CR, Resnekov L, Shick JFE, Krasnegor NA, Fennell W, Freedman DX. Cardiovascular and subjective effects of intravenous cocaine administration in humans. Archives of General Psychiatry, 1976, (33), 983–989.]

BOX 4.5

WHAT IS A NARCOTIC?

Strictly speaking, narcotics are drugs such as morphine that blunt, rather than excite, brain activity and produce narcosis (sleepiness), but the term has been more widely used in the legal sense to refer to any drug or substance that affects mood or behavior and is sold for nonmedical, illegal purposes.

---

producing smokeable cocaine because it is simpler and safer than the ether extraction method. Today, most of the available crack cocaine in the United States is produced this way.

Amphetamines were first synthesized in 1887 in Germany and had widespread medical use in the treatment of narcolepsy and a variety of other disorders from 1936 to the mid-1940s.

D-Amphetamine was sold over-the-counter in Europe until the 1960s when many cases of acute psychotic schizophrenia-like episodes began to occur. The term *amphetamine* originates from the chemical name α-methylphenethylamine and includes dextroamphetamine (D-amphetamine) and levoamphetamine (L-amphetamine). The D-isomer is five to 10 times more potent than the L-isomer in producing central nervous system effects. Methamphetamine was first synthesized in Japan in 1893 and is the methylated derivative of amphetamine, in which a methyl group is added to the amphetamine base structure. The methyl group increases amphetamine's ability to cross the blood–brain barrier, thus hypothetically facilitating its psychoactive effects.

There are two isomers, D and L, and the D isomer is much more psychoactive than the L isomer. The L isomer is still the active ingredient in nasal decongestant inhalers like Vicks Vapor inhaler. Although rarely prescribed, methamphetamine (D-methamphetamine; Desoxyn) is approved in the United States for the treatment of attention-deficit/hyperactivity disorder and as a short-term adjunct treatment in a regimen for weight loss based on caloric restriction.

Methamphetamine came into widespread use during World War II to increase the endurance and performance of military personnel. Methamphetamine was sold over-the-counter in Japan as Philopin and Sedrin as a product to fight sleepiness and enhance vitality. At the end of World War II (1945–1955), an epidemic of methamphetamine use occurred in Japan, attributed to dumping military stockpiles of stimulant agents on the open market. Japan had an estimated 550,000 methamphetamine abusers in 1954. Sweden also witnessed an epidemic of abuse of phenmetrazine, an amphetamine-like stimulant, in the 1950s and 1960s. Illegal diversion of amphetamines in the 1960s paralleled the increased use of the drugs on the street, resulting in a cyclical pattern of abuse by users who were known as "speed freaks" (habitual users of amphetamines).

In the 1960s, methamphetamine was synthesized illegally and called "crank," and it dominated the "speed" (generic term for psychostimulants in the amphetamine grouping) market. Manufacture shifted to the San Diego area in the 1980s with the production of "crystal meth." Crystal meth is synthesized from ephedrine and iodine and has a crystalline-like appearance when it is pure. The high-purity crystalline form is also termed "ice" because of its resemblance to shards of ice crystals. Both the powdered and crystal forms of methamphetamine are the hydrochloride salt, and in contrast to cocaine, the salt form of methamphetamine can be smoked. Freebase methamphetamine is an oily liquid at room temperature. Smoking methamphetamine became a popular route of administration in the 1980s in Hawaii, the Pacific Coast of the United States, and southern California and subsequently spread to the rest of the United States.

The 2011 United States *National Survey on Drug Use and Health* from the Substance Abuse and Mental Health Services Administration estimated that 36.9 million people aged 12 and older (14.6%) had ever engaged in cocaine use, and 18.5 million (7.2%) people aged 12 and older had ever engaged in stimulant use. Of those 12 and older, 3.9 million were last-year users of cocaine (1.5%), and 2.7 million were last-year users of stimulants (1.0%). Of these, 11.9 million (4.6%) had used methamphetamine, and 1.0 million (0.4%) were last-year users of methamphetamine. Notable statistics from the survey included the following. In 2011, of those people aged 12 or older who ever used in the last year, 0.82 million (21.1%) showed cocaine abuse or dependence, and 0.33 million (12.9%) showed stimulant abuse or dependence (Substance Use Disorder based on the *Diagnostic and Statistical Manual of Mental Disorders*, 5th edition [DSM-5], criteria), 0.58 million (14.5%) of those who ever used in the last year showed cocaine dependence, and 0.25 million (9.3%) of those who ever used in the last year showed stimulant dependence (DSM-IV criteria; see Chapter 1).

PHYSIOLOGICAL EFFECTS

Both cocaine and amphetamine increase systolic and diastolic blood pressure. In humans, a dose of 10 mg of D-amphetamine administered intravenously produces an increase in blood pressure that is equal to that produced with a dose of 32 mg of intravenous cocaine (Figure 4.3). In addition to increasing blood pressure, cocaine and amphetamines also stimulate the heart rate, but amphetamines may cause less of an effect than one would expect based on other physiological measures because of a reflexive slowing of heart rate. These drugs also produce bronchial dilation, pupillary dilation, and decreases in glandular secretions, all of which are effects observed after activation of the sympathetic nervous system.

The mechanism of action for the autonomic effects of indirect sympathomimetics such as amphetamines and cocaine has long been known. Both drugs indirectly release norepinephrine and epinephrine by either blocking reuptake (cocaine) or stimulating release (amphetamines). Conversely, chemical or physical destruction of noradrenergic (norepinephrine) fibers or pharmacological treatment with drugs that decrease the levels of catecholamines (e.g., norepinephrine and dopamine) abolishes the autonomic effects of cocaine and amphetamine. The exact mechanism by which psychostimulants directly affect various neurochemical and neurocircuitry systems to produce their psychostimulant effects is discussed in greater detail below.

BEHAVIORAL EFFECTS

Cocaine administered intranasally produces stimulant effects similar to those of amphetamines, but with a much shorter duration of action (20–45 min), including feelings of having much energy, fatigue reduction, a sense of well being, increased confidence, and increased talkativeness. Intoxication includes a euphoric effect that has been described as exhilarating, with a kind of rush that "goes straight to one's brain," mild elation, and an enhanced ability to concentrate. Sigmund Freud wrote:

> "The psychic effect of cocaine in doses of 50–100 mg consists of exhilaration and lasting euphoria, which does not differ in any way from the normal euphoria of a healthy person."

In a letter to his fiancée Martha, dated June 2, 1884, he wrote:

> " ... a small dose lifted me to heights in a wonderful fashion" (Jones E. The Life and Work of Sigmund Freud. Basic Books, New York, 1961).

When taken intravenously or smoked, cocaine produces an intense euphoria, sometimes followed by a crash (a very sudden drop in mood and energy). William Burroughs wrote in 1959:

> "When you shoot coke in the mainline there is a rush of pure pleasure to the head...Ten minutes later you want another shot...intravenous C is electricity through the brain, activating cocaine pleasure connections." (Burroughs WS. The Naked Lunch. Grove Press, New York, 1959).

Cocaine has many of the same stimulant effects as amphetamines, including sustained performance in situations of fatigue. A study with normal, healthy volunteers tested with a wide range of intravenous doses of cocaine or D-amphetamine showed that cocaine produced many of the same subjective and physiological effects as D-amphetamine, although D-amphetamine was more potent (Figure 4.4, Box 4.6).

Amphetamines in recreational dose ranges produce stimulant effects, but the most dramatic effects are observed in situations of fatigue and boredom. Such stimulant effects can translate into enhanced performance in these situations and include increased stimulation, improved coordination, increased strength and endurance, increased mental and physical activation, and improved subjective sensations of fatigue. Mood changes include boldness, elation, and friendliness. Amphetamines also enhance performance in simple motor and cognitive tasks, including

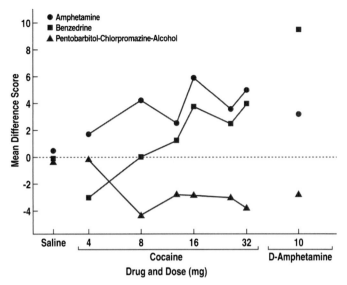

FIGURE 4.4 **Mean change in scores on five separate scales of the Addiction Research Council Inventory (ARCI).** A short form of the ARCI was answered prior to drug or saline injection and again 15 min after the injection. The scales included amphetamine, benzedrine, and pentobarbital-chlorpromazine-alcohol. [*Taken with permission from Fischman MW, Schuster CR, Resnekov L, Shick JFE, Krasnegor NA, Fennell W, Freedman DX. Cardiovascular and subjective effects of intravenous cocaine administration in humans.* Archives of General Psychiatry, *1976, (33), 983–989.*] *These data show that cocaine and D-amphetamine are identified by subjects as euphoric, amphetamine-like, and not sedative. The morphine–benzedrine scale is a measure of euphoria. The pentobarbital–chlorpromazine–alcohol scale is a measure of sedation. The amphetamine scale is a measure of "amphetamine-like." See page 247 of Martin WR, Sloan JW, Sapira JD, Jasinski DR. Physiologic, subjective, and behavioral effects of amphetamine, methamphetamine, ephedrine, phenmetrazine, and methylphenidate in man.* Clinical Pharmacology and Therapeutics, *1971, (12), 245–258.*

measures of reaction time, speed, attention, and performance (Figure 4.5). Amphetamines can also improve athletic performance by small amounts (0.5–4%), and these superficially negligible improvements might be sufficient in highly competitive situations (Table 4.3).

Nonetheless, stimulants such as the amphetamines and cocaine can also fail to improve performance in well-functioning, motivated subjects, and little evidence suggests that amphetamines can enhance intellectual functioning in complex tasks or tests of intelligence. One study found that methamphetamine failed to improve performance on a complex attention task, although it did increase the rate at which a visual display was scanned. An inverted U-shaped dose–response function that inversely relates stimulant dose to cognitive performance has been hypothesized, in which lower doses

may improve performance, but higher doses decrease performance (Figure 4.6). As the dose of stimulant increases, behavior becomes progressively more constricted and repetitive, resulting in both cognitive and behavioral perseveration. However, the effects of the drug depend on initial conditions. The memory-enhancing effects of methylphenidate (or Ritalin, a stimulant used to treat attention-deficit/hyperactivity disorder), for example, depend on healthy subjects' baseline performance on the same memory task in an undrugged state, such that greater improvement was observed in subjects with lower baseline memory capacity.

Other acute actions of amphetamines and cocaine include a decrease in appetite, for which these drugs have been used therapeutically and to which tolerance develops (Table 4.4). Trials over 4 weeks reported significant weight loss;

BOX 4.6

CASE REPORT: ACUTE ANXIETY RESPONSE TO COCAINE

A 19-year-old white male had been experimenting with a variety of drugs, including snorting cocaine, for approximately two years. He had used cocaine exclusively in a recreational setting and indicated that he found nothing but pleasure in the drug experience and never had any problem, nor had he escalated his dose. One day a group of friends were injecting cocaine and they persuaded him to try this route of administration. As he had had no difficulty with cocaine previously, and as a result of curiosity and peer group pressure, he decided that he would experiment with injection. Following the intense stimulation and rush he became acutely anxious and frightened. Upon arrival at the Medical Section of the Haight-Ashbury Free Medical Clinic, he was found to have a very rapid pulse rate as well as a hyperventilation administered anxiety. He was treated with 10 mg of i.v. Valium(R) administered slowly with reassurance. To cease

the carpopedal spasms he had developed as a consequence of his hyperventilation syndrome, he was told to breathe into a paper bag which increased his carbon dioxide levels. The acute anxiety and its subsequent sequelae faded in approximately three hours. Follow-up indicated no recurrences or further experimentation with intravenous injection of cocaine by this individual. This use of intravenous sedative hypnotic medication is controversial and some critics of this approach use oral medication only while others stress reassurance alone without medication. We would recommend intravenous Valium(R) only after nonpharmacological intervention has failed.

Wesson DR, Smith DE, Cocaine: its use for central nervous system stimulation including recreational and medical uses. In: Petersen RC, Stillman RC (Eds.), Cocaine: 1977, (series title: NIDA Research Monograph, vol. 13), National Institute on Drug Abuse, Rockville MD, 1977, pp. 137–152.

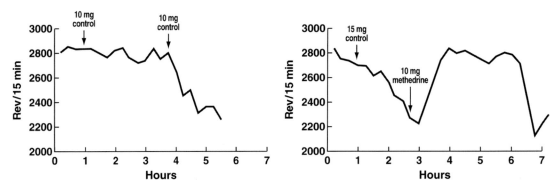

FIGURE 4.5   **Performance on a cycle ergometer in humans after treatment with the psychostimulant methedrine.** *[From: Cuthbertson DP, Knox JAC. The effects of analeptics on the fatigued subject. Journal of Physiology, 1947, (106), 42–58.] This very early study showed that administration of methedrine (methamphetamine) to a human sustained performance on a stationary bicycle long past when a placebo-treated individual fatigued.*

TABLE 4.3 Comparative Effects of Amphetamine Sulfate and Placebo on Swimming Performance Times in Subjects* Under Rested and Fatigued Conditions

| Swim Style | Swim Time (sec) | | |
	Placebo	Amphetamine (0.2 mg/kg)	Improvement
Rested			
Freestyle (100 yard)	57.47	56.87	1.04%
Butterfly (100 yard)	70.96	69.36	2.25%
Freestyle (200 yard)	136.88	135.94	0.69%
Backstroke (200 yard)	159.80	158.32	0.93%
Breaststroke (200 yard)	171.87	170.22	0.96%
Fatigued			
Freestyle (100 yard)	59.31	58.53	1.32%
Butterfly (100 yard)	76.06	74.80	1.66%
Freestyle (200 yard)	144.24	142.38	1.29%
Backstroke (200 yard)	166.48	167.19	–
Breaststroke (200 yard)	175.14	176.87	–

* Three subjects performed each of the swim tasks specified, under both the rested (1st swim) and fatigued (2nd swim) conditions. The 2nd swim occurred 15 min after the 1st swim.
[Data from Smith GM, Beecher HK. Amphetamine sulfate and athletic performance: I. Objective effects. Journal of the American Medical Association, 1959, (170), 542–557.]

trials over 6 months reported no significant effects. Amphetamines also decrease sleepiness, increase the latency to fall asleep, increase the latency to the onset of rapid-eye-movement (REM) sleep, and reduce total REM sleep.

Finally, amphetamines and cocaine have long been reported to heighten sexual interest and prolong orgasm. In some instances, such delays in ejaculation have led to marathon bouts of intercourse that last for hours and may reflect some of the behavioral psychopathology produced by these drugs. However, with chronic amphetamine and cocaine abuse, psychostimulants can lead to significant decreases in sexual performance with prolonged use of the drug.

MEDICAL USES

Cocaine was recognized as early as 1884 as a local anesthetic in ophthalmology, and the only currently accepted medical uses today for cocaine are for mucous membrane anesthesia and vasoconstriction. These indications ultimately led to the discovery of procaine (Novocain), which produces local anesthesia but does not produce cocaine's euphoric or vasoconstrictor effects. Amphetamines were originally synthesized as possible alternative drugs for the treatment of asthma and were the principal component of the original benzedrine inhalers (Figure 4.7). The United States military continues to use amphetamines today to allay fatigue, and amphetamines are currently legally available for medical use as adjuncts for short-term weight control. Amphetamines are also effective treatments for narcolepsy and attention-deficit/hyperactivity disorder in both children and adults (Box 4.7).

PHARMACOKINETICS

The nature of the stimulant effects of cocaine and amphetamines depends on the route of administration. These drugs can be smoked (crack) or administered intravenously (shooting up), intranasally (snorted), or orally. As noted above, intravenous or inhaled freebase preparations produce intense, pleasurable sensations characterized as a "rush" that users have likened to sexual orgasm. Such extreme euphoria has

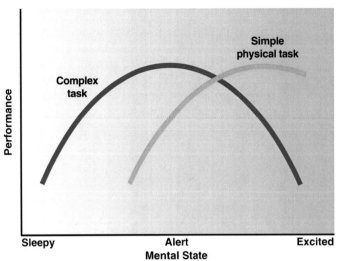

FIGURE 4.6 **Effects of psychostimulants on performance.** The figure shows hypothetical inverted U-shaped functions that relate the dose of psychostimulant to performance, depending on the complexity of the task. For a more complex task, the entire dose-effect function shifts to the left (think of a neurosurgeon or watch maker doing a delicate task). For simpler tasks (like chopping wood), the dose–effect function shifts to the right. [*From: Hart CL, Ksir C, Ray O. Drugs, Society and Human Behavior, 13th edn. McGraw-Hill, Boston, 2009.*]

TABLE 4.4   Weight Loss (in Pounds) Induced by Benzphetamine and D-Amphetamine

Medication	Week 0	Week 1	Week 2	Week 3	Week 4
Benzphetamine*	1.84 ± 0.23 (n = 20)	0.86 ± 0.1 (n = 19)	0.70 ± 0.24 (n = 16)	0.49 ± 0.20 (n = 14)	0.53 ± 0.23 (n = 9)
D-Amphetamine	1.53 ± 0.16 (n = 19)	0.93 ± 0.16 (n = 17)	0.56 ± 0.14 (n = 12)	0.54 ± 0.24 (n = 11)	0.29 ± 0.25 (n = 8)

Benzphetamine, a phenylalkylamine, is chemically and pharmacologically related to amphetamine. [Taken with permission from Simkin B, Wallace L. A controlled clinical comparison of benzphetamine and D-amphetamine in the management of obesity. American Journal of Clinical Nutrition, 1961, (9), 632–637.]

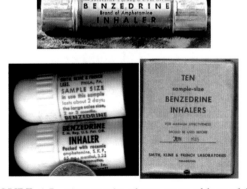

FIGURE 4.7 **Photographs of two types of benzedrine inhaler, first introduced to the market in 1932 by Smith, Kline & French Co.**

been shown to be a powerful motivational factor for abusing these drugs. The intravenous doses that produce these subjective effects are approximately 8–16 mg cocaine and 10 mg of D-amphetamine. Peak cocaine levels in the bloodstream after intravenous administration appear almost immediately and rapidly decrease over the next 2 h (Figure 4.8). Smoked cocaine in the freebase form is absorbed into the bloodstream at a rate very similar to intravenous administration, and 50 mg of freebase produces cardiovascular effects approximately equivalent to 32 mg cocaine administered intravenously. Intranasal doses of 20–30 mg cocaine produce euphoric and stimulant effects that are short-lived and

BOX 4.7

HOW DOES ONE EXPLAIN THE SEEMING PARADOX THAT PSYCHOSTIMULANTS SUCH AS AMPHETAMINES AND METHYLPHENIDATE CAN TREAT ADHD?

Although seemingly counterintuitive, psychostimulants are indeed one of the primary treatments for attention-deficit/hyperactivity disorder (ADHD). One may question this paradox: How does a stimulant drug treat someone who already appears to be highly stimulated? The answer lies in the fact that psychostimulants not only increase arousal; they also focus attention. A person with ADHD has difficulty controlling impulsive behavior – that is, their attention can rapidly shift from one thing to another. A psychostimulant, such as Adderall, helps focus attention and tune out distractions that would otherwise cause the person to lose focus on the task at hand.

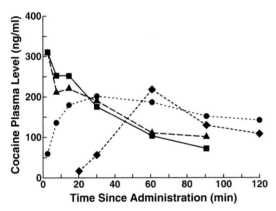

FIGURE 4.8 **Cocaine plasma levels in blood after administration via intravenous, smoked, intranasal, and oral routes.** These data show that the route of cocaine administration determines the profile of absorption over time. Notice that the peak levels of cocaine in the blood are delayed with oral administration compared with intravenous and smoked cocaine and that the peak levels in the blood are higher for intravenous and smoked cocaine. Notice also that the profile of absorption of intravenous cocaine is virtually identical to smoked cocaine. [*From: Fischman MW. Behavioral pharmacology of cocaine.* Journal of Clinical Psychiatry, *1988, 49(2 suppl): 7–10.] © 1988, Physicians Postgraduate Press. Reprinted by permission.*

last for approximately 30 min. Cocaine levels in the blood after intranasal administration start low, build quickly, and then slowly taper off. Cocaine administered orally has less powerful effects than cocaine administered intravenously, presumably because of a much slower absorption rate. Peak blood levels after oral administration occur after about 60 min. South American Indians have used an oral coca leaf preparation combined with ash for centuries to promote absorption. They recognized that coca leaves were effective as a stimulant to reduce hunger and fatigue, and chewing the leaves (or drinking tea preparations) did not have any obvious major negative physical or psychic effects. Intranasal or oral administration of D-amphetamine in the dose range of 2.5–15 mg produces stimulant effects which are similar to cocaine. People report feelings of alertness, energetic vitality, confidence, assertiveness, and decreases in appetite and fatigue. Intranasal absorption is faster than oral administration and has more intense effects (Box 4.8). Compared with cocaine's effects, which last for about 30 min, the stimulant effects of amphetamines last much longer – up to 4–6 h.

Amphetamine is metabolized in the liver, and approximately 30% is excreted unchanged in urine. Amphetamine has a relatively long half-life of approximately 12 h, but the half-life can depend on the pH of urine (for a definition of "half-life," see Chapter 2). Alkaline urine can extend the half-life to over 16 h; acidic urine can shorten it to just 8 h. Methamphetamine's

---

BOX 4.8

WHICH ROUTE OF ADMINISTRATION PRODUCES THE FASTEST ACCESS TO THE BRAIN?

Intravenous administration produces the quickest, nearly instantaneous, psychopharmacological effects, paralleled by smoking, the effects of which appear within seconds. The intranasal route is also very fast, with effects beginning to appear almost immediately and peak effects occurring after about 20 min. The oral route, similar to all drugs of abuse, is the slowest because of the time needed for absorption.

BOX 4.9

BEHAVIORAL MECHANISM OF ACTION

In this book, a "behavioral mechanism of action" refers to a unifying and integrating principle of order and predictability at the behavioral level for a given drug. Although the addiction process for each drug class has certain common neurobiological elements, each class of drugs is also unique and engages the addiction cycle at different points. Each drug class has different behavioral effects that define a phenotype. This behavioral mechanism may derive from medical use or behavioral pathology that informs medical use.

---

metabolism and excretion are similar to amphetamine. Methamphetamine has a half-life of 11 h for the smoked route and 12 h for the intravenous route. Cocaine, in contrast, is rapidly and efficiently metabolized (half-life of just 48–75 min), and less than 10% is excreted unchanged in urine.

BEHAVIORAL MECHANISM OF ACTION

High doses of amphetamines and cocaine or prolonged use/abuse can lead to significant behavioral pathology (Box 4.9). Amphetamine abusers persist in repetitive thoughts or actions for hours. These behaviors can include repetitively cleaning the house or car, bathing in a tub all day, elaborately sorting small objects, or endlessly dismantling and putting back together items such as clocks or radios. Termed "punding" by Rylander (1971), this behavior was described as "organized, goal-directed, but meaningless activity." Such repetitive behavior under the influence of amphetamines and cocaine is called "stereotyped behavior" and can be defined as "integrated behavioral sequences that acquire a stereotyped character, being performed at an increasing rate in a repetitive manner." (Randrup A, Munkvad I. Biochemical, anatomical and psychological investigations of stereotyped behavior induced by amphetamines. In: Costa E, Garattini S (eds.) *International Symposium on Amphetamines and Related Compounds.* Raven Press, New York, 1970, pp. 695–713). Stereotyped behavior is observed in many animal species. Monkeys will pick at their skin, exhibit mouth and tongue movements, and stare. Rats will sniff intensely in one location.

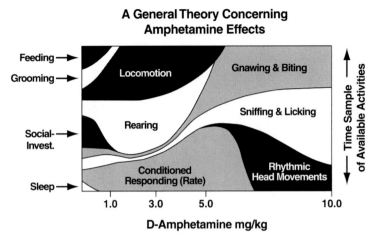

A General Theory Concerning Amphetamine Effects

FIGURE 4.9 Schematic drawing depicting the relative distribution of varying behavioral activities within a given time sample relative to increasing doses of D-amphetamine. Notice that as the dose increases, the number of activities decreases, but the rate of behavior within a given behavioral activity increases. [From: Lyon M, Robbins TW. The action of central nervous system stimulant drugs: a general theory concerning amphetamine effects. In: Essman WB, Valzelli L (eds.) Current Developments in Psychopharmacology, vol. 2. Spectrum Publications, New York, 1975, pp. 79–163.]

Pigeons will repetitively peck at one location on a stimulus display.

Insights into the nature and behavioral mechanism of action of amphetamine-like drugs derived from further experimental and theoretical analysis of stereotyped behavior (Figure 4.9). Lyon and Robbins (1975) hypothesized that as the dose of amphetamine increases, the repetition rate of all motor activity increases, with the result that the organism will exhibit "increases in response rates within a decreasing number of response categories." This type of analysis makes a number of predictions. Complex behavioral ensembles are the first to be eliminated as the response categories decrease. Behaviors capable of repetition without long pauses then dominate, and shorter and shorter response sequences result. As a result, high rates of responding in operant situations decrease and locomotor activity decreases. Thus, the classic inverted U-shaped (i.e., ∩-shaped) dose-response function that relates amphetamines to locomotor activity (or any other high rate behavior) – in which the dose is plotted on the X-axis and the behavior is plotted on the Y-axis – may reflect the competitive nature of that activity and stereotyped behavior. The inverted U-shaped function that relates the psychostimulant dose to performance is also reflected in the famous behavioral pharmacological principle of "rate

dependency." One of the strong propositions associated with rate dependency is that general differences in the rates of responding will determine differences in the effects of a drug. High rates of responding are decreased and low rates of responding are increased with administration of psychostimulants, and this effect generalizes to a broad range of behaviors. Some aspects of the behavioral principle for stimulants outlined above, in which the increasing rates of behavior combine with a decreasing number of response categories, can be considered a form of rate dependency. In rodents, as the psychostimulant dose increases, high rates of behavior in operant situations decrease, locomotor activity decreases, and rearing, head bobbing, and other forms of stereotyped behavior that have an initially low frequency increase. Such stereotyped behavior may actually contribute to the cycle of abuse associated with the compulsive use of these drugs by narrowing an individual's behavioral repertoire toward the singular act of drug use.

USE, ABUSE, AND ADDICTION

Amphetamines and cocaine have high abuse potential and have been unequivocally shown to produce clinically defined Dependence (ICD-10), Substance Use Disorders (DSM-5), and

Binge Cycle

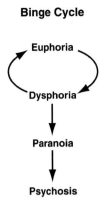

FIGURE 4.10 **Different stages of the binge cycle associated with cocaine.** Some individuals experience these stages in a single cocaine smoking episode with high doses; others experience them with low-dosage, chronic use patterns. Stage 1 (*Euphoria*) is marked by euphoria, affective lability, increased cognitive and motor performance, hyperalertness, hyperactivity, anorexia, and insomnia. Stage 2 (*Dysphoria*) is marked by sadness, melancholia, apathy, difficulty concentrating, anorexia, and insomnia. Stage 3 (*Paranoia*) is marked by suspiciousness, paranoia (both grandiosity and persecutory), hallucinations, and insomnia. Stage 4 (*Psychosis*) is marked by anhedonia, hallucinations, stereotyped behavior, paranoid delusions, insomnia, loss of impulse control, and disorientation. *[From: Koob GF, Le Moal M. Neurobiology of Addiction. Academic Press, London, 2006. For further reading, see Siegel, 1982.]*

addiction by most modern definitions. Compulsive use results in an exaggeration of the *binge/intoxication* stage of the addiction cycle (see Chapter 1), in which a user characteristically re-administers the drug regularly for days and then stops. A typical pattern of dependent cocaine use follows a cycle that appears to loop back on itself (Figure 4.10). Intense *euphoria* occurs first, which can be enhanced by increasing the speed at which the drug enters the brain (e.g., by the intravenous or smoked routes). Euphoria is followed immediately by *dysphoria*. The onset and intensity of the "high" and the subsequent dysphoria depend on the route of administration, with a more rapid and intense high and more rapid onset of dysphoria from smoked cocaine than from either the intranasal or oral routes. Repetitive movements (called stereotyped behavior

or stereotypy), such as teeth grinding and pacing, may appear, as well as hyperactivity, rapid and frenzied speech (called "pressure speech"), and emotional instability. High doses can cause paranoia and hallucinations in some users, and heavy users may experience outright psychotic symptoms similar to the acute psychosis of paranoid schizophrenia. Within a binge, euphoria is followed by dysphoria and then more drug use. As this cycle continues, paranoia and psychosis ultimately develop in some people as the dose increases or the binge duration lengthens.

With chronic psychostimulant use, the dose required to produce euphoria increases, and the subjective high decreases. Tolerance to the euphoric effects can also occur in subjects with one bout of cocaine administration. Human subjects show increases in the subjective sensations of intoxication during the rising phase of plasma cocaine levels (ascending limb) after smoking coca paste, but mood shifts dramatically to a negative state rapidly afterward. In fact, the mood state falls into a zone of dysphoria while plasma cocaine levels are still quite high (see Figure 1.9 in Chapter 1). Similar results have been seen in animal studies, in which a bout of 10 intravenously administered injections of cocaine lowered brain reward thresholds (reflecting increased brain reward function) immediately after the bout, but 80 injections only elevated brain reward thresholds (reflecting decreased brain reward function) immediately post-bout (see Figure 1.11 in Chapter 1). Thus, as cocaine use and duration increase, the positive reinforcing effects are diminished while the resulting dysphoria increases. Oral administration of regularly spaced doses is less likely to produce tolerance to the subjective effects of psychostimulants, but intravenous or smoked administration can produce rapid acute tolerance. Tolerance does not develop into stereotyped behavior or psychosis induced by stimulants; rather, these effects show sensitization (i.e., an increase with repeated administration). Similar results have been found in animal studies, with tolerance developing to the anorexic and lethal

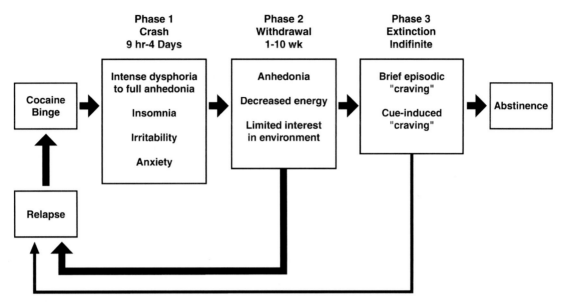

FIGURE 4.11   **Phases of cocaine withdrawal following a binge.** The duration and intensity of symptoms vary based on binge characteristics and diagnosis. Binges can range from under 4 hours to six or more days. *[Modified from: Gawin FH, Kleber HD. Abstinence symptomatology and psychiatric diagnosis in cocaine abusers: clinical observations. Archives of General Psychiatry, 1986, (43), 107–113.]*

effects of amphetamine but not to stereotyped behavior.

A possible understanding of how amphetamines produce paranoid ideation and psychosis in humans can be derived from extending the analysis of overt motor effects of these drugs to their effects on cognitive function. Amphetamines are well known to produce paranoid psychotic episodes in individuals who abuse stimulants chronically or take large doses acutely. In one study of nine physically healthy volunteers who had previously administered large doses of amphetamine (and three who had previously experienced episodes of amphetamine-induced psychoses), repeated oral administration of 5–10 mg D-amphetamine produced paranoid delusions, often with blunted emotion in all subjects when a cumulative dose range of 55–75 mg was reached. Psychosis can also develop during withdrawal from an abuse cycle of amphetamine. This paranoid psychosis induced by stimulants, in its most severe form,

is indistinguishable from nondrug-induced paranoid psychosis. Such paranoia can also produce actual physical toxicity, in which subjects believe that bugs (known as "crank bugs") are crawling under their skin and need to be gouged out.

Withdrawal from chronic or high-dose cocaine use in humans is associated with relatively few overt physical signs but numerous motivationally relevant symptoms, such as dysphoria, depression, anxiety, anergia (lack of energy), insomnia, and drug craving. Three distinct withdrawal phases have been identified in outpatient studies of compulsive users (Figure 4.11). *Phase 1* consists of a "crash" that lasts up to 4 days, with a rapid lowering of mood and energy and the acute onset of both agitation and depressive symptoms. Craving for the drug, anxiety, and paranoia peak during this phase and then are replaced by hyperphagia (increased energy) and insomnia. *Phase 2* is characterized by prolonged dysphoria, anhedonia, lack of motivation, and increased craving that can last up to 10 weeks. Relapse is highly likely during this phase. *Phase 3* is characterized by episodic craving that can last indefinitely. The withdrawal syndrome contributes to a cycle in which abstinence leads to withdrawal symptoms, and the associated dysphoria and craving, in turn, lead to relapse. Hospital inpatients, however, do not show these three withdrawal phases; instead, inpatients begin with high scores of mood-distress and craving that decrease gradually and steadily over several weeks, suggesting an important role for the environment in eliciting the cocaine withdrawal syndrome (Boxes 4.10 – 4. 12).

NEUROBIOLOGICAL EFFECTS

Endogenous Brain Dopamine Systems

At the neuropharmacological level, indirect sympathomimetics, such as amphetamine and

---

BOX 4.10

CASE REPORT: COCAINE-INDUCED DEPRESSION

A 24-year-old white female worked as a secretary and had no history of significant prior depression. She periodically used cocaine by the intranasal route, and, at one point, was given an unusually large quantity of cocaine. (The material was professionally analyzed by a street drug analysis laboratory in the San Francisco Bay Area, which found it to contain 93 percent cocaine.) After "snorting" five to eight lines of the cocaine per night for several days, she began waking up feeling depressed. To overcome this depression, and go to work, she snorted one to two lines of cocaine in the morning. By the end of the second week, she was progressively developing severe anxiety, depression and increasing irritability which was interfering with her interpersonal relationships. Her concern over this drug-induced depression and anxiety faded in approximately two days and she re-established her usual level of positive affect and mood. Since this occurrence, she periodically uses cocaine in social-recreational settings; however, she is careful to keep her dosage at a low enough level to avoid recurrence of this drug-induced depression.

Wesson DR, Smith DE, Cocaine: its use for central nervous system stimulation including recreational and medical uses. In: Petersen RC, Stillman RC (Eds.), Cocaine: 1977, (series title: NIDA Research Monograph, vol. 13), National Institute on Drug Abuse, Rockville MD, 1977, pp. 137–152.

BOX 4.11

WHAT ARE THE KEY SYMPTOMS OF PSYCHOSTIMULANT WITHDRAWAL?

Phase 1 (the "crash") – Day 1 to 4
    dysphoria, decreased energy, agitation, depressive symptoms, craving, anxiety, paranoia, hyperphagia (dramatically increased appetite), insomnia

Phase 2 – Week 1 to 10
    prolonged dysphoria, anhedonia, lack of motivation, craving
Phase 3 – Indefinite
    episodic craving

BOX 4.12

CASE REPORT: COCAINE ADDICTION

A 31-year-old white male law student in his fourth year of law school had a long history of experimental drug use including alcohol (his first drug), marijuana and LSD; but at no time had he abused a psychoactive drug. Approximately two years ago he was introduced to cocaine in a social setting by a group of friends and fellow law students. He became a regular recreational user of cocaine and in a social setting during an evening would chop up and snort between 10 and 20 lines of cocaine in the usual fashion. (Often, as with this case, cocaine is used in a recreational setting along with alcohol and marihuana.) With this law student, the pattern of recreational cocaine use continued for some time, but moved to a more daily pattern when he found that the inhalation of cocaine stimulated his performance and ability to study at night, something he found desirable because he had begun to prepare for the bar examinations. One evening, a female friend with whom he was periodically having sexual relations produced a needle and syringe and indicated that the injection of cocaine produced a pleasurable, orgasmic-like "rush." The law student injected the cocaine simultaneously with his female sexual acquaintance and found the orgasmic "rush" quite desirable. Over a several month period he escalated his intravenous cocaine use on a daily basis, injecting from approximately 10 p.m. until 7 a.m., on a 15 minute to 1 hour repeated schedule, using approximately 2 g of cocaine per night. Despite the fact that the law student was independently wealthy as a result of a family inheritance, he found that he was rapidly consuming his inheritance as his cocaine habit was costing him $50–150 per day. As a consequence he began dealing cocaine to his friends in order to help support his own habit. While the injection of cocaine involved both male and female figures,

he would almost invariably inject with a woman in a sexual context, although he reported that as he became more deeply involved with cocaine, his libido dropped dramatically; for both he and his female sexual partners, the orgasmic effects of the cocaine injection became a substitute for actual sexual intercourse. One evening he injected a female friend in his usual fashion (he would first inject the woman and then himself). She suddenly had a series of seizures, became comatose, required mouth-to-mouth resuscitation and was subsequently transported to an emergency room. During this particular cocaine run, he also experienced the first evidence of a cocaine psychosis, with auditory and visual hallucinations and extreme paranoia. The negative effects both on himself and on his girlfriend were quite shocking, because he had believed cocaine to be as free of adverse consequences as marihuana. Because of these two episodes, he decided to quit cocaine use and seek treatment. During the "withdrawal period" he experienced difficulty sleeping and a severe drug-induced depression associated with anxiety that lasted for approximately one week. Most depressive symptoms gradually abated; however, the anxiety continued along with an urge to use cocaine late in the evening at the time for his previous cocaine runs. To help with the anxiety, depression and sleep disorder, 10 mg of Valium(R) p.o. was administered each night. As there was no evidence of a prolonged underlying depression which preceded the cocaine abuse or that lasted following the "fade out" period of the drug-induced depression, no tricyclic antidepressants were administered. He made a decision to self-medicate the lethargy and reactive depression with the intranasal use of cocaine which he resumed on a daily basis.

Continued

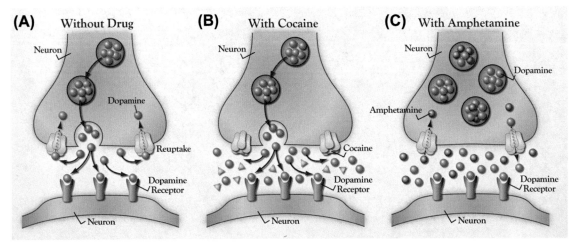

FIGURE 4.12   **Cocaine increases the quantity of dopamine present in the synapse by blocking neurotransmitter reuptake.** Amphetamine increases the quantity of dopamine present in the synapse by increasing neurotransmitter release. (A) Normal release and reuptake of dopamine from the presynaptic terminal. (B) Blockade of reuptake by cocaine increases dopamine in the synaptic cleft. (C) Increased dopamine release is produced by amphetamine, in which amphetamine reverses the action of the dopamine transporter.

cocaine, enhance the amount of monoamines available within the synaptic cleft in the central nervous system, but for the psychotropic actions related to psychostimulant addiction the effects are largely mediated by the monoamine dopamine. Numerous ways exist to enhance neurotransmission and increase levels of neurotransmitters: enhance synthesis, enhance release from presynaptic vesicles, block reuptake of the neurotransmitter back into the presynaptic terminal, and block enzymes that metabolize the neurotransmitters (see Chapter 2; Figure 4.12). Amphetamine and cocaine, for example, block the reuptake of the neurotransmitters norepinephrine, dopamine, and serotonin, but each drug affects each neurotransmitter in different ways and to differing degrees. The rank order of potency for cocaine's ability to block monoamine reuptake is *serotonin > dopamine > norepinephrine*, and for methamphetamine and D-amphetamine the rank order for their ability to block reuptake and facilitate release is *norepinephrine ≥ dopamine > serotonin*. Amphetamine inhibits monoamine oxidase to some extent. All of these actions contribute to the psychomotor stimulant and reinforcing effects of indirect sympathomimetics, but a key neurotransmitter for the psychostimulant effects of all of these drugs is dopamine.

Dopamine neurons are organized into major pathways in the brain which originate in the midbrain and project to numerous forebrain and cortical regions (see Chapter 2). Each projection is responsible for particular psychomotor stimulant actions. The *mesocorticolimbic dopamine system* originates in the ventral tegmental area and projects to the ventral forebrain, including the nucleus accumbens, olfactory tubercle, septum, and frontal cortex. It mediates exploratory activity, incentive salience, and locomotor activity induced by indirect sympathomimetics. The *nigrostriatal dopamine system* originates in the substantia nigra and projects to the corpus striatum and is associated with motor function and response initiation and mediates stereotyped behavior produced by psychostimulants. Degeneration or destruction of the nigrostriatal and mesocorticolimbic dopamine systems (by disease, trauma, or experimental lesions) results in the severe motor disturbances observed in Parkinson's disease

patients, including tremor, dystonic involuntary movements, and akinesia. Large bilateral lesions of the midbrain dopamine system using the selective dopamine neurotoxin 6-hydroxydopamine reproduce many of these Parkinsonian-like deficits. Rats become akinetic to the point of aphagia (won't eat) and adipsia (won't drink) and will die unless intubated by the experimenter. These rats also exhibit severe learning deficits in a conditioned avoidance task, in which an animal learns to avoid an aversive stimulus (such as a footshock) by responding to a cue that precedes the aversive stimulus. The motor and learning impairments can be successfully treated with L-DOPA (3,4-dihydroxy-L-phenylalanine, also called levodopa), a dopamine precursor for dopamine synthesis that makes more dopamine available in the synapse (Box 4.13).

Destruction of the mesocorticolimbic dopamine system with 6-hydroxydopamine blocks amphetamine- and cocaine-stimulated

---

BOX 4.13

BRAIN LESIONS: ELECTROLYTIC, CELL BODY, AND PATHWAY LESIONS

Historically in neuroscience, the technique of destroying neurons to observe functional deficits has been used extensively to delineate function. Conceptually, such techniques have proved significant when positive results have been obtained, with the proper controls and interpretations. However, negative results with lesion studies have always been suspect because of the issue of redundancy. Three types of lesion techniques have been used. With electrolytic lesions, sufficient current is passed through the tip of an electrode to destroy the tissue in the immediate area around the tip of the electrode. The amount of tissue destroyed is directly related to the current intensity and size of the electrode. With cell body-specific lesions, a drug such as ibotenic

acid is used that overexcites the cell to the extent that the cell dies. Such lesions are specific to cell bodies and in theory do not destroy fibers of passage. Lesions of the terminal projections of specific neurochemical systems can be effected using neurotoxins that are taken up by the nerve terminals and selectively destroy them. 6-Hydroxydopamine is selectively taken up by dopamine and norepinephrine nerve terminals and has been shown to selectively deplete either pathways or terminal areas of dopamine and norepinephrine, respectively. To selectively destroy dopamine neurons, a noradrenergic reuptake inhibitor can be concomitantly administered to spare uptake of 6-hydroxydopamine into the norepinephrine projections.

locomotor activity, and similar effects have been observed following injections of selective dopamine receptor antagonists into the nucleus accumbens. Functional disruption of the nigrostriatal dopamine system blocks the stereotyped behavior associated with high-dose D-amphetamine. Specific 6-hydroxydopamine lesions of the dorsal striatum block the intense, restricted, repetitive behavior produced by high-dose amphetamine, resulting in more robust locomotor activity. Notably, however, the functions of the mesocorticolimbic or nigrostriatal dopamine system largely depend on their specific connections and not any intrinsic functional attributes.

Incentive Salience – Synaptic Plasticity in the Mesocorticolimbic System, Nucleus Accumbens, and Dorsal Striatum

Much work in the nondrug state has shown that the firing rate of midbrain dopamine neurons changes in response to reward as an animal learns. A novel reward produces the transient firing of dopamine neurons and phasic release of dopamine in the nucleus accumbens (ventral striatum). As the animal learns to recognize the cues that predict a reward, the response of dopamine neurons changes. The response to the reward itself decreases or habituates, and dopamine neurons begin to fire in response to the cues that predict the reward. These data support the hypothesis that one function of dopamine release in the nucleus accumbens is to serve as an error-detection signal or learning signal. Such a change in firing pattern requires that midbrain dopamine neurons (or the postsynaptic medium spiny neurons that the dopamine neurons innervate) receive important information from the prefrontal cortex and other regions, such as the hippocampus (external context), insula (internal states), and basolateral amygdala, presumably from glutamate neurons. One term that has become synonymous with this process is "incentive salience," which has been defined as a mechanism that explains the motivational value of specific learned stimuli (Pavlovian conditioned stimuli) and associated natural rewards (unconditioned stimuli) in humans and animals. One formulation defines incentive salience as a motivational magnet quality that makes the conditioned or unconditioned stimulus a desirable and attractive goal (for further reading, see Zhang et al., 2009).

Binge/Intoxication Stage

Psychostimulants increase dopamine release in a phasic manner at a level 10 times the normal release of dopamine. Thus, drug-induced synaptic plasticity in the nucleus accumbens (ventral striatum) and dorsal striatum exaggerates the cue-induced drug seeking outlined above. In humans, positron emission tomography (PET) imaging studies have confirmed that all major classes of drugs increase dopamine in the nucleus accumbens (ventral striatum) and dorsal striatum, and the drug-induced increases in dopamine in the striatum are proportional to the intensity of the subjective experience of euphoria or "high" (for further reading, see Volkow et al., 2009). Human studies also show that prefrontal cortex regions become activated when cocaine abusers are exposed to craving-inducing stimuli (either drugs or cues), thus supporting the concept of the plasticity of the neurocircuitry.

Repeated treatments with amphetamine or cocaine in animals increase dendritic spine density and the number of branched spines in the nucleus accumbens and prefrontal cortex, which can last for weeks. Multiple cellular mechanisms have been identified to account for this structural plasticity. Previously silent synapses that involve the expression of N-methyl-D-aspartate receptors are observed with repeated psychostimulant administration in the shell of the nucleus accumbens, and withdrawal and protracted abstinence involve the overexpression of AMPA receptors. Drugs that block AMPA receptors also block the cue-induced reinstatement of cocaine-seeking behavior, linking this synaptic plasticity with incentive salience (Box 4.14; for further reading, see Grueter et al., 2012).

BOX 4.14

SYNAPTIC PLASTICITY

Synaptic plasticity is the capacity for continuous alteration of the neural circuits and synapses of the living brain and nervous system in response to experience or injury. Plasticity includes long-term potentiation (LTP) and has been observed at the cellular level in the ventral tegmental area and nucleus accumbens with repeated psychostimulant exposure. LTP occurs when neurons are turned on and take longer than usual to turn off. Cellular plasticity also includes changes in synaptic strength (signals may be stronger or weaker than normal) that require activation of N-methyl-D-aspartate glutamate receptors from excitatory inputs that originate in prelimbic cortical areas and do not depend on dopamine receptors (for further reading, see Thomas and Malenka, 2003).

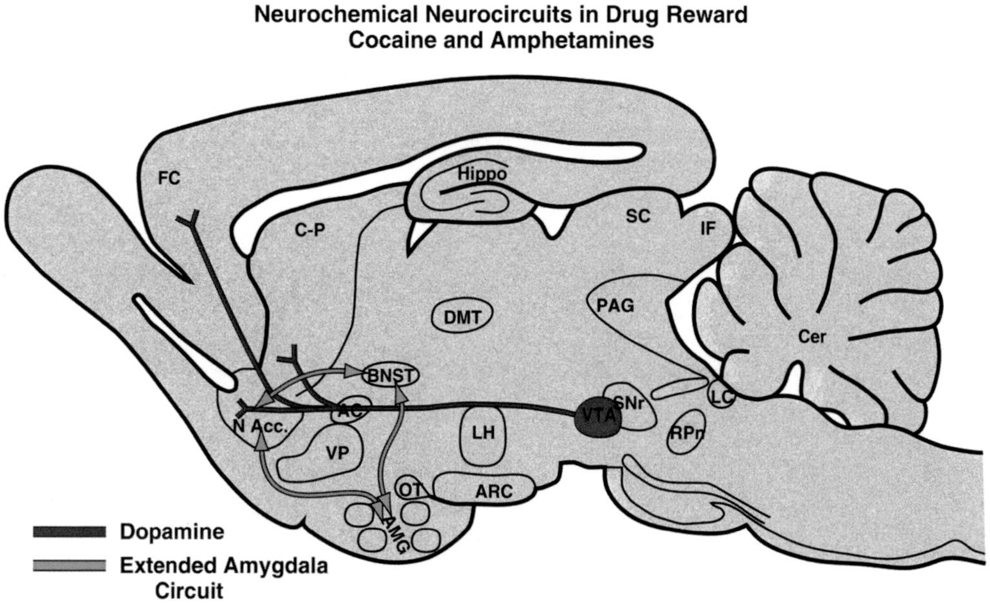

Neurochemical Neurocircuits in Drug Reward
Cocaine and Amphetamines

Dopamine
Extended Amygdala Circuit

FIGURE 4.13 **Sagittal section through a representative rodent brain illustrating the pathways and receptor systems implicated in the acute reinforcing actions of cocaine and amphetamines.** Cocaine and amphetamines activate release dopamine in the nucleus accumbens and amygdala via direct actions on dopamine terminals. The blue arrows represent the interactions within the extended amygdala system hypothesized to have a key role in psychostimulant reinforcement. AC, anterior commissure; AMG, amygdala; ARC, arcuate nucleus; BNST, bed nucleus of the stria terminalis; Cer, cerebellum; C-P, caudate putamen; DMT, dorsomedial thalamus; FC, frontal cortex; Hippo, hippocampus; IF, inferior colliculus; LC, locus coeruleus; LH, lateral hypothalamus; N Acc., nucleus accumbens; OT, olfactory tract; PAG, periaqueductal gray; RPn, reticular pontine nucleus; SC, superior colliculus; SNr, substantia nigra pars reticulata; VP, ventral pallidum; VTA, ventral tegmental area. *[From Koob GF, Le Moal M, 2006. Neurobiology of Addiction. Academic Press, London.]*

The acute reinforcing actions of cocaine, amphetamines, and methamphetamine are mediated by the release of dopamine in the terminal areas of the mesocorticolimbic dopamine system (Figure 4.13). Lesions of the mesocorticolimbic dopamine system with 6-hydroxydopamine block the reinforcing effects of cocaine and D-amphetamine, assessed by drug

TABLE 4.5   Effects of Specific Lesions of the Midbrain Dopamine Systems on Behavior

System	Effect
Mesocorticolimbic and nigrostriatal dopamine systems	↑ Parkinsonian-like symptoms ↓ Spontaneous activity ↓ Eating ↓ Drinking ↓ Performance in conditioned avoidance task
Mesocorticolimbic dopamine system	↓ Amphetamine-induced locomotor activity ↓ Cocaine-induced locomotor activity ↓ Cocaine self-administration ↓ D-amphetamine self-administration
Nigrostriatal dopamine system	↓ D-amphetamine-induced stereotypy
Dorsal striatum	↑ Locomotor activity ↓ Amphetamine-induced stereotyped behavior
Nucleus accumbens	↓ Cocaine self-administration ↓ Amphetamine self-administration

self-administration. Rats that are trained to self-administer cocaine or amphetamine intravenously and then subjected to 6-hydroxydopamine lesions of the nucleus accumbens show an extinction-like response pattern that consists of a high level of responding (lever-presses) at the beginning of the test session followed by a gradual decline over subsequent sessions and a long-lasting decrease in responding (Table 4.5, Figure 4.14). Lesions of the dorsal striatum do not block cocaine self-administration. Much of the work on the acute reinforcing effects of psychostimulants has focused on the medial subregion of the nucleus accumbens, termed the shell of the nucleus accumbens (see Chapter 2). Early *in vivo* microdialysis studies in awake, freely moving animals showed preferential activation of dopamine in the shell of the nucleus accumbens with administration of all drugs of abuse (for further reading, see Di Chiara 2002). Injections of a dopamine D_1 receptor antagonist directly into the shell of the nucleus accumbens, central nucleus of the amygdala, and bed nucleus of the stria terminalis also decrease the reinforcing effects of cocaine and block the motivation to work for intravenous cocaine (that is, animals are not willing to press a lever as many times to receive a drug injection). Knockout studies show that D_1 receptors, D_2 receptors, and the dopamine transporter play important roles in psychostimulant actions (for example, D_1 knockout mice do not self-administer cocaine; Table 4.6). Thus, the mesocorticolimbic dopamine system is clearly critical for psychostimulant activation and reinforcement, and it also plays a major role in the reinforcing actions of other drugs of abuse (for further reading, see Koob, 1992). The heterogeneity of connectivity within subregions of the nucleus accumbens, for example, suggests that the nucleus accumbens shell may provide a link between the terminals of the mesocorticolimbic dopamine system and other forebrain areas involved in psychostimulant reinforcement.

More specifically, the reinforcing effects of psychostimulants involve output systems that engage striatal–pallidal–thalamic–cortical loops that have been hypothesized to interact within the topographical connections of the basal ganglia (see Chapter 2). While the initial acute reinforcing actions of psychostimulants engage the ventral part of the basal ganglia, such as the shell of the nucleus accumbens, as drug self-administration becomes more habit-like (a more regular and stereotyped pattern), the dorsal part of the basal ganglia becomes engaged. Some have argued that these circuits play a key role in the compulsive-like responding associated with psychostimulant addiction (for further reading, see Everitt and Wolf, 2002; Belin and Everitt, 2008).

Individual differences in response to psychostimulant drugs are determined by many factors, but a key factor is activation of the hypothalamic–pituitary–adrenal (HPA) axis and the release of glucocorticoids. In normal

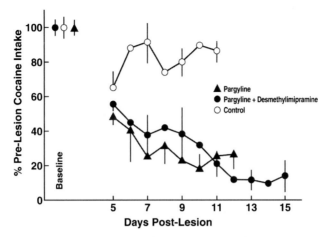

FIGURE 4.14 **Effect of 6-hydroxydopamine lesions of the nucleus accumbens on cocaine self-administration in rats.** The data-points represent mean (± SEM) daily intake for each group. One group received the monoamine oxidase inhibitor pargyline (50 mg/kg) prior to 6-hydroxydopamine treatment (filled triangles). Another group received both pargyline and the tricyclic antidepressant desmethylimipramine (25 mg/kg) prior to 6-hydroxydopamine (filled circles). The control group received pargyline and desmethylimipramine prior to vehicle infusions (rather than 6-hydroxydopamine infusions) into the nucleus accumbens. Cocaine was not available for self-administration until day 5 post-lesion. A significant difference was found between the two lesion groups and the control group. No difference was observed between the 6-hydroxydopamine groups. *These data show that removal of dopaminergic terminals in the mesocorticolimbic dopamine system in the nucleus accumbens with a neurotoxin that selectively destroys monoamine axons and terminals causes rats to stop taking cocaine. In other words, the rats extinguished their drug seeking behavior although cocaine was readily available (see* Chapter 3 *for a definition of extinction). [From: Roberts DCS, Koob GF, Klonoff P, Fibiger HC. Extinction and recovery of cocaine self-administration following 6-hydroxydopamine lesions of the nucleus accumbens.* Pharmacology Biochemistry and Behavior, 1980, (12), 781–787.]

situations and during the rodent's active period in the light/dark cycle, glucocorticoids increase dopaminergic function, especially in mesocorticolimbic regions. The interaction between glucocorticoids and the mesocorticolimbic dopamine system may have a significant impact on the vulnerability to self-administer psychostimulant drugs. Rats that have a high initial propensity to explore a novel environment also have a high initial corticosterone response (corticosterone is the rodent equivalent to human cortisol) and are much more likely to self-administer psychostimulant drugs. Additionally, rats with normal initial sensitivity that receive repeated injections of corticosterone acquire cocaine self-administration at a much lower dose than rats that receive vehicle injections. Corticosterone administration causes rats that would not initially self-administer amphetamine at low doses

to self-administer the drug (Figure 4.15; for further reading, see Piazza and Le Moal, 1996).

Electrophysiological recordings in awake, freely moving animals during intravenous cocaine self-administration have identified several types of neurons in the nucleus accumbens that respond to drug infusion and reinforcement, and these studies emphasize the key role of the nucleus accumbens in the acute reinforcing actions of cocaine and, by extrapolation, psychostimulants in general. One group of neurons in the nucleus accumbens shows anticipatory neuronal responses, as if the neurons "sense" the coming reinforcement. Another group of neurons increases or decreases firing following the response to cocaine and represents a direct effect of reinforcement. Much data have been generated with *in vivo* electrophysiology to show that neuronal firing in the

TABLE 4.6 Dopamine Receptor Subtype-Specific Knockouts and Psychostimulant-Induced Behavior in Mice

Locomotor Response	Dopamine Receptor Knockout	Rewarding Effects
↓ Amphetamine ↓ Cocaine ↓ Amphetamine sensitization ↓ Cocaine sensitization	D₁	↓ Amphetamine-induced conditioned place preference ↓ Cocaine-induced conditioned place preference ↓ Amphetamine self-administration ↓ Cocaine self-administration
↓ Amphetamine ↓ Cocaine	D₂	↑ Cocaine self-administration (descending limb)
↑ Amphetamine ↑ Cocaine	D₃	No significant effects
↑ Amphetamine ↑ Cocaine ↑ Amphetamine sensitization	D₄	↓ Methamphetamine-induced conditioned place preference
No significant effects	D₅	No significant effects

nucleus accumbens can also follow the acquisition, extinction, and maintenance of cocaine self-administration.

In humans, acute infusions of cocaine have been shown to selectively increase brain metabolic activity in reward structures in functional magnetic resonance imaging studies. In cocaine-dependent subjects who were abstinent for 18h, the brain was imaged for 5 min before and 13 min after infusion of either cocaine or saline while the subjects rated their subjective feelings of *rush*, *high*, *low*, and *craving*. The *high*

only appeared in the drug group, followed by dysphoria 11 min post-infusion, whereas peak craving occurred 12 min post-infusion. Prior to both infusions (saline and cocaine), within 5 min a positive signal change was observed in the ventral region of the nucleus accumbens and subcallosal cortex. After the cocaine infusion, the signal increased in some areas, such as the nucleus accumbens, subcallosal cortex, caudate putamen, thalamus, insula, hippocampus, cingulate, lateral prefrontal cortex, temporal cortex, ventral tegmentum, and pons. The

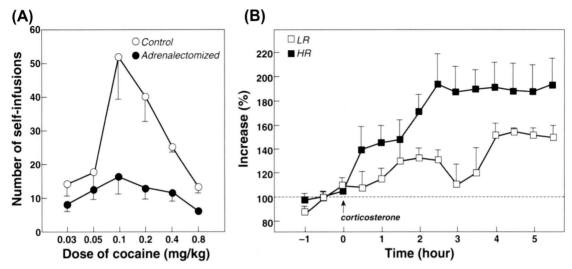

FIGURE 4.15 **Corticosteroids and behavioral effects of psychostimulants.** (A) Effects of adrenalectomy on cocaine self-administration in rats. Animals were trained to self-administer cocaine by nosepoking and then subjected to several doses of cocaine. Adrenalectomy produced a flattening of the dose-effect function, with decreases in cocaine intake at all doses. (B) Corticosterone-induced changes in extracellular concentrations of dopamine in rats bred for either high-responsiveness (HR) or low-responsiveness (LR) to stress and psychostimulant drugs. High-responding animals that drank the corticosterone solution (100 mg/ml) in the dark period showed a faster and higher increase in nucleus accumbens dopamine than low-responding animals. *These data show that removal of the adrenal glands and the source of circulating glucocorticoids block the reinforcing effects of cocaine and that the glucocorticoid corticosterone increased the release of dopamine measured by* in vivo *microdialysis in rats selected for a high response to novelty. Thus, glucocorticoids facilitate the dopaminergic response to cocaine and its consequent reinforcing effects.*

[Panel A. Modified from: Deroche V, Marinelli M, Le Moal M, Piazza PV. Glucocorticoids and behavioral effects of psychostimulants: II. Cocaine intravenous self-administration and reinstatement depend on glucocorticoid levels. Journal of Pharmacology and Experimental Therapeutics, *1997, (281), 1401–1407.]*

[Panel B. From: Piazza PV, Rouge-Pont F, Deroche V, Maccari S, Simon H, Le Moal M. Glucocorticoids have state-dependent stimulant effects on the mesencephalic dopaminergic transmission. Proceedings of the National Academy of Sciences USA, *1996, (93), 8716–8720.]*

signal actually decreased in some subjects in the amygdala, temporal pole, and medial frontal cortex. Saline infusion produced a limited set of significant activation, such as frontal and temporal-occipital cortices, to match some of the activation seen in the cocaine group. The activation correlated with the degree of emotional ratings (Figure 4.16; for further reading, see Koob and Le Moal, 2006).

Withdrawal/Negative Affect Stage

Cocaine withdrawal in animal studies is characterized by significant motivational changes

measured by changes in reward thresholds but few physical or somatic symptoms. Elevations in brain reward thresholds reflect decreases in reward (that is, more stimulation is required for the individual to sense the stimulus as rewarding). During an acute 12h binge of intravenous cocaine self-administration in rats that were tested for brain reward thresholds, a dose-dependent elevation in these thresholds in the medial forebrain bundle occurred when the self-administration session ended (Figure 4.17). Rats that had access to cocaine for 48h showed elevations in thresholds that lasted for 5 days after cocaine self-administration ended. Similar

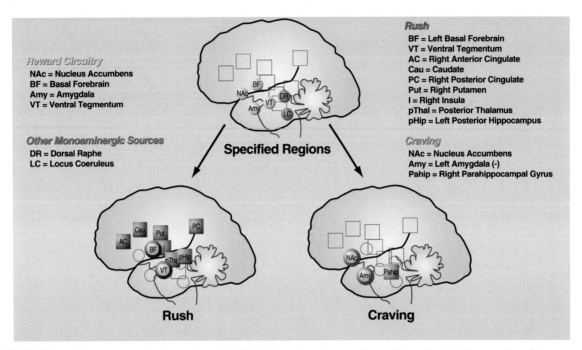

FIGURE 4.16 **Summary of limbic and paralimbic brain regions that correlate with euphoria (*red*) *vs.* regions that correlate with craving (*green*).** Above these schematics are indications of the brain regions (*yellow*) predicted to be active after an infusion of cocaine. Two other brainstem monoaminergic regions, potentially encompassed in pontine activation seen in a baseline vs. post-infusion comparison, are illustrated in *blue*. This pontine activation correlated with behavioral ratings of "rush." *[From: Breiter HC, Gollub RL, Weisskoff RM, Kennedy DN, Makris N, Berke JD, Goodman JM, Kantor HL, Gastfriend DR, Riorden JP, Mathew RT, Rosen BR, Hyman SE. Acute effects of cocaine on human brain activity and emotion. Neuron, 1997, (19), 591–611.]*

results have been observed with cocaine and D-amphetamine. Elevations in brain reward thresholds (decreased reward) temporally preceded and were highly correlated with escalation in cocaine intake with extended access (Figure 4.18). Post-session elevations in reward thresholds failed to fully return to baseline levels in rats that had extended access to cocaine before the onset of each subsequent self-administration session, thereby progressively deviating more and more from baseline levels. These results provide compelling evidence that brain reward dysfunction occurs with escalated cocaine intake.

With cocaine and amphetamines, the neurochemical basis of the motivational significance of withdrawal involves both a decrease in the function of neurotransmitters related to reward function and recruitment of brain stress systems. Dopamine and serotonin release in the basal forebrain (e.g., nucleus accumbens), measured by *in vivo* microdialysis, decreases during withdrawal in animal studies. Animals that underwent escalation of drug intake had enhanced sensitivity to the mixed D_1/ D_2 receptor antagonist *cis*-flupenthixol, with a leftward shift of the dose-response function, suggesting that escalation in cocaine self-administration may be mediated, at least partially, by decreased function of dopamine receptors or transduction mechanisms. The initial "crash" experienced immediately after a binge by human cocaine users may reflect a decrease in extracellular dopamine that can persist for months after chronic high-dose use.

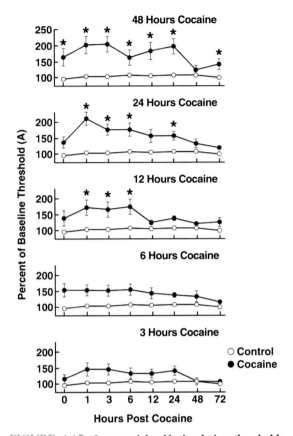

FIGURE 4.17 **Intracranial self-stimulation thresholds in rats following 3–48 h of cocaine self-administration at several time-points post-cocaine (0, 1, 3, 6, 12, 24, 48, and 72 h).** Data are expressed as a percent change from baseline threshold levels. Asterisks (*) indicate statistically significant differences between the control and experimental groups. *These data show that animals that are allowed extended access to cocaine show elevations in reward thresholds measured by intracranial self-stimulation (see Chapter 3 for details of intracranial self-stimulation). These increases can be interpreted as dysphoric-like effects and clearly are dose-related. More self-administration is associated with a greater increase in thresholds and longer duration of the increase in thresholds. [From: Markou A, Koob GF. Post-cocaine anhedonia: an animal model of cocaine withdrawal. Neuropsychopharmacology, 1991, (4), 17–26.]*

Chronic cocaine administration decreased dopamine neuron firing in the mesocorticolimbic system, consistent with results from microdialysis studies during acute withdrawal. The change in dopamine transmission is dose- and time-dependent. Decreases in neuronal excitability and firing rates in the nucleus accumbens also predominate with repeated cocaine self-administration. Interestingly, nucleus accumbens neurons that increase firing in response to limited or intermittent cocaine self-administration show a resistance to decreased firing during a prolonged, continuous self-administration session. A decrease in ventral tegmental area and nucleus accumbens nondrug-reward-related activity occurs with repeated cocaine administration, consistent with neuropharmacological studies of decreased nondrug (e.g., food) reward with repeated administration.

Few human imaging studies have been done during acute withdrawal from drugs of abuse. However, imaging studies of protracted or prolonged withdrawal, once the signs and symptoms of acute withdrawal have subsided, have documented hypofunction in dopamine pathways, reflected by decreases in D_2 receptor expression and decreases in dopamine release, which may contribute to the hypohedonia (i.e., decreased sensitivity to rewarding stimuli) and amotivation reported by subjects with addiction during protracted withdrawal (Figure 4.19).

At the molecular level, the dysphoria and motivational symptoms of withdrawal from cocaine appear to result from downstream signal transduction adaptations in response to excessive drug intake. Early studies in rats demonstrated that chronic cocaine administration (15 mg/kg twice daily for 14 days) upregulated the cyclic adenosine monophosphate (cAMP) pathway in the nucleus accumbens for 16 h after the last injection. Stimulation of protein kinase A (PKA; which activates cAMP response element binding protein [CREB] in the nucleus accumbens) decreased cocaine self-administration. Elevated CREB levels in the nucleus accumbens also decreased cocaine self-administration. Blockade of PKA activity and CREB antagonism in the nucleus accumbens increased cocaine reward in the form of

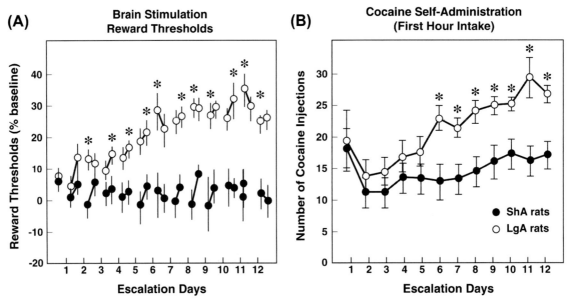

FIGURE 4.18 **Relationship between elevations in intracranial self-stimulation (ICSS) reward thresholds and cocaine intake escalation.** (A) Percentage change from baseline ICSS thresholds. (B) Number of cocaine injections earned during the first hour of each session. Rats were first prepared with bipolar electrodes in either the right or left posterior lateral hypothalamus. One week after surgery, they were trained to respond for electrical brain stimulation. ICSS thresholds (measured in μA) were then assessed. During the screening phase, the rats tested for self-administration were allowed to self-administer cocaine during only 1 h on a fixed-ratio 1 schedule of reinforcement, after which two balanced groups with the same weight, cocaine intake, and ICSS reward thresholds were formed. During the escalation phase, one group had access to cocaine self-administration for only 1 h per day (short access or ShA rats), and the other group had access for 6 h per day (long-access or LgA rats). ICSS reward thresholds were measured in all rats twice per day, 3 h and 17–22 h after each daily self-administration session (ShA and LgA rats). Each ICSS session lasted approximately 30 min. Asterisks (*) indicate a significant difference from drug-naive or ShA rats. *These data show that the overall increase over days in thresholds associated with extended access to cocaine parallels the overall increase over days in drug taking (termed escalation; see* Chapter 3) *associated with extended access. Notice that the increases in thresholds are generally greater 17–22 h after each daily self-administration session compared with 3 h after each daily session and that rats with short access do not show an overall increase in reward thresholds.* [From: Ahmed SH, Kenny PJ, Koob GF, Markou A. Neurobiological evidence for hedonic allostasis associated with escalating cocaine use. Nature Neuroscience, 2002, (5), 625–626.]

conditioned place preference and increased self-administration.

CREB regulates dynorphin gene expression *in vitro* and *in vivo*. Elevated CREB in the nucleus accumbens produces dysphoria-like responses and increases dynorphin expression, and dynorphin is a neuropeptide associated with decreased function of the mesocorticolimbic dopamine system. Psychostimulants also increase the expression of the opioid peptide dynorphin in the nucleus accumbens. Elevated CREB in the nucleus accumbens increased the aversion to

cocaine in a conditioned place preference test and produced a depression-like profile in the forced swim test. This "depressive" state in rodents was reversed by a κ opioid receptor antagonist (κ is one of the three opioid receptors: κ preferentially binds the opioid dynorphin, δ preferentially binds the opioid enkephalin, and μ preferentially binds the opioid endorphin; see Chapter 5). These results suggest that CREB and dynorphin in the nucleus accumbens contribute to the dysphoria associated with withdrawal from chronic cocaine (see Chapter 2; Figure 4.20).

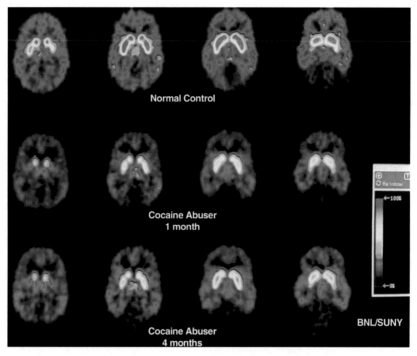

FIGURE 4.19   Brain imaging of a normal control subject and cocaine abuser tested 1 and 4 months after the last cocaine use. The images correspond to the four sequential planes where the basal ganglia are located. The color scale has been normalized to the injected dose. Notice the lower uptake of the image tracer in the cocaine abuser compared with the normal control. Notice also the persistence of the decreased uptake even 4 months after cocaine discontinuation. BNL, Brookhaven National Laboratory; SUNY, State University of New York. *[From: Volkow ND, Fowler JS, Wang GJ, Hitzemann R, Logan J, Schlyer DJ, Dewey SL, Wolf AP, Decreased dopamine D2 receptor availability is associated with reduced frontal metabolism in cocaine abusers,* Synapse, *1993, (14),169–177.]*

Much research has focused on a monoamine deficiency hypothesis to explain the decreased reward (and by extrapolation, dysphoria in humans) associated with acute psychostimulant withdrawal, but more recent theories have invoked the activation of other brain systems that may act in opposition to brain reward systems. At least two neuropeptide systems, dynorphin (see above) and corticotropin-releasing factor (CRF; see below), are recruited during acute cocaine withdrawal and may contribute to the negative emotional state.

Stressors and the state of stress contribute to acute withdrawal, protracted abstinence, and vulnerability to relapse. As noted above, the HPA axis is activated during psychostimulant dependence and acute withdrawal, and its dysregulation can persist long after the acute withdrawal period. An acute binge of cocaine dramatically increases adrenocorticotropic hormone (ACTH), corticosterone, and CRF in the hypothalamus. In a parallel fashion, brain CRF function outside of the HPA axis in the extended amygdala is activated during acute withdrawal and may mediate the behavioral aspects of stress associated with abstinence. Rats treated repeatedly with cocaine show significant anxiety-like responses following the cessation of chronic administration that are reversed by intracerebroventricular administration of a CRF receptor antagonist. CRF levels increase in the central nucleus of the amygdala during acute

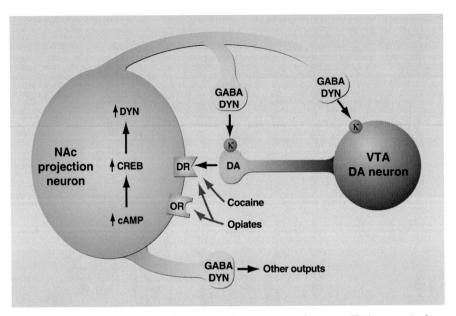

FIGURE 4.20   **Regulation of CREB by drugs of abuse.** The figure shows a dopamine (DA) neuron in the ventral tegmental area (VTA) innervating a class of γ-aminobutyric acid (GABA) projection neurons from the nucleus accumbens (NAc) that expresses dynorphin (DYN). Dynorphin constitutes a negative feedback mechanism in this circuit: dynorphin, released from terminals of the NAc neurons, acts on κ-opioid receptors located on nerve terminals and cell bodies of the dopamine neurons to inhibit their functioning. Chronic exposure to cocaine or opiates upregulates the activity of this negative feedback loop through upregulation of the cAMP pathway, activation of CREB, and induction of dynorphin. cAMP, cyclic adenosine monophosphate; CREB, cyclic adenosine monophosphate response element binding protein; DR, dopamine receptor; OR, opioid receptor. *[Modified from: Carlezon WA Jr, Nestler EJ, Neve RL. Herpes simplex virus-mediated gene transfer as a tool for neuropsychiatric research.* Critical Reviews in Neurobiology, *2000, (14), 47–67; see also Nestler EJ. Molecular basis of long-term plasticity underlying addiction.* Nature Reviews Neuroscience, *2001, (2),119–128.]*

withdrawal from drugs of abuse in rodents, and animals that self-administer cocaine continuously for 12h show a time-related increase in CRF in the amygdala (Figure 4.21). The opioid peptide dynorphin has also been implicated in the anti-reward, dysphoric-like effects of withdrawal from repeated cocaine exposure, in which dynorphin levels increase in the nucleus accumbens and then in turn decrease dopamine release.

Preoccupation/Anticipation Stage

To study the neurocircuitry of the *preoccupation/anticipation* stage, animal models have been characterized extensively using drug-, cue-, and

stress-induced reinstatement (see Chapter 3). In animal models of cocaine-induced reinstatement, the neuropharmacological circuits have focused largely on dopaminergic and glutamatergic mechanisms (Figure 4.22; for further reading, see Shaham et al., 2003). Activation of the mesocorticolimbic dopamine system is clearly implicated in cocaine-induced reinstatement, based on studies of dopamine agonists that mimic the effects of cocaine and studies of dopamine receptor antagonists that block the effects of cocaine, depending on which brain region is targeted. Dopamine antagonism in the dorsal prefrontal cortex but not the nucleus accumbens blocked cocaine-induced reinstatement. Cocaine-induced reinstatement was facilitated by glutamatergic agonists and

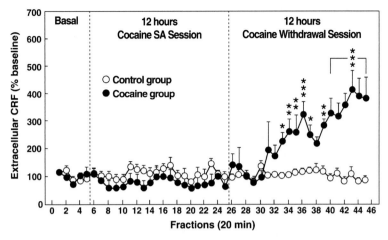

FIGURE 4.21 Mean (± SEM) dialysate corticotropin-releasing factor (CRF) concentrations collected from the central nucleus of the amygdala of rats during baseline, a 12h cocaine self-administration session, and a subsequent 12h withdrawal period (cocaine group). CRF levels in animals with the same history of cocaine self-administration training and drug exposure, but not given access to cocaine on the test day, are shown for comparison (control group). Dialysate samples were collected over 2h periods alternating with 1h nonsampling periods. During cocaine self-administration, dialysate CRF concentrations in the cocaine group were decreased by about 25% compared with control animals. In contrast, termination of access to cocaine significantly increased CRF efflux, which began approximately 5h post-cocaine and reached about 400% of presession baseline levels at the end of the withdrawal session. The asterisks (*) indicate significant differences between the cocaine and control groups, with multiple asterisks indicating more pronounced differences. [From: Richter RM, Weiss F. In vivo CRF release in rat amygdala is increased during cocaine withdrawal in self-administering rats. Synapse, 1999, (32), 254–261.]

inhibited by glutamatergic antagonists at various levels of the mesocorticolimbic dopamine system, including the nucleus accumbens, prefrontal cortex, and ventral tegmental area.

Cue-induced reinstatement involves stimuli that were previously associated with cocaine reinforcement that can then elicit the reinstatement of cocaine self-administration. This cue-induced responding involves basal forebrain projections and connections with the origins and terminal areas of the mesocorticolimbic dopamine system. Cocaine-predictive stimuli activated Fos protein in the basolateral amygdala and medial prefrontal cortex (Box 4.15). With regard to cue-induced reinstatement, Fos activation in the amygdala in rats parallels findings in humans of neural activation within the amygdala and anterior cingulate during cue-induced craving for cocaine. The medial prefrontal cortex/nucleus accumbens glutamate connection appears to be critical for cue-induced reinstatement, in a similar way to cocaine-induced reinstatement (Figure 4.22; for further reading, see Kalivas and McFarland 2003; See et al., 2003).

Using in vivo electrophysiological measures, neurons in the nucleus accumbens also seem to respond to stimuli paired with cocaine reinforcement. Cells in the nucleus accumbens that exhibit a post-response change in firing within seconds of the reinforced response can be controlled by the stimulus that was paired with cocaine delivery. Similarly, neurons in the basolateral amygdala that exhibited increased firing immediately after the cocaine response can be activated by an audio/visual cue paired with cocaine. In a particularly intriguing study, neurons in both the nucleus accumbens and medial prefrontal cortex were recorded simultaneously in rats that self-administered cocaine. These neurons "anticipated" a cocaine infusion and increased their firing a few seconds before

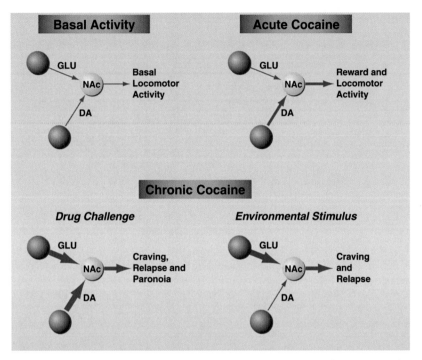

FIGURE 4.22 **The role of glutamate (GLU) and dopamine (DA) transmission in the relapse to drug-seeking behavior.** During baseline neurotransmission, tonic dopamine and glutamate transmission equally modulate the output of the nucleus accumbens (NAc) to allow normal locomotor activity. Following acute cocaine administration, dopamine levels in the nucleus accumbens are elevated, with little effect on glutamatergic tone, to increase locomotor activity and stimulate reward processes. After withdrawal from chronic drug intake, a single cocaine administration may induce relapse to drug taking or paranoia through increased dopamine release associated with and dependent on increased glutamate transmission which may be a consequence of interoceptive cues (that is, internal cues within the body or brain) associated with drug taking. However, in the absence of cocaine administration, an environmental cue may induce craving and relapse through enhanced glutamate transmission with little dopamine involvement. *[From: Cornish JL, Kalivas PW. Cocaine sensitization and craving: differing roles for dopamine and glutamate in the nucleus accumbens.* Journal of Addictive Diseases, 2001, (20), 43–54.]*

BOX 4.15

FOS PROTEIN AND THE C-FOS GENE

Fos protein and its gene, c-*fos*, are common markers of brain activation used in neurobiological research. Fos detection tells researchers which brain regions have neurons that are activated by a particular manipulation, so this procedure is often used to narrow the field of regions that are likely candidates for further investigation.

the lever press. Inter- and intraregional correlations in firing patterns were found between pairs of simultaneously recorded neurons in these two distinct brain areas.

Stress-induced reinstatement involves activation of the brain stress neurotransmitter CRF outside of the HPA axis in the extended amygdala. CRF receptor antagonists block the footshock-induced reinstatement of cocaine-seeking behavior in rats. The bed nucleus of the stria terminalis, an area rich in CRF receptors, terminals, and cell bodies, appears to play a significant role. An asymmetric lesion technique functionally dissected a critical, but not exclusive, role of the CRF pathway that originates in the central nucleus of the amygdala and projects to the bed nucleus of the stria terminalis. Similarly, microinjection studies revealed a role for the ventral noradrenergic (norepinephrine) pathway that projects to the bed nucleus of the stria terminalis in the stress-induced reinstatement of cocaine seeking behavior (Figure 4.23). These observations are consistent with major reciprocal connections of CRF and norepinephrine in the basal forebrain and brainstem, in which CRF activates brainstem norepinephrine, and norepinephrine activates forebrain CRF (for further reading, see Aston-Jones and Harris, 2004; Koob and Kreek, 2007). Such an hypothesized loop might explain the intensified stress responses that occur with repeated drug exposure that could lead to psychopathology and addiction.

Vulnerability to relapse continues for weeks, months, and even years after acute withdrawal, and long-term molecular changes in the brain circuits described above are thought to mediate such vulnerability. One hypothesized mechanism for long-term molecular changes in cellular function is the induction of transcription factors (proteins that bind to specific parts of DNA and control the transfer or transcription of genetic information from DNA to RNA). Acute administration of cocaine induces the expression of the transcription factor c-*fos*, but the expression is short-lived and returns to normal levels within 12 h of drug exposure. Chronic cocaine administration reduced the ability of cocaine to induce c-*fos* expression, suggesting tolerance to this effect. However, chronic cocaine caused an accumulation of another transcription factor, activator protein 1 (AP-1), which is composed of proteins from the Fos family, specifically ΔFosB. The induction of ΔFosB in the nucleus accumbens is long-lived after chronic cocaine exposure, and ΔFosB overexpression increases the sensitivity to the locomotor-activating and rewarding effects of cocaine, increases cocaine self-administration, and increases progressive-ratio responding for cocaine. ΔFosB, therefore, has a potential role in initiating and maintaining an addictive state by increasing the drive for drug reward, even weeks and months after the last drug exposure (for further reading, see Nestler, 2005).

In parallel, during protracted abstinence, imaging studies have reported that enhanced sensitivity to conditioned cues also occurs during detoxification. The brain sites that mediate such responses include basal forebrain projections and connections with the mesocorticolimbic dopamine system and hippocampus, including the basolateral amygdala, medial prefrontal cortex, nucleus accumbens, and ventral pallidum. These conditioned responses can help sustain the cycle of abstinence and relapse that is a hallmark of substance use disorders. Imaging studies that evaluated markers of brain function have also shown that drug abusers who are tested during protracted detoxification have disrupted activity of frontal brain regions, including dorsolateral prefrontal regions, the cingulate gyrus, and the orbitofrontal cortex. This dysfunction may underlie impaired inhibitory control and impulsivity and contribute to relapse (for further reading, see Jentsch and Taylor 1999; Goldstein and Volkow, 2002; Volkow et al., 2003).

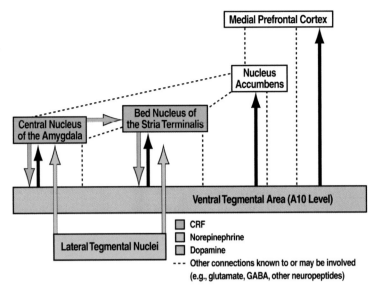

FIGURE 4.23 **Overview of the circuitry that comprises and integrates the extended amygdala and mesocorticolimbic systems and that forms the basis for a neuroanatomical model of stress-induced reinstatement of cocaine seeking.** The extended amygdala circuitry extends from a transition area in the shell of the nucleus accumbens to the bed nucleus of the stria terminalis and central nucleus of the amygdala. The mesocorticolimbic dopamine system originates in the ventral tegmental area and comprises a system of dopamine neurons that provide projections between the ventral tegmental area, nucleus accumbens, and prefrontal cortex. The bed nucleus of the stria terminalis and central nucleus of the amygdala receive major noradrenergic (that is, norepinephrine) innervation from neurons of the lateral tegmental nuclei, which give rise to the ventral norepinephrine pathway. Although the extended amygdala is also innervated by the dorsal noradrenergic pathway originating in the locus coeruleus, it is the ventral pathway that has been specifically implicated in the effects of norepinephrine on stress-induced reinstatement of drug seeking and the aversive effects of opiate withdrawal. The central nucleus of the amygdala and bed nucleus of the stria terminalis are also innervated by dopamine neurons originating in regions of the midbrain, including the ventral tegmental area. Both norepinephrine and dopamine neurons synapse with, or in close proximity to, corticotropin-releasing factor (CRF) neurons in the central nucleus of the amygdala and bed nucleus of the stria terminalis. CRF neurons in the central nucleus of the amygdala are hypothesized to project to the bed nucleus of the stria terminalis and ventral tegmental area, and CRF neurons in the bed nucleus of the stria terminalis provide a local source of CRF and also project to the ventral tegmental area. CRF in the ventral tegmental area may initially have an excitatory effect on dopamine and glutamate transmission in the region. Based on this circuitry, a neuroanatomical model of stress-induced reinstatement of cocaine seeking has been proposed, whereby footshock stress initially activates lateral tegmental (but not locus coeruleus) norepinephrine neurons, which in turn activate CRF projection neurons from the central nucleus of the amygdala to the bed nucleus of the stria terminalis and local CRF interneurons in the bed nucleus of the stria terminalis. Subsequently, CRF-induced activation of excitatory projection neurons from the bed nucleus of the stria terminalis (which possibly contain CRF as a neurotransmitter or cotransmitter) in turn act in distal brain areas (including dopamine or non-dopamine ventral tegmental area neurons) to initiate the approach behaviors involved in reinstatement. *[From: Erb S. Evaluation of the relationship between anxiety during withdrawal and stress-induced reinstatement of cocaine seeking. Progress in Neuropsychopharmacology and Biological Psychiatry, 2010, (34), 798–807.]*

SUMMARY

Indirect sympathomimetics, such as cocaine and amphetamines, have a long history of being used in tonics and other preparations to allay fatigue and sustain performance. These drugs have an equally long history of abuse and dependence, with episodic, collective social amnesia about the behavioral toxicity associated with excessive use. Cocaine and amphetamines have a characteristic abuse cycle that consists of binge administration and withdrawal dysphoria, paranoia, and psychosis-like symptoms as the cycle continues and intensifies. The abuse potential varies with the availability of the drug, both environmentally and physiologically. Intravenous and smoked forms of both cocaine and amphetamines produce much more severe addiction than other routes of administration. Cocaine and amphetamines produce euphoria, increase activity, facilitate performance (particularly in situations of fatigue), and decrease appetite. Amphetamines have medical uses as adjuncts for short-term weight control, in the treatment of attention-deficit/hyperactivity disorder, and in the treatment of narcolepsy. Cocaine has been used as a local anesthetic for mucous membrane anesthesia and vasoconstriction. An inverted U-shaped dose-response function relates the performance-enhancing effects of psychostimulants to dose. The behavioral mechanism of action reflects a behavioral principle in which increases in response rates occur for a given behavior, with a concomitant decrease in the number of response categories. This principle has significant explanatory power not only for the acute stimulant effects of the drugs but also for their pathophysiology.

Significant advances have been made in our understanding of the mechanism of action of psychomotor stimulant drugs at the behavioral, neuropharmacological, and molecular levels that have important implications for understanding the neurobiology of addiction. In the *binge/intoxication* stage of the addiction cycle, the mesocorticolimbic dopamine system is critically important for the acute reinforcing effects of cocaine and D-amphetamine. Dopamine release in the nucleus accumbens is necessary for intravenous cocaine self-administration. Neural elements in the nucleus accumbens at the cellular level respond to both the self-administration of the drug and the *anticipation* of drug self-administration. Molecular neuropharmacological studies have revealed important roles for dopamine D_1, D_2, and D_3 receptors. In the *withdrawal/negative affect* stage, acute psychostimulant withdrawal produces major elevations in brain reward thresholds that may play a critical role in driving the escalation to dependence.

At the neurochemical level, decreases in mesocorticolimbic dopamine and serotonin function and increases in the brain stress neurotransmitters CRF and dynorphin appear to be involved in this acute motivational withdrawal syndrome. Stimulation of cAMP-dependent protein kinase and activation of CREB with concomitant expression of dynorphin in the nucleus accumbens may provide one mechanism for motivational tolerance and dependence; the activation of brain stress systems in the amygdala may provide another mechanism. In the *preoccupation/anticipation* stage of the addiction cycle, animal models of relapse have revealed important roles for the basolateral amygdala and medial prefrontal cortex connections to the nucleus accumbens and extended amygdala, with the neurotransmitters dopamine, glutamate, and CRF all playing important roles. How these circuits are altered by molecular and cellular events following the chronic administration of cocaine and amphetamines to produce the neuroadaptive changes associated with addiction is the subject of intense investigations. Several molecular sites in the medial prefrontal cortex/nucleus accumbens glutamate projection have been proposed to mediate the enhanced glutamatergic signal involved in cocaine-induced reinstatement. Another long-term molecular change that may lead to increased sensitivity to cocaine long after abstinence is increased expression of ΔFosB. Such studies provide key insights into our understanding of the vulnerability to psychostimulant addiction and vulnerability to relapse.

Suggested Reading

Aston-Jones, G., Harris, G.C., 2004. Brain substrates for increased drug seeking during protracted withdrawal. Neuropharmacology 47 (suppl 1), 167–179.

Belin, D., Everitt, B.J., 2008. Cocaine seeking habits depend upon dopamine-dependent serial connectivity linking the ventral with the dorsal striatum. Neuron 57, 432–441.

Di Chiara, G., 2002. Nucleus accumbens shell and core dopamine: differential role in behavior and addiction. Behav. Brain. Res. 137, 75–114.

Everitt, B.J., Wolf, M.E., 2002. Psychomotor stimulant addiction: a neural systems perspective. J. Neurosci. 22, 3312–3320. [erratum: 22(16): 1a].

Goldstein, R.Z., Volkow, N.D., 2002. Drug addiction and its underlying neurobiological basis: neuroimaging evidence for the involvement of the frontal cortex. Am. J. Psychiatry. 159, 1642–1652.

Grueter, B.A., Rothwell, P.E., Malenka, R.C., 2012. Integrating synaptic plasticity and striatal circuit function in addiction. Curr. Opin. Neurobiol. 22, 545–551.

Jentsch, J.D., Taylor, J.R., 1999. Impulsivity resulting from frontostriatal dysfunction in drug abuse: implications for the control of behavior by reward-related stimuli. Psychopharmacology 146, 373–390.

Kalivas, P.W., McFarland, K., 2003. Brain circuitry and the reinstatement of cocaine seeking behavior. Psychopharmacology 168, 44–56.

Koob, G.F., 1992. Drugs of abuse: anatomy, pharmacology, and function of reward pathways. Trends. Pharmacol. Sci. 13, 177–184.

Koob, G.F., Kreek, M.J., 2007. Stress, dysregulation of drug reward pathways, and the transition to drug dependence. Am. J. Psychiatry. 164, 1149–1159.

Koob, G.F., Le Moal, M., 2006. Neurobiology of Addiction. Academic Press, London.

Lyon, M., Robbins, T.W., 1975. The action of central nervous system stimulant drugs: a general theory concerning amphetamine effects. In: Essman, W.B., Valzelli, L. (Eds.), Current Developments in Psychopharmacology, vol. 2. Spectrum Publications, New York, pp. 79–163.

Nestler, E.J., 2005. Is there a common molecular pathway for addiction? Nat. Neurosci. 8, 1445–1449.

Piazza, P.V., Le Moal, M., 1996. Pathophysiological basis of vulnerability to drug abuse: role of an interaction between stress, glucocorticoids, and dopaminergic neurons. Annu. Rev. Pharmacol. Toxicol. 36, 359–378.

Rylander, G., 1971. Stereotype behavior in man following amphetamine abuse. In: Baker, S.B.C. (Ed.), The Correlation of Adverse Effects in Man with Observations in Animals. series title: International Congress Series, vol. 220. Excerpta Medica, Amsterdam, pp. 28–31.

See, R.E., Fuchs, R.A., Ledford, C.C., McLaughlin, J., 2003. Drug addiction, relapse, and the amygdala. In: Shinnick-Gallagher, P., Pitkanen, A., Shekhar, A., Cahill, L. (Eds.), The Amygdala in Brain Function: Basic and Clinical Approaches. series title: Annals of the New York Academy of Sciences, vol. 985. New York Academy of Sciences, New York, pp. 294–307.

Shaham, Y., Shalev, U., Lu, L., de Wit, H., Stewart, J., 2003. The reinstatement model of drug relapse: history, methodology and major findings. Psychopharmacology 168, 3–20.

Siegel, R.K., 1982. Cocaine smoking. J. Psychoactive Drugs 14, 271–359.

Thomas, M.J., Malenka, R.C., 2003. Synaptic plasticity in the mesolimbic dopamine system. Trans. R. Soc. Lond. B Biol. Sci. 358, 815–819.

Volkow, N.D., Fowler, J.S., Wang, G.J., 2003. The addicted human brain: insights from imaging studies. J. Clin. Invest. 111, 1444–1451.

Volkow, N.D., Fowler, J.S., Wang, G.J., Baler, R., Telang, F., 2009. Imaging dopamine's role in drug abuse and addiction. Neuropharmacology 56 (suppl 1), 3–8.

Zhang, J., Berridge, K.C., Tindell, A.J., Smith, K.S., Aldridge, J.W., 2009. A neural computational model of incentive salience. PLoS Comput. Biol. 5, e1000437.

Opioids

DEFINITIONS

Opioids are drugs with major medical uses, including the treatment of pain and diarrhea, and have been used throughout human history for both the relief of human suffering and their psychotropic properties (Box 5.1).

Opioids are the most potent and effective analgesics known to man. Opiates, such as morphine and codeine, together with 20 other alkaloids were originally derived from the extracts of the juice of the opium poppy (*Papaver somniferum*; Figure 5.1). An opiate drug was defined as any natural or semi-synthetic derivative that has morphine-like effects. Because of the development of synthetic drugs with morphine-like actions and the discovery of morphine-like acting substances in the brain, the term *opioid* came into use and can be defined as all drugs, both natural and synthetic, with morphine-like actions. The term "opioids" also encompasses endogenous opioid peptides

---

BOX 5.1

SYNOPSIS OF THE NEUROPHARMACOLOGICAL TARGETS FOR OPIOIDS

Opioid drugs – natural, semisynthetic, and synthetic – all have pharmacological actions similar to morphine and bind as direct agonists to the opioid receptors in the brain to produce their behavioral effects. Opioid drugs mimic the actions of endogenous opioid peptides that also bind as agonists to the opioid receptors, including β-endorphin (which has cell bodies in the hypothalamus) and enkephalins and dynorphins (which are widely distributed throughout the brain and have high concentrations in reward- and pain-related neurocircuits). The behavioral effects of opioids are transduced by three transmembrane G-protein-coupled opioid receptors – μ, δ, and κ – and subsequent second-messenger gene transcription changes. The μ opioid

receptor is responsible for the pain-relieving and intoxicating effects of opioids, in addition to a wide range of other behavioral and physiological effects. The intoxicating effects of opioids are largely mediated by actions on μ opioid receptors in the origin and terminal areas of the mesocorticolimbic dopamine system, including the nucleus accumbens and extended amygdala (central nucleus of the amygdala, bed nucleus of the stria terminalis, and a transition zone in the shell of the nucleus accumbens). The addiction potential of opioids largely derives from powerful within-system neuroadaptations (signal transduction mechanisms) and between-system neuroadaptations (neurocircuitry changes) in the brain motivational and stress systems.

(i.e., neuropeptides found naturally in the body that have morphine-like actions), such as enkephalins, dynorphins, and endorphins, that bind to the same receptors as opioid receptor agonists and antagonists. For simplicity, this book generally uses the term "opioids."

HISTORY OF OPIOID USE

One of the first references to the medical use of opium was by the Greek, Theophrastus, who, at the beginning of the third century B.C., spoke of *meconium*, which was composed of the extracts of the stems, leaves, and fruit of *Papaver somniferum*. Parcelus (1490–1540 A.D.), a famous physician from the Middle Ages, used opium often, and his followers were equally enthusiastic. Thomas Sydenham, a well-known physician of the 17th century, described the treatment of

a series of dysentery epidemics that occurred in 1669–1672:

"And here I cannot but break out in praise of the great God, the giver of all good things, who hath granted to the human race, as a comfort in their affliction, no medicine of the value of opium, either in regard to the number of diseases it can control, or its efficiency in extirpating them." *(Latham RG, The Works of Thomas Sydenham, Syndenham Society, London, 1848.)*

However, just as early as the description of the beneficial medical effects of opioids, the phenomenon of opioid withdrawal was described. Dr. John Jones was very candid in his account from 1700: "A return of all diseases, pains and disasters, must happen generally, because the opium takes them off by a bare diversion of the sense thereof by pleasure." Such a description presaged the ultimate

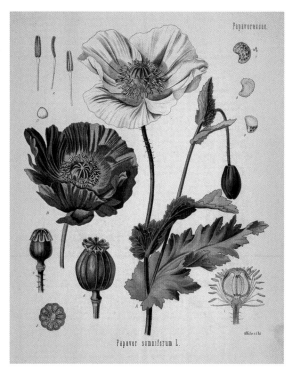

FIGURE 5.1 *Papaver somniferum* L. *[From: Bentley R, Trimen H. Medicinal plants: being descriptions with original figures of the principal plants employed in medicine and an account of the characters, properties and uses of their parts and products of medicinal value. Churchill, London, 1880.]*

dilemma with opioids. They have tremendous beneficial medical effects accompanied by significant side effects, the most devastating of which are opioid addiction and chronic uncontrolled use.

The history of opioid abuse in the Western world began with the spread of opium from the Middle East to Europe and the Orient. Europeans traded opium for tea from China through the British East India Company. British merchants smuggled opium into China to balance their purchases of tea for export to Britain. The Chinese realized the marked addictive properties of opium and attempted to stop the trade practice, ultimately resulting in the Opium Wars of the 1840s, the outcome of which was a British victory. The British were ceded Hong Kong from the Chinese, and the Chinese ports were opened to the opium trade. As a result, the importation of opium to China was legalized. Opium use then spread to the United States and elsewhere with the immigration of Chinese laborers. Unlimited opium use in the United States contributed to the passage of the Harrison Narcotics Act in 1914 and, the social marginalization of opioid use and development of heroin addiction.

Heroin addiction remains a substantial medical problem in the United States, and prescription opioids present a growing medical problem. The 2011 United States *National Survey on Drug Use and Health* from the Substance Abuse and Mental Health Services Administration estimated that 4.2 million people aged 12 and older had ever engaged in heroin use (1.7%), and 34.6 million people aged 12 and older had ever engaged in the use of analgesics (13.5%). Additionally, 0.62 million people aged 12 and older were last-year users of heroin (0.2%), and 11.1 million people aged 12 and older were last-year users of analgesics (4.3%). Notable statistics from the survey included the following. In 2011, of those people aged 12 or older who ever used in the last year, 0.43 million (65.5%) showed heroin abuse or dependence, and 1.8 million (16.5%) showed analgesic abuse or dependence (Substance Use Disorder based on the *Diagnostic and Statistical Manual of Mental Disorders*, 5th edition [DSM-5], criteria). Of those who ever used in the last year, 0.37 million (57%) showed heroin dependence, and 1.4 million (12.7%) showed analgesic dependence (DSM-IV criteria; see Chapter 1).

PHYSIOLOGICAL EFFECTS

In non-tolerant adults at analgesic doses, morphine decreases body temperature, decreases the release of stress hormones via its action on the pituitary gland, decreases respiration, suppresses the cough reflex, and can induce nausea.

Opioids at therapeutic doses have little effects on blood pressure or heart rate but can cause orthostatic hypotension (commonly known as dizzy spells or head rushes), particularly in the elderly. Opioids decrease gastrointestinal secretions and gastrointestinal motility, reflecting their well-known anti-diarrheal properties. Opioids can also produce pruritis (itching) and suppress the immune system. At toxic doses, morphine and its derivatives can produce coma, constricted (pinpoint) pupils, and respiratory depression.

BEHAVIORAL EFFECTS

Opioids have pronounced behavioral effects in two domains – pain relief and intoxication (profound euphoria or "high") – both of which are described below in detail. The intensity of the euphoric effect varies with the route of administration. Intravenous and smoked opioids produce a dramatic and intense pleasurable effect. Opioids can also impair cognitive function, block memory formation, and impair performance of cognitive and skilled tasks. Other behavioral effects of opioids are related to their non-central nervous system actions, many of which are considered side effects, such as pruritis (itching) and constipation.

MEDICAL USES

Opium contains 10% morphine but also other opiate alkaloids, such as thebaine and codeine. Morphine was first isolated from opium by Serturner in 1804 and named after Morpheus, the God of Dreams, or Morphina, the God of Sleep – both very appropriate reflections of opium's effects. Codeine was first isolated from opium in 1832 by Robiquet and subsequently used in the United States as a tonic for various problems and ailments. It is still the most widely prescribed legal opioid used largely for analgesic, antitussive, and anti-diarrheal effects. Thebaine is stimulatory instead of sedative and at higher doses produces convulsions. Thebaine was mainly used to produce semi-synthetic derivatives of opiates, such as naloxone (an opioid antagonist) and oxycodone (a powerful opioid agonist; Figure 5.2). Heroin (diacetylmorphine) was developed by the Bayer Company in 1898 as an effective cough suppressant with alleged stimulant action on the respiratory system. Although heroin does appreciably inhibit the cough reflex, the latter assertion

FIGURE 5.2 **The four sources of opioids.** (1) Opium is the natural source of opiates, such as morphine, codeine, and thebaine. (2) The semi-synthetic opioids are derivatives of the natural opiates. (3) The synthetic opioids are not derived from natural opiates. (4) Endogenous opioid peptides are found in the body and brain.

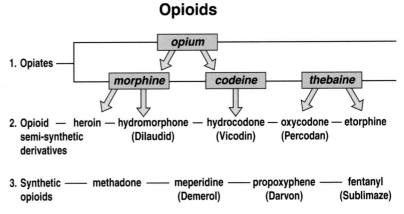

of a stimulant-like effect was later proven false (Figure 5.3). As mentioned above, another well-known (and often undesirable in the context of pain management) effect of opioids is their anti-diarrheal effects, which in the management of chronic pain must also be managed with the use of other drugs that help prevent or reverse the blockade of gastrointestinal motility.

However, the most common indication for the prescription of opioids is their unmatched effectiveness in pain relief (Box 5.2). Opioids are the most powerful and effective drugs known to man for the relief of pain. Pain relief from

morphine at a standard dose of 10 mg administered intramuscularly or subcutaneously lasts up to 3–4 h. Opioid analgesia has been described as the selective suppression of pain without effects on other sensory modalities at reasonable analgesic doses. Opioid analgesia also distinguishes between different types of pain. Opioids have minimal effects on the initial sharp sensation produced by noxious stimuli but are very effective against the dull continuous ache that continues after a noxious stimulus. Presumably, this distinction has survival value. The selective suppression of continuous pain by endogenous

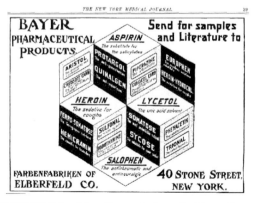

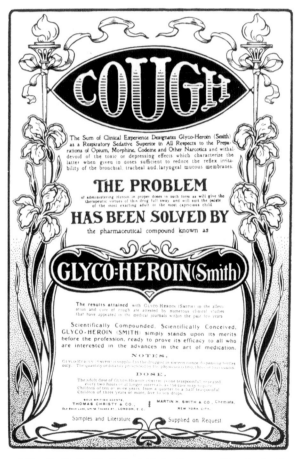

FIGURE 5.3 **Advertisements from the Bayer Company and Martin M. Smith & Co. Ltd. for the use of heroin for the treatment of cough, circa early 1900s.**

BOX 5.2

TYPES OF PAIN

Somatic Pain

Also called "nociceptive pain," somatic pain refers to the sensation caused by peripheral nerve fiber stimulation. Such pain can be further classified as either mechanical or thermal.

Neuropathic Pain

Neuropathic pain can result from injury to the nerves of the central nervous system. The pain can be described as a burning sensation or "pins and needles," such as a person experiences when their leg "falls asleep." Dysesthesia is the global

term used to describe such abnormal sensations. Neuralgia refers to pain that occurs in nerves without specific stimulation of nociceptors. Allodynia is another form of neuropathic pain, referred to as pain elicited by normally innocuous stimuli.

Affective Dimension of Pain

The moment-to-moment unpleasantness of pain is made up of emotional feelings that pertain to the present or short-term future, such as distress or fear.

---

opioids allows for relief from the pain of a previous injury but does not eliminate one's awareness of the immediate danger of a new injury. Opioids are less effective in reducing the neuropathic pain that results from nerve injury. Perhaps more importantly for the neurobiology of addiction, opioids also effectively reduce the "affective dimension of pain" (for further reading, see Gutstein and Akil, 2001).

Opioids also produce analgesia when administered into the periphery or at local sites, and opioid receptors are present on peripheral nerves. Opioids are commonly administered epidurally (into the outermost space of the spinal canal) for the management of obstetric pain during delivery. Both the epidural and intrathecal (under the arachnoid membrane that surrounds the brain) routes of administration have been used for chronic pain states, such as lower back pain, neuralgia, and limb pain. With intrathecal administration, the drug can access cerebrospinal fluid and thus avoid the blood-brain barrier. With epidural administration, opioids bind to opioid receptors in the spinal cord and produce analgesia without causing impairments

in motor or sensory function. Drugs with high selectivity for the μ opioid receptor and high lipid solubility, such as fentanyl, are taken up rapidly into the spinal cord and have a fast onset of action.

Opioids are often used to relieve pain during general anesthesia. However, they also are a component of "balanced anesthesia," in which a balance of agents is used to produce the different components of anesthesia, including analgesia, amnesia, muscle relaxation, and the abolition of autonomic reflexes. Currently, fentanyl and its congeners alfentanil and remifentanil are used as components of balanced anesthesia because of their rapid onset of action. The inclusion of an opioid into general anesthesia can also reduce preoperative pain and anxiety, decrease adverse responses to manipulations of the airways, lower the requirements for inhaled anesthetics, and provide immediate postoperative pain relief.

Patient-controlled analgesia is a method of opioid administration in which the patient can carefully titrate the rate of opioid administration to meet their individual pain relief needs. Although such titration can be achieved with oral dosing, specifically designed infusion pumps can deliver a continuous infusion with bolus doses by the intravenous, subcutaneous, or epidural routes. The pumps are programmed to the needs of the patient, with limits set to prevent overdose. This method of delivery can provide a consistent level of analgesia and is associated with greater patient compliance.

Table 5.1 shows the equivalent doses of commonly prescribed opioids required to produce analgesia similar to a standard 10 mg dose of morphine. Numerous natural and synthetic opioids are available for mild to moderate pain relief. Codeine, a natural component of opium, is the most commonly used opioid analgesic for the management of mild to moderate pain and is often combined with aspirin or acetaminophen. It is significantly less potent than morphine. Oxycodone (oxycontin) is a synthetic derivative of morphine that is used for the management of mild to moderate pain and is nearly equipotent with morphine when given orally and slightly more potent than morphine via the intravenous route.

The use of prescription opioids for pain is steadily increasing in the United States, paralleled by an increasing prevalence of chronic pain syndromes. The prevalence of prescription opioids in the United States, according to the Institute of Medicine 2011, is estimated to be 70–116 million. As will be seen below, in some individuals with chronic pain, the use of chronic opioids leads to opioid-induced hyperalgesia, adding to the difficulty of the differential diagnosis of chronic pain and opioid withdrawal.

PHARMACOKINETICS

Heroin is among the most well-known abused semi-synthetic derivatives of opium. Heroin injected intravenously rapidly enters the blood. After smoking, heroin blood levels peak in just 1–5 min and then decrease quickly, reaching the minimum limits of detection in 30 min.

Intravenous heroin has a half-life of only 3 min and is rapidly converted to 6-monacetylmorphine

TABLE 5.1   Dosing Data for Opioid Analgesics

Drug	Approximate Equianalgesic Oral Dose	Approximate Equianalgesic Parenteral Dose
Morphine[1]	30 mg q 3–4 h (around-the-clock dosing) 60 mg every 3–4 h (single or intermittent dose)	10 mg q 3–4 h
Codeine[2]	130 mg every 3–4 h	75 mg every 3–4 h
Hydromophone[1] (Dilaudid)	7.5 mg every 3–4 h	1.5 mg every 3–4 h
Hydrocodone (Lorcet, Lortab, Vicodin, others)	30 mg every 3–4 h	not available
Levorphanol (Levo-Dromoran)	4 mg every 6–8 h	2 mg every 6–8 h
Meperidine (Demerol)	300 mg every 2–3 h	100 mg every 3 h
Methadone (Dolophine, others)	20 mg every 6–8 h	10 mg every 6–8 h
Oxycodone (Roxicodone, Percocet, Percodan, Tylox, others)[3]	30 mg every 3–4 h	not available
Oxymorphine[1]	not available	1 mg every 3–4 h
Propoxyphene (Darvon)	130 mg[4]	not available
Tramadol[5] (Ultram)	100 mg[4]	100 mg

[1] For morphine, hydromorphone, and oxymorphone, rectal administration is an alternate route for patients unable to take oral medications, but equianalgesic doses may differ from oral and parenteral doses because of pharmacokinetic differences.

[2] Caution: Codeine doses above 65 mg often are not appropriate due to diminishing incremental analgesia with increasing doses but continually increasing constipation and other side effects.

[3] Oxycontin is an extended-release preparation containing up to 160 mg of oxycodone per tablet and is recommended for use every 12 h.

[4] Doses for moderate pain not necessarily equivalent to 30 mg oral or 10 mg parenteral morphine.

[5] Risk of seizures; parenteral formulation not available in the United States. [Taken with permission from Gutstein HB, Akil H. Opioid analgesics. In: Hardman JG, Limbird LE, Goodman-Gilman A (eds.) Goodman and Gilman's The Pharmacological Basis of Therapeutics, 10th edition. McGraw-Hill, New York, 2001, pp. 569–619.]

and then more slowly to morphine. The elimination half-life by the smoked route is approximately 3.3 min for heroin, 5.4 min for 6-monoacetylmorphine, and 18.8 min for morphine. Morphine is then metabolized to morphine 3-β-glucuronide and morphine 6-β-glucuronide. Oxycodone has a relatively short half-life of 2–3 h and is excreted mainly via the kidneys. See Table 5.1 for equivalent doses and half-lives for commonly prescribed opioid drugs.

Heroin is basically a prodrug, which is a drug or substance that by itself would have no pharmacological activity. It can exert its biological or psychotropic effects only after it is converted to its active metabolites. Heroin must first be metabolized to 6-monoacetylmorphine and then to morphine (Figure 5.4). These two metabolites then bind to μ opioid receptors, producing the characteristic behavioral and neurobiological effects attributed to heroin. The conversion of heroin to 6-monacetylmorphine is very rapid, occurring via esterase enzymes in the brain and blood and virtually every tissue, including the liver. The wide availability of these enzymes accounts for the more rapid onset of action and potency of heroin compared to morphine. 6-Monacetylmorphine eventually becomes converted to morphine, further contributing to the duration of heroin's effects.

Morphine 6-β-glucuronide is pharmacologically active and binds to μ opioid receptors, but its potency is so low that it is unlikely to contribute to the analgesic effects of morphine. This was demonstrated in a study in which the analgesic effects of morphine and morphine 6-β-glucuronide were tested in a transcutaneous electrical pain model in healthy volunteers. The subjects were stimulated with an electrical current that produced pain, and morphine 6-β-glucuronide did not contribute significantly to the analgesic effects. Morphine 3-β-glucuronide, another morphine metabolite, does not bind to opioid receptors but has some excitatory effects when injected directly into the brain. In a controlled clinical trial, morphine 3-β-glucuronide was found to be devoid of opioid-like activity and also had no anti-morphine effects.

BEHAVIORAL MECHANISM OF ACTION

The behavioral mechanism most associated with opioids is their effects on pain processing and the relief of pain and suffering. Pain relief takes on many forms in several parts of the central nervous system and outside it. Within this book, a behavioral mechanism of action refers to a unifying principle of order and predictability at the behavioral level. Each drug class has behavioral effects that define its phenotype. This behavioral mechanism may derive from medical use, behavioral pathology, or some combination of both.

Opioids can also relieve emotional pain, and this is one of the behavioral mechanisms strongly implicated in the addiction cycle (see Chapter 1). A unique aspect of heroin addiction has been described as:

> "The special role the drug comes to play in the personality organization of these patients. They have not successfully established familiar defensive, neurotic, characterological or other common adaptive mechanisms as a way of dealing with their distress. Instead, they have resorted to the use of opioids as a way of coping with a range of problems including ordinary human pain, disappointment, anxiety, loss, anguish, sexual frustration, and other suffering." (Khantzian EJ, Mack JE, Schatzberg AF. Heroin use as an attempt to cope: clinical observations. American Journal of Psychiatry, 1974, (131), 160–164 [p. 162].)

This aspect of drug addiction has been extended to an overall hypothesis of self-medication, in which patients are purported to experiment with various classes of drugs to discover the one that is particularly well-suited for that individual because it changes the emotional states that the patient finds particularly problematic, painful, or desirable. Opioids have been hypothesized to be preferred by many

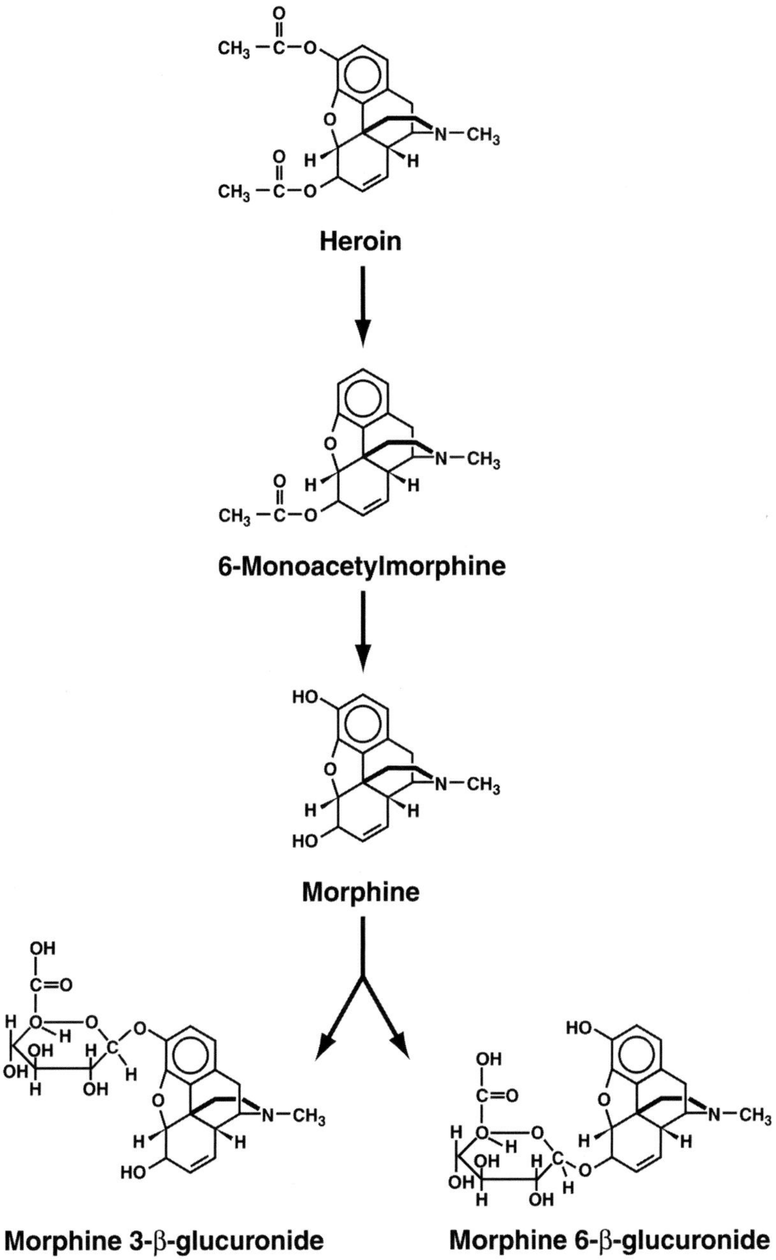

FIGURE 5.4 **Biotransformation pathway for heroin in humans.** *[Taken with permission from Pichini S, Altieri I, Pellegrini M, Zuccaro P, Pacifici R. The role of liquid chromatography-mass spectrometry in the determination of heroin and related opioids in biological fluids. Mass Spectrometry Reviews, 1999, (18), 119–130.]*

individuals because of their powerful actions in diminishing the disorganizing and threatening effects of rage and aggression. Subjects who experienced or expressed physical abuse and violent behavior have described the way that opioids helped them feel normal, calm, mellow, soothed, and relaxed.

Paradoxically, opioids can also *induce* pain as a result of counteradaptive processes. Patients who receive long-term opioid therapy that lasts from weeks to years can develop unexpectedly abnormal pain and hyperalgesia upon withdrawal from the opioid treatment. In a review of the clinical experiences of over 750 patients who received epidural or spinal morphine over an average of 124 days, it was reported that many of these developed increased sensitivity to sensory stimuli (hyperesthesia) and that normally innocuous sensory stimulations elicited pain (allodynia).

USE, ABUSE, AND ADDICTION

Opioids are probably the classic drugs of addiction. A pattern of drug taking evolves, including an intense intoxication via the intravenous or smoked routes for heroin and via the oral or intravenous routes for opioid analgesics (Box 5.3). Tolerance develops, and intake escalates, with profound dysphoria, physical discomfort, and somatic withdrawal signs during abstinence. Intense preoccupation with obtaining opioids (craving) develops that often precedes the somatic signs of withdrawal, and this preoccupation is linked not only to stimuli associated with obtaining the drug but also to stimuli associated with withdrawal and internal and external states of stress. The drug must be obtained to avoid the severe dysphoria and discomfort of abstinence.

However, a popular, virtually universal misconception about opioid use is that any opioid use within or outside medical settings inevitably leads to intractable physiological dependence and addiction. Extensive work has established a wide variety of patterns of non-medical opioid consumption, ranging from non-problematic to abusive. Three modes of opioid use have been described: controlled subjects or "chippers," marginal subjects or abusers, and compulsive subjects with addiction. Controlled use is generally recognized as occasional use and most often indicates a non-addictive pattern of opioid use. A marginal user could have possibly met the criteria for Substance Abuse defined by the *Diagnostic and Statistical Manual of Mental Disorders*, 4th edition (DSM-IV), and may meet the criteria for Substance Use Disorder for Opioids as defined by the DSM-5. A person with addiction, in contrast, definitely meets the criteria for Substance Dependence as defined by the DSM-IV and will probably meet the criteria for severe Substance Use Disorder for Opioids as defined by the DSM-5. Controlled opioid use has several characteristics that differ from the other extreme of a compulsive user.

Controlled substance users ("chippers") limit their use of the drug, often to amounts or periods of time that do not interfere with social and occupational functioning. To do this, they develop elaborate rules, such as refusing to inject intravenously, planning for use, budgeting money for only a certain amount of use, and deferring use when opioids are not available. Controlled use patterns can be stable and last as long as 15 years (Table 5.2).

An example of controlled opioid use is the following:

> "Arthur, a 'controlled user,' was a forty-year-old white male who had been married for 16 years and was the father of three children. He had lived in his own home in a middle-class suburb for 12 years. He had been steadily employed as a union carpenter with the same construction firm for five years. During the ten years prior to the first interview, Arthur used heroin on weekends, occasionally injecting during the week, but during the previous five years mid-week use had not occurred." (Harding WM, Zinberg NE. *Occasional opiate use.* Advances in Substance Abuse, *1983, (3), 27–61).*

BOX 5.3

It is so long since I first took opium, that if it had been a trifling incident in my life, I might have forgotten its date: but cardinal events are not to be forgotten; and from circumstances connected with it, I remember that it must be referred to the autumn of 1804. During that season I was in London, having come thither for the first time since my entrance at college. And my introduction to opium arose in the following way. From an early age I had been accustomed to wash my head in cold water at least once a day: being suddenly seized with toothache, I attributed it to some relaxation caused by an accidental intermission of that practice; jumped out of bed: plunged my head into a basin of cold water; and with hair thus wetted went to sleep. The next morning, as I need hardly say, I awoke with excruciating rheumatic pains of the head and face, from which I had hardly any respite for about twenty days. On the twenty-first day, I think it was, and on a Sunday, that I went out into the streets; rather to run away, if possible, from my torments, than with any distinct purpose. By accident I met a college acquaintance who recommended opium. Opium! dread agent of unimaginable pleasure and pain! I had heard of it as I had of manna or of ambrosia, but no further: how unmeaning a sound was it at that time! what solemn chords does it now strike upon my heart! what heart-quaking vibrations of sad and happy remembrances! Reverting for a moment to these, I feel a mystic importance attached to the minutest circumstances connected with the place and the time, and the man (if man he was) that first laid open to me the Paradise of Opium-eaters. It was a Sunday afternoon, wet and cheerless: and a duller spectacle this earth-of-ours has not to show than a rainy Sunday in London.

Arrived at my lodgings, it may be supposed that I lost not a moment in taking the quantity prescribed. I was necessarily ignorant of the whole art and mystery of opium-taking: and, what I took, I took under every disadvantage. But I took it: and in an hour, oh! heavens! what a revulsion! what an upheaving, from its lowest depths, of the inner spirit! what an apocalypse of the world within me! That my pains had vanished, was now a trifle in my eyes: this negative effect was swallowed up in the immensity of those positive effects which had opened before me – in the abyss of divine enjoyment thus suddenly revealed. Here was a panacea – a *φαρμαχον νηπενθες* for all human woes [literally a "drug of forgetfulness"]: here was the secret of happiness, about which philosophers had disputed for so many ages, at once discovered: happiness might now be bought for a penny, and carried in the waistcoat pocket: portable ecstasies might be had corked up in a pint bottle: and peace of mind could be sent down gallons by the mail coach. But, if I talk in this way, the reader will think I am laughing: and I can assure him, that nobody will laugh long who deals much with opium: its pleasures even are of a grave and solemn complexion; and in his happiest state, the opium-eater cannot present himself in the character of *l'Allegro*: even then, he speaks and thinks as becomes *Il Penseroso*. Nevertheless, I have a very reprehensible way of jesting at times in the midst of my own misery: and, unless when I am checked by some more powerful feelings, I am afraid I shall be guilty of this indecent practice even in these annals of suffering or enjoyment. The reader must allow a little to my infirm nature in this respect: and with a few indulgences of that sort, I shall endeavour to be as grave, if not drowsy, as fits a theme like opium, so antimercurial as it really is, and so drowsy as it is falsely reputed.

the elevation of spirits produced by opium is necessarily followed by a proportionate depression, and that the natural and even immediate consequence of opium is torpor and stagnation,

Continued

BOX 5.3   *(Cont'd)*

animal and mental. The first of these errors I shall content myself with simply denying; assuring my reader, that for ten years, during which I took opium at intervals, the day succeeding to that on which I allowed myself this luxury was always a day of unusually good spirits.

Thus I have shown that opium does not, of necessity, produce inactivity or torpor; but that, on the contrary, it often led me into markets and theatres. Yet, in candour, I will admit that markets and theatres are not the appropriate haunts of the opium-eater, when in the divinest state incident to his enjoyment. In that state, crowds become an oppression to him; music even, too sensual and gross. He naturally seeks solitude and silence, as indispensable conditions of those trances, or profoundest reveries, which are the crown and consummation of what opium can do for human nature.

One day a Malay knocked at my door. What business a Malay could have to transact amongst English mountains, I cannot conjecture: but possibly he was on his road to a sea-port about forty miles distant.

He lay down upon the floor for about an hour, and then pursued his journey. On his departure, I presented him with a piece of opium. To him, as an Orientalist, I concluded that opium must be familiar: and the expression of his face convinced me that it was. Nevertheless, I was struck with some little consternation when I saw him suddenly raise his hand to his mouth, and (in the school-boy phrase) bolt the whole, divided into three pieces, at one mouthful. The quantity was enough to kill three dragoons and their horses: and I felt some alarm for the poor creature: but what could be done? I had given him the opium in compassion for his solitary life, on recollecting that if he had travelled on foot from London, it must be nearly three weeks since he could have exchanged a thought with any human being. I could not think of violating the laws of

hospitality, by having him seized and drenched with an emetic, and thus frightening him into a notion that we were going to sacrifice him to some English idol. No: there was clearly no help for it: he took his leave: and for some days I felt anxious: but as I never heard of any Malay being found dead, I became convinced that he was used to opium: and that I must have done him the service I designed, by giving him one night of respite from the pains of wandering.

However, as some people, in spite of all laws to the contrary, will persist in asking what became of the opium-eater, and in what state he now is, I answer for him thus: The reader is aware that opium had long ceased to found its empire on spells of pleasure; it was solely by the tortures connected with the attempt to abjure it, that it kept its hold.

I saw that I must die if I continued the opium: I determined, therefore, if that should be required, to die in throwing it off. How much I was at that time taking I cannot say; for the opium which I used had been purchased for me by a friend who afterwards refused to let me pay him; so that I could not ascertain even what quantity I had used within the year. I apprehend, however, that I took it very irregularly: and that I varied from about fifty or sixty grains, to 150 a-day. My first task was to reduce it to forty, to thirty, and, as fast as I could, to twelve grains.

I triumphed: but think not, reader, that therefore my sufferings were ended; nor think of me as of one sitting in a *dejected* state. Think of me as of one, even when four months had passed still agitated, writhing, throbbing, palpitating, shattered.

From: De Quincey T, Confessions of an English Opium Eater, *Penguin Books, New York, 1986.*

TABLE 5.2 Characteristics of Controlled vs. Compulsive Chippers

	Controlled Subjects (*n* = 61)	Compulsive Subjects (*n* = 30)
Age (mean)	25.9 years	25.9 years
Male	77%	67%
Female	23%	33%
Duration of current style of use (months)	53.4 months	59.5 months
Average frequency of use (last 12 months):		
>2 times daily	–	23%
once every 1–2 days	–	23%
2 times weekly	41%	47%
1–3 times monthly	36%	3%
<once monthly	23%	3%
Length of use (mean)	7.2 years	6.8 years
Peak frequency of use:		
>2 times daily	23%	87%
once every 1–2 days	54%	13%
2 times weekly	16%	–
1–3 times monthly	5%	–
<once monthly	2%	–
Percentage who selected rules for use:		
never use in strange place	20%	13%
never use with strangers	31%	28%
never inject	13%	–
special schedule for use	34%	20%
special schedule for use	30%	–
plan for use	28%	31%
never share needles	26%	10%
never use alone	53%	20%
caution in "copping"	48%	23%
budgets for use		
History of adverse reactions	36%	45%

[Data from Harding WM, Zinberg NE. *Occasional opiate use.* Advances in Substance Abuse, *1984, (3), 105–118.*]

In contrast, many individuals report "controlled, recreational" opioid use prior to eventual compulsive use. The person may experiment with various drugs and then snort or smoke heroin. Subsequently, the person is often initiated into using heroin intravenously, which produces a pronounced high, but repeated use leads to the negative effects of withdrawal symptoms. The transition to the intravenous route of administration signals the beginning of the addiction cycle of regular injections, withdrawal, and craving. An example of a compulsive opioid user is the following:

> "Bob, a 'compulsive user,' was a twenty-six-year-old white male who lived alone, a college graduate with a degree in psychology. Following separation from his wife and child three years before interview, he had worked sporadically in part-time jobs. Dealing drugs had become his major source of income. He had used heroin at least three to four times per week since beginning use 30 months before interview, and had had many periods of daily use lasting for as long as two weeks." (*Harding WM, Zinberg NE. Occasional opiate use.* Advances in Substance Abuse, *1983, (3), 27–61*).

One can ask what constitutes the difference, from a clinical perspective, between a "chipper" and a "junkie." Clearly, personality deficits and physiological states induced by the drug itself interact. Limited access will not produce the neuroadaptations that drive compulsive opioid abuse, but personality factors can increase the vulnerability to engage in the compulsive use that then evokes those same neuroadaptations, leading to the vicious cycle of opioid addiction (see Chapter 1).

The natural history of opioid addiction reflects a disorder that is remarkably stable over time. Although repeated cycles of remission and resumption of use occur, these patterns extend over long periods of time. Longitudinal studies have shown that heroin addiction, at least for some individuals, is a lifelong condition. Similar results were obtained in a longitudinal study of 581 males with heroin addiction admitted to the California Civil Addict Program during the years 1962–1964 and followed for 33 years. In 1995–1997,

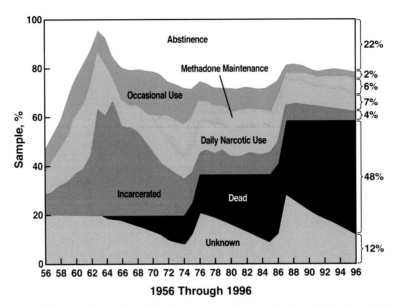

FIGURE 5.5 **The natural history of narcotics addiction among a sample of male individuals with heroin addiction (n = 581) admitted to the California Civil Addict Program, a compulsory drug treatment program for heroin-dependent criminal offenders, during the years 1962 through 1964.** This 33-year follow-up study updated information previously obtained from admission records and two face-to-face interviews conducted in 1974–1975 and 1985–1986. In 1996–1997, at the latest follow-up, 284 were dead and 242 were interviewed. The mean age of the 242 interviewed subjects was 57.4 years. Age, disability, years since first heroin use, and heavy alcohol use were significant correlates of mortality. Of the 242 interviewed subjects, 20.7% tested positive for heroin. The group also reported high rates of health problems, mental health problems, and criminal justice system involvement. Long-term heroin abstinence was associated with less criminality, morbidity, psychological distress, and higher employment. While the number of deaths increased steadily over time, heroin use patterns were remarkably stable for the group as a whole. For some, heroin addiction had been a lifelong condition associated with severe health and social consequences. *[Taken with permission from Hser YI, Hoffman V, Grella CE, Anglin MD. A 33-year follow-up of narcotic addicts.* Archives of General Psychiatry, *2001, (58), 503–508.]*

33 years later, 21% of the subjects tested positive for heroin, 10% refused urine analysis, and 14% were incarcerated. This was very similar to the data from 1974–1975, in which 23% had positive urine, 6% refused urine analysis, and 18% were incarcerated (Figure 5.5). The rate of abstinence in 1996–1997 was related to the amount of time previously abstinent, and most subjects (75%) who reported abstinence for longer than five years were still abstinent in 1996–1997. The number of negative urine samples was also relatively stable, but the number of deaths progressively increased. The most common causes of death were overdose, chronic liver disease, cancer, and cardiovascular disease. By age 50–60, only about half of the interviewed subjects tested negative

for heroin, which argues against the hypothesis that drug addiction lessens with age.

Opioid Intoxication

Intoxication for a person with opioid addiction after an intravenous self-injection or smoking has been described as consisting of four different states that can overlap over time: "rush," "nod," "high," and "being straight" (Table 5.3). These states typically occur with 1–3 mg heroin or 3–15 mg morphine. Profound euphoria, termed the "rush," occurs first, which has been described as occurring approximately 10 s after the beginning of the injection. The rush includes a wave

TABLE 5.3 States of Opiate Intoxication After Administering 1–3 mg Heroin or 3–15 mg Morphine

State	Duration	Effects
Rush	45 s	Intense pleasure, with waves of intense euphoria likened to sexual orgasm. In this first state, visceral sensations occur, with facial flushing and deepening of the voice. Although other effects show tolerance with chronic use, the rush is resistant to tolerance.
Nod	15–20 min	A state of escape from reality that can range from sleepiness to virtual unconsciousness. Addicts are described as calm, detached, and very uninterested in external events.
High	Several hours	This state follows the rush. It is a general feeling of well-being that can extend several hours beyond the rush and shows tolerance.
Being straight	Up to 8 h	This is the point at which the user is no longer experiencing the rush, nod, or high but also is not yet experiencing withdrawal. This state can last up to 8 h following an injection or smoking of heroin.

of euphoric feelings, frequently characterized in sexual terms:

> "So I snort again and *holy f___ing s__t!* I felt like I died and went to heaven. My whole body was like one giant f___ing incredible orgasm." *(Inciardi JA. The War on Drugs: Heroin, Cocaine, Crime, and Public Policy. Mayfield, Palo Alto CA, 1986, p. 61.)*

> "After a while she asks me if I want to try the needle and I say no, but then I decide to go halfway and *skin-pop* [injecting into the muscle just beneath the skin]. Well, man, it was wonderful. Popping was just like snorting, only stronger, finer, better, and faster." *(ibid, p. 62.)*

> "Travelin' along the mainline was like a grand slam home run f___, like getting a blow job from Miss America. The rush hits you instantly, and all of a sudden you're up there on Mount Olympus talking to Zeus." *(ibid, p. 62.)*

In this first state, visceral sensations are also experienced, including facial flushing and a deepening of the voice. Although other effects show tolerance with chronic use, the rush is resistant to tolerance. The second state is the "nod," which is a state of escape from reality that can range from sleepiness to virtual unconsciousness and lasts 15–20 min. Individuals in this state are described as calm, detached, and noticeably uninterested in external events.

Following the nod, the third state occurs, called the "high." The high is described as a general feeling of well-being and can last several hours beyond the rush. In contrast to the rush, however, the high shows tolerance. The fourth and final state is characterized as "being straight." The user no longer experiences the rush, nod, or high but is also not yet experiencing withdrawal. This state can last up to 8 h following intravenous or smoked heroin.

The route of administration and infusion rate of that administration have profound effects on the subjective and physiological effects of opioids. In one study, healthy volunteers received intravenous injections of two doses of morphine at three different infusion rates. Faster infusions produced greater positive subjective effects than slower infusions on ratings of "good drug effect," "drug liking," and "high" (Figure 5.6). In experimental studies of heroin addiction, detoxified individuals with opioid addiction were allowed to intravenously self-administer heroin with self-regulated access to increasing doses over a 10 day period in a residential laboratory setting in a locked unit of a large psychiatric hospital. The early phase of heroin self-administration was accompanied by elated mood and decreased "somatic concern." The later stages were characterized by a profound shift toward dysphoria, with notable increases in somatic concern, anxiety, depression, social isolation, and motor retardation. Initially, the reinforcing properties of heroin stemmed primarily from its ability to relieve tension and produce euphoria. However, as the frequency of drug self-administration increased, tolerance quickly developed

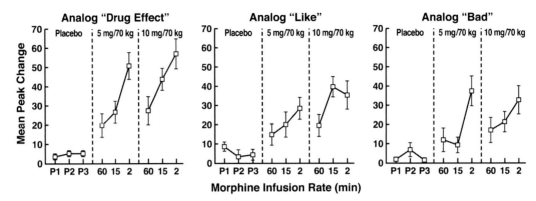

FIGURE 5.6 **Mean peak change scores for the drug effect, drug liking, and high effects of morphine on a Visual Analog Scale (VAS) for different infusion rates and dosing conditions.** Infusions were made over 2, 15, or 60 min in a blinded fashion. Subjects in all conditions received an hour-long infusion composed of drug and/or saline (depending on their infusion rate and dose condition). Three separate pumps were set to be activated by a nurse at time 0, 45, and 53 min for subjects in the 60, 15, and 2 min infusion rate conditions, respectively. Thus, subjects who received an hour-long infusion of drug received drug at all three time points. The subjects in the 15 min drug infusion condition received saline at time 0 min and drug at times 45 and 58 min. The subjects in the 2 min bolus drug infusion condition received saline at times 0 and 45 min and drug at time 58 min. *VAS:* On this measure, subjects rated the extent to which they experienced multiple effects (but only three are shown here: drug effect, drug liking, and drug-induced high). The analog scales consisted of a line approximately 100 mm in length, anchored at each end by "not at all" and "severe." Subjects were instructed to move a cursor along the line reflecting the degree to which they were currently experiencing each of the six drug effects. Responses were recorded as a score ranging from 0 to 100. *ARS:* Self-reports of drug effects were rated on a modified version of an adjective rating scale listing 32 items describing typical opioid drug effects and withdrawal effects. Subjects were instructed to move a cursor along a line anchored at each end by "not at all" and "severe" for each symptom they had experienced. Responses were recorded as a score ranging from 0 to 9. Opioid drug effects included nodding, rush, loaded/high, coasting, itchy skin, etc., and withdrawal effects included such items as irritability, chills/gooseflesh, runny nose, yawning, etc. *These data indicate a faster infusion rate is associated with more intense subjective effects of the drug. This supports the hypothesis that intravenous infusion of a drug may have more "addiction potential" than other routes of administration for which the infusion rate is slower.* [Taken with permission from Marsch LA, Bickel WK, Badger GJ, Rathmell JP, Swedberg MD, Jonzon B, Norsten-Hoog C. *Effects of infusion rate of intravenously administered morphine on physiological, psychomotor, and self-reported measures in humans.* Journal of Pharmacology and Experimental Therapeutics, 2001, (299), 1056–1065.]

to the euphorigenic effects, although single injections remained capable of producing brief periods of positive mood that lasted 30–60 min. This tolerance was accompanied by a distinct shift in the direction of psychopathology and dysphoria. Symptoms included sleep disturbances, social isolation, belligerence, irritability, less motivation for sexual activity, and motor retardation.

Opioid Withdrawal

The characteristic withdrawal syndrome associated with withholding opium derivatives from chronic users was described over a half century

ago by C.K. Himmelsbach (1942). The symptoms of withdrawal included yawning, lacrimation (tearing eyes), rhinorrhea (runny nose), perspiration, gooseflesh, tremor, dilated pupils, anorexia, nausea, emesis, diarrhea, restlessness, insomnia, weight loss, dehydration, hyperglycemia, elevations of temperature and blood pressure, and alterations in pulse rate. Although many of these symptoms were recognized at that time as manifestations of disturbances in the function of the autonomic nervous system, a negative emotional state was also acknowledged as accompanying these physical signs of opioid withdrawal (see Box 5.3). A negative emotional or affective state is defined as a dysphoric state accompanied by depressive-like and anxiety-like symptoms that do not fully meet the criteria of a major mental disorder, such as a major depressive episode or generalized anxiety disorder. Individuals with opioid addiction were described as attempting to obtain sufficient drug to "prevent the dysphoria associated with the [opioid] withdrawal syndrome." (Reichard JD. Can the euphoric, analgetic and physical dependence effects of drugs be separated? I. With reference to euphoria. *Federation Proceedings*, 1943, (2), 188–191.)

Subsequent descriptions of acute opioid withdrawal included two types of symptoms: purposive symptoms and non-purposive symptoms. Purposive symptoms were defined as symptoms that are goal-oriented (i.e., directed at getting more drug) and included complaints, pleas, demands, and manipulations. Purposive symptoms significantly decreased in a hospital setting where such efforts to obtain more drug had no consequences. In contrast, non-purposive symptoms were defined as those that are not goal-oriented and are relatively independent of the observer, the patient's will, and the environment. A more modern framework probably would consider purposive symptoms as "craving" or motivational symptoms and non-purposive symptoms as physical or somatic.

The symptoms of opioid withdrawal also change significantly over time since the last administration (Table 5.4). In the early stages of withdrawal from heroin (6–8h after the last dose), purposive, goal-oriented behavior is prominent and peaks 36–72h after the last dose. Non-purposive, peripheral autonomic signs appear 8–12h after the last dose and include yawning and sweating, runny nose, and watery eyes. These mild autonomic signs increase in intensity during the first 24h and then level off. Additional non-purposive, physical symptoms then appear, peak at 36–48h, and continue up to 72h. These symptoms include pupillary dilation, gooseflesh, hot and cold flashes, loss of appetite, muscle cramps, tremor, and insomnia. Other autonomic signs include elevated blood pressure, increased heart rate, increased respiratory rate, increased body temperature, nausea, and vomiting.

Withdrawing individuals complain of feeling chilled, alternating with a flushing sensation and excessive sweating. Waves of gooseflesh (goose bumps) are prominent, resulting in skin that looks like a plucked turkey. Interestingly, this symptom is the basis of the expression "quitting cold turkey." Accompanying these symptoms are also the subjective symptoms of aches and pains and general misery, mimicking a flu-like state. Muscle spasms, uncontrollable muscle twitching, and kicking movements may be the basis of the expression "kicking the habit." At 24–36h, diarrhea and dehydration may occur. The peak of the physical withdrawal syndrome appears to be approximately 48–72h after the last dose. Without treatment, the physical syndrome completes its course in 7–10days. However, residual, subclinical signs may persist for many weeks after withdrawal.

The persistent signs of abstinence in detoxified subjects, including hyperthermia, mydriasis (pupillary dilation), increased blood pressure, increased respiratory rate, increased pain and stress sensitivity, and dysphoria can continue for months after opioid withdrawal and have been termed "protracted abstinence." Protracted abstinence includes signs of drug abstinence that persist after the acute withdrawal syndrome subsides. Metabolic changes have been reported during an even later stage of protracted abstinence, in which the direction of the changes is *opposite* of the acute signs of abstinence (for example, hypothermia instead of hyperthermia, miosis [pupil constriction] instead of mydriasis, hypotension instead of hypertension, etc.). This protracted abstinence state also has a motivational component, with individuals reporting a "gray" mood state in which few stimuli or activities produce pleasure:

> "It's staying off that is the hard part. It takes a lot of willpower. But seeing smack eats away at your willpower; it makes it very hard. When I stop I just feel vacant with no direction or energy and that lasts for months." (Stewart T. The Heroin Users. *Pandora, London, 1987, p. 166.*)

TABLE 5.4   Abstinence Signs in Sequential Appearance after Last Dose of Narcotic

Grade of Abstinence	Withdrawal Signs	Hours after Last Dose		
		Methadone	Morphine	Heroin
Grade 0	craving for drug anxiety	12	6	4
Grade 1	yawning perspiration runny nose lacrimation	34–48	14	8
Grade 2	increase in above signs mydriasis gooseflesh piloerection tremors muscle twitches hot and cold flashes aching bones and muscles anorexia	48–72	16	12
Grade 3	increased intensity of above insomnia increased blood pressure increased temperature increased respiratory rate and depth increased pulse rate restlessness nausea	n/a	24–36	18–24
Grade 4	increased intensity of above facial flushing curled up position on hard surface vomiting diarrhea weight loss spontaneous ejaculation or orgasm hemoconcentration leucocytosis eosinopenia increased blood sugar	n/a	36–48	24–36

na, not applicable.
[*Modified with permission from Blachly PH. Management of the opiate abstinence syndrome.* American Journal of Psychiatry, *1966, (122), 742–744.*]

Other opioid drugs show qualitatively similar opioid withdrawal effects that vary in duration and intensity, depending on pharmacokinetics. Methadone is a well-known, long-acting opioid that is used as a replacement for heroin in users who are attempting to quit.

Methadone withdrawal, even after large doses, is slower to develop than heroin withdrawal and is less intense and more prolonged. Few or no withdrawal symptoms are observed for almost two days, and peak withdrawal intensity is reached on about the sixth day. In contrast, the

TABLE 5.5   Time Course of Withdrawal from Various Narcotic Agents

	Non-purposive Withdrawal Symptoms (hours)	Peak (hours)	Time in which Majority of Symptoms Terminate (days)
Morphine	14–20	36–48	5–10
Heroin	8–12	48–72	5–10
Methadone	36–72 (second day)	72–96 (sixth day)	14–21
Codeine	24		
Dilaudid	4–5		
Meperidine	4–6	8–12	4–5

Purposive symptoms are goal-oriented, highly dependent on the observer and environment, and directed at getting more drugs. *Non-purposive symptoms* are not goal-oriented, are relatively independent of the observer and of the patient's will and the environment.
The purposive phenomena, including complaints, pleas, demands, and manipulations, and symptom mimicking are as varied as the psychodynamics, psychopathology, and imagination of the drug-dependent person. In a hospital setting, these phenomena are considerably less pronounced when the patient becomes aware that this behavior will not affect the decision to give him a drug.
[Taken with permission from Kleber H. Detoxification from narcotics. In: Lowinson JH, Ruiz P (eds.) Substance Abuse: Clinical Problems and Perspectives. Williams and Wilkins, Baltimore, 1981, 317–338.]

TABLE 5.6   Conditioned Positive and Negative Reinforcement

Conditioned positive reinforcement	• *Resistance to extinction* Drug cues are paired with drug effects such that they begin to predict the onset of positive feelings Extinction means that the drug cues are no longer predictive of drug availability However, if drug cues are always present, then they will continue to predict drugs, and the person will be less likely to discontinue drug use in the presence of drug-associated cues Less likely to withhold drug taking cues that were always present during drug taking • *Blockade of withdrawal* Drug paraphernalia can alleviate malaise ("Needle freak" phenomenon) • *Relapse* Drug cues can serve as "triggers"
Conditioned negative reinforcement	• *Conditioned withdrawal* Drug cues can elicit withdrawal signs (when interviewing Vietnam war veterans about wartime opiate use, they began to sweat and feel withdrawal) • *Motivated state* The cues remind them that drug taking alleviates painful or aversive events • *Relapse* The negative feelings that the cues elicit can lead to drug seeking

meperidine (Demerol) withdrawal syndrome usually develops quickly, within three hours of the last dose, reaches a peak within 8–12 h, and then decreases. These differences in the time course and intensity of opioid withdrawal with different opioids reflect the general principle that long-acting drugs produce a withdrawal syndrome with a longer onset, longer duration, and less intensity compared to short-acting opioids (Table 5.5).

Stimuli paired with opioid withdrawal or opioids themselves can have motivational significance by eliciting drug taking or alleviating withdrawal, respectively (Table 5.6). Environmental stimuli can be conditioned both to the acute reinforcing effects of opioids and the withdrawal associated with opioids, and both have been suggested to contribute to craving. These phenomena may contribute to the maintenance and relapse associated with opioid addiction. In humans, stimuli paired with a morphine injection have also been shown to alleviate withdrawal:

"Further evidence that the picture of withdrawal symptoms has its basis in an emotional state is the response on the part of one of our addicts at the end of a 36 hour withdrawal period to the hypodermic injection of sterile water. Despite his obvious suffering, he immediately went to sleep and slept for eight hours. Addicts frequently speak about the 'needle habit,' in which the single prick of the needle brings about relief. It is not uncommon for one addict to give another a hypodermic injection of sterile water and the recipient to derive a 'kick' and become quiet. On the other hand, it has been our experience just as frequently to have the addict know that he was given a hypodermic injection of sterile water and to have him fail to respond to its effect. Paradoxical as it may seem, we believe that the greater the craving of the addict and the severity of the withdrawal symptoms, the better are the chances of substituting a hypodermic injection of sterile water to obtain temporary relief." (Light AB, Torrance EG. Opium addiction: VI. The effects of abrupt withdrawal followed by readministration of morphine in human addicts, with special reference to the composition of the blood, the circulation and the metabolism. Archives of Internal Medicine, 1929, (44) 1–16.)

Later studies of this phenomenon described these individuals as "needle freaks." At least part of the relief and pleasure they experienced from injecting the drug resulted from a conditioned positive response to the heroin injection procedure. In an experimental laboratory setting under double-blind conditions, subjects were administered an opioid antagonist and then allowed to self-administer vehicle or an opioid. All of the self-injections were rated as pleasurable at first. After three to five injections, the subjects reported neutral effects.

In contrast, conditioned withdrawal can be observed in humans, setting up a condition of negative reinforcement (see Table 5.6). A physician described the experience of an individual with opioid addiction upon returning to an environment where he had previously experienced opioid withdrawal:

"For example, one patient who was slowly detoxified after methadone maintenance went to visit relatives in Los Angeles after receiving his last dose. Since he knew that he would be away from the clinic in Philadelphia for three weeks, he saved one take-home bottle of methadone in case he got sick while in California. To his surprise, he felt no sickness while in this new environment and never even thought about the bottle of methadone in his suitcase. He felt healthy over the three-week, drug-free period, but

as soon as he arrived in the Philadelphia airport, he began to experience craving. By the time he reached his home, there was yawning and tearing. He immediately took the methadone he had been saving and felt relieved, but the symptoms re-occurred the next day. After three weeks of being symptom-free in Los Angeles, he experienced regular withdrawal in Philadelphia." (O'Brien CP, Ehrman RN, Ternes JM. Classical conditioning in human opioid dependence. In: Goldberg SR, Stolerman IP (eds.) Behavioral Analysis of Drug Dependence. Academic Press, Orlando FL, 1986, pp. 329–356.)

Conditioned withdrawal has been experimentally induced in the laboratory. Methadone-maintained volunteers were subjected to repeated episodes of opioid withdrawal induced by a very small dose of the opioid receptor antagonist naloxone associated with a tone and peppermint smell in a specific environment. Naloxone administration alone elicited tearing, rhinorrhea, yawning, decreased skin temperature, increased respiratory rate, and subjective feelings of drug sickness and craving. After repeated pairings of naloxone with the peppermint smell, a simple injection of physiological saline accompanied by the peppermint smell and tone also elicited reliable signs and symptoms of opioid withdrawal that were similar to precipitated withdrawal, although the symptoms were less severe.

Thus, "needle freak" behavior is an excellent example of conditioned positive reinforcement, and "conditioned withdrawal" is an excellent example of conditioned negative reinforcement (see Table 5.6).

Opioid Tolerance

Tolerance can be defined as a decreased response to a drug with repeated administration or the requirement for larger doses of a drug to produce the same effect. Tolerance develops to the analgesic, euphorigenic, sedative, and other central nervous system depressant effects of opioids. Tolerance also develops to the lethal effects of opioids. Individuals with opioid addiction can increase their intake to enormous doses, such as 2 g of morphine administered intravenously over a period of 2–3 h with no significant changes in blood pressure or heart rate. To put this in perspective, the lethal dose of morphine in a non-tolerant person is approximately 30 mg parenterally or 120 mg orally (a 20- to 70-times difference).

Opioid tolerance is also characterized by a shortening of the duration of action. The rate of tolerance development is dependent on not only the dose of the drug but also the pattern of use and setting. With doses in the therapeutic range and appropriate intermittent use, obtaining the desired analgesic effect for an indefinite period is possible. When the opioid is taken continuously, significant tolerance develops rapidly. Cross-tolerance between opioids also develops as long as the mechanism of action of the opioids occurs through the same opioid receptor subtype.

Tolerance can be both dramatic and differential. Subjects may become very tolerant to the lethal or respiratory depressant effects of opioids but still continue to show sedation, miosis, and constipation. Constipation can continue for up to 8 months with daily use in many methadone-maintained individuals. Insomnia is observed in 10–20% of patients, and excessive sweating is observed in 50% of patients.

Tolerance can derive from two mechanisms: dispositional and pharmacodynamic. Dispositional tolerance is the decreased response to a drug with repeated administration caused by a reduction of the amount of drug at its pharmacological site of action. Pharmacodynamic tolerance refers to changes in the response to a drug that result from neuroadaptive changes, excluding changes in drug disposition (see Chapter 2). Although some evidence indicates that drug metabolism may be enhanced in tolerant animals, most opioid tolerance is thought to have a pharmacodynamic basis.

Acute and chronic tolerance and acute and chronic withdrawal also have important associative bases. Drug administration produces disturbances in the body (largely via the brain to cause the drug's psychotropic effects), and these disturbances can then elicit unconditioned responses that compensate for the perturbation produced by the drug. For example, individuals with opioid addiction are more likely to overdose in a novel context associated with obtaining a drug:

"[One example is] a case report of a patient, suffering with pancreatic cancer, who was receiving about four morphine injections in his home every day for pain relief. The patient stayed in his bedroom (which was dimly lit and contained apparatus necessary for his care), and received his injection in this environment. For some reason, after staying in this bedroom for about a month, the patient left his bed and went to the living room (which was brightly lit and different in many ways from the bedroom/sickroom). He was in considerable pain in the living room, and, as it was time for his next scheduled morphine administration, he was administered his usual dose of the drug. The patient quickly displayed signs of opiate overdose (constricted pupils, shallow breathing), and died a few hours later." *(Siegel S, Elsworth DW. Pavlovian conditioning and death from apparent overdose of medically prescribed morphine: a case report.* Bulletin of the Psychonomic Society, *1986, (24), 278–280.)*

The unconditioned stimulus is the drug effect, and the unconditioned responses are responses that compensate for the drug effect. These compensatory responses are ultimately elicited by drug-associated cues in a Pavlovian conditioning process. Such conditioned compensatory responses are often opposite in direction to the unconditioned effects of a drug and can mediate tolerance in the presence of the drug and withdrawal in the absence of the drug. Pavlovian conditioning and learning in general contribute to the development of tolerance.

Conditioned compensatory responses are observed most clearly by presenting the pre-drug cues that have been paired with the effects of the drug in the absence of the drug. Opioids produce conditioned compensatory responses under such conditions, which can be studied in animal models. Rats are assigned to a paired or unpaired condition. For the paired animals, morphine injections are signaled by an audiovisual cue. Unpaired animals are exposed to the same cues and injections but in an unpaired manner. When subsequently tested in the presence of the cue, paired animals are more tolerant than unpaired animals. Conditioned compensatory responses produced in the absence of drugs are also reflected by conditioned withdrawal-like effects.

The role of associative mechanisms in opioid tolerance, withdrawal, and relapse impacts their neurobiological substrates, which has important practical implications for the treatment of opioid addiction. Opioid-tolerant patients or addicted individuals who administer drugs in a different context or via a different route of administration may be at risk of overdose because conditioned compensatory responses will not be triggered.

Pain in Opioid Withdrawal and Protracted Abstinence

Increased sensitivity to pain has been observed in individuals with opioid addiction during abstinence. Individuals with former opioid addiction either maintained on methadone or maintained on the partial agonist buprenorphine showed increased sensitivity to cold pressor pain. Such a hyperalgesic-like state can persist for up to 5 months in abstinent individuals with a history of opioid addiction. Individuals with addiction and heightened pain sensitivity also displayed greater cue-induced craving at this time point, and pain is one of the main triggers of relapse to addiction in methadone-maintained individuals. Thus, opioid-addicted individuals with poor pain tolerance may suffer a more severe form of addiction, have difficulty tolerating the discomfort (pain) inherent in detoxification and early abstinence, and be more likely to relapse.

Neonatal Opioid Abstinence Syndrome

When a newborn infant is born to a mother with opioid addiction, the child is at risk of opioid withdrawal. The constellation of withdrawal symptoms that present at delivery with the discontinuation of drugs from the maternal circulation can lead to a syndrome known as the neonatal abstinence syndrome. All drugs of abuse can produce such a syndrome, but the prominent presentation is the neonatal abstinence syndrome with opioids. The newborn with opioid withdrawal will show central nervous system excitability, vasomotor signs, and gastrointestinal signs. Infants can be assessed with a standardized scoring system that evaluates excessive crying, shortened episodes of sleep, an exaggerated Moro reflex (which is a hyperactive response with excessive abduction at the shoulder and extension at the elbow, with or without tremors), tremors, increased muscle tone, redness of the skin or broken/bleeding skin that results from rubbing an extremity or face on a linen-covered surface due to excessive and uncontrolled movements of the extremities (tremors) or head (rooting), generalized seizures, hyperthermia, and excessive yawning, sweating, and sneezing. The time of symptom onset varies, but infants exposed to heroin or other short-acting opiates will typically show symptoms within the first 48–72 h after birth. Similarly to adults, infants who are prenatally exposed to methadone or buprenorphine will show symptoms later but usually within the first 4 days (for further reading, see Jansson et al., 2009).

NEUROBIOLOGICAL EFFECTS

Endogenous Opioids

The neurobiological research community greeted with great excitement the discovery of endogenous opioid-like substances in the brain that bind to the same receptors as morphine. Before the discovery of endorphins, dynorphins, and enkephalins, physiological studies showed

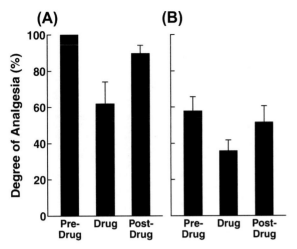

(A)   **(B)**

FIGURE 5.7   The effects of naloxone (1 mg/kg) on stimulation-produced analgesia in (A) rats showing an initial degree of analgesia of 100% and (B) animals showing a mean initial degree of analgesia of 58%. *These data show that the opioid antagonist naloxone can reverse stimulation-induced analgesia in rodents. The stimulation was in the periaqueductal gray, producing analgesia. Naloxone reversed analgesia, suggesting that there must be an endogenous opioid-like compound in the brain, which of course we now know there is. [Taken with permission from Akil H, Mayer DJ, Liebeskind JC. Antagonism of stimulation-produced analgesia by naloxone, a narcotic antagonist. Science, 1976, (191), 961–962.]*

TABLE 5.7   Opioid Receptors are G-Protein-Coupled Receptors with Seven Transmembrane-Spanning Regions

Receptor Subtype	Endogenous Opioids	Receptor Agonists and Partial Agonists	Receptor Antagonists
μ	β-endorphin* Enkephalin	Morphine Hydromorphone Meperidine Methadone Fentanyl Oxycodone Codeine	Naloxone Cyprodine
δ	Enkephalin* β-endorphin	ADL5859 AZD2327	Naltrindole Naloxone
κ	Dynorphin	Butorphanol U50,488	Norbinaltorphimine Naloxone

* *higher affinity*

that animals that received electrical stimulation directly in the central gray exhibited analgesia that was reversed by the opioid antagonist naloxone (Figure 5.7). Methionine and leucine enkephalin were first shown to bind to the opioid receptor and exert opioid-like activity *in vivo*. β-endorphin and dynorphin were then isolated, and the precursor molecules for enkephalins and endorphins were identified. Three distinct families of peptides have so far been identified: enkephalins, endorphins, and dynorphins. Each of these peptides has a distinct polypeptide precursor and a distinct but overlapping neuroanatomical distribution (Table 5.7, Figure 5.8). These endogenous opioid peptides produce self-administration, analgesia, locomotor activation, and place preference when administered directly into the brain.

Opioid peptides produce analgesia when injected directly into the raphe, periaqueductal gray, nucleus reticularis gigantocellularis of the medulla, and spinal cord, among other sites. Microinjection of an enkephalinase inhibitor into the brain, which blocked the degradation of enkephalin, had analgesic effects when injected into the central nucleus of the amygdala, periaqueductal gray, and ventral medulla.

Endogenous opioid peptides and non-peptide opioids, such as morphine, injected directly into the nucleus accumbens and ventral tegmental area produce locomotor activation, and animals will also self-administer them both intracerebroventricularly (which is a nonspecific injection into the ventricles of the brain that does not target any particular brain site) and directly into several brain sites, notably the lateral hypothalamus and nucleus accumbens. β-endorphin injected intracerebroventricularly produced conditioned place preference in rats, and enkephalin injected into the ventral tegmental area

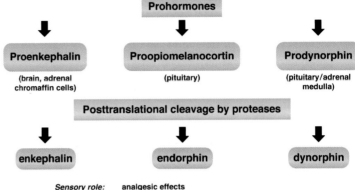

produced conditioned place preference. Another opioid peptide, endomorphin-1 (this peptide is hypothesized to be an endogenous compound, but the gene and synthetic pathway have yet to be discovered) has high selectivity for μ opioid receptors and produces locomotor activity when injected into the ventral tegmental area but not the nucleus accumbens.

One question that remains to be answered is the way that opioids act at the cellular level to engage reward circuits. One hypothesis is that opioids excite neurons by disinhibiting inhibitory interneurons. For example, μ opioid agonists inhibit the firing of a subgroup of neurons (likely γ-aminobutyric acid [GABA] neurons) in the central nucleus of the amygdala.

Pharmacologists initially identified three putative opioid receptors – μ, δ, and κ – based on differential pharmacological actions, differential antagonism, and ultimately radioligand binding. Differential opioid receptor density was localized to different brain areas using autoradiography. High concentrations were found in regions that overlap with the endogenous opioid and are associated with pain, such as the periaqueductal gray, medial thalamus, and amygdala (Figure 5.9).

The subsequent cloning and characterization of the genes that encode the μ, δ, and κ receptors confirmed the pharmacological categories. The amino acid sequences of these three receptors are very similar and share approximately 70% sequence identity. However, each receptor is derived from different chromosomes, suggesting high conservation and a lack of divergence in recent evolutionary history. A nociceptin receptor was discovered later, culminating in a four-member gene subfamily of the G-protein-coupled receptor family. The endogenous peptide nociceptin binds to the nociceptin receptor, but rather than having opioid effects it appears to have more anti-stress like effects (see Chapter 2).

Mouse strains that lack the genes of the opioid system have been generated by utilizing homologous recombination technology. Molecular studies have provided important confirmation and extension of pharmacological studies of the molecular basis of the effects of opioids. The most important receptor for the effects of opioids in relation to addiction is the μ receptor. Morphine reinforcement, measured by conditioned place preference and self-administration, is absent in μ receptor knockout mice. These mice also fail to exhibit the development of somatic signs of morphine dependence. In fact, all of the effects of morphine tested so far, including analgesia, hyperlocomotion, respiratory depression, and inhibition of gastrointestinal motility, are abolished in μ knockout mice (Figure 5.10).

Studies of δ opioid receptor knockout mice found increased levels of anxiety-like behavior in numerous behavioral tests. δ Opioid receptor knockout mice also show less tolerance to the analgesic effects of morphine, suggesting that these receptors may contribute to this adaptive aspect of chronic opioid exposure. κ Opioid receptor knockout mice, in contrast, show effects that support the hypothesis that activation of the dynorphin-κ receptor systems in the brain can produce dysphoric-like actions.

Binge/Intoxication Stage

Opioid drugs are profoundly reinforcing in animal models, independent of pain or discomfort. Opioid drugs, such as heroin, are readily self-administered intravenously by mice, rats, monkeys, and humans. If provided limited access, rats will maintain stable levels of daily drug intake without any major signs of physical dependence, similar to "chipping" in humans. This heroin self-administration pattern typically involves rapid responding at the beginning of a test session, followed by more regular interinjection intervals. This model has been used to study the neurobiological basis of heroin reward, independent of the confounds of dependence or negative reinforcement as elaborated in the *International Statistical Classification of Diseases and Related Health Problems*, 10th revision (ICD-10), or the compulsive-like state now described within the category of Substance Use Disorders of the *Diagnostic and Statistical Manual of Mental Disorders*, 5th edition (DSM-5; see Chapter 1). Decreases in the dose of heroin available to the animal change the pattern of self-administration. The animals will decrease their interinjection interval and increase the number of injections.

The animals will also attempt to compensate for opioid antagonism (for example, when they also receive an injection of naloxone) by increasing the amount of drug injected.

Neural elements in the region of the ventral tegmental area and nucleus accumbens are responsible for the activational and reinforcing properties of opioids, with both dopamine-dependent and -independent mechanisms (Figure 5.11). Direct intracerebral administration of opioid antagonists into the nucleus accumbens and ventral tegmental area block the locomotor-activating effects and intravenous self-administration of opioids in rats. Such studies indicate that opioid receptors in both the ventral tegmental area and nucleus accumbens are important for the acute reinforcing actions of opioids. Strong evidence of the role of the ventral tegmental area in the acute reinforcing effects of opioids in nondependent rats has also been found in place conditioning studies.

Intracranial self-administration studies, in which opioids are directly self-administered into the brain, showed a significant overlap with the sites identified with opioid receptor antagonists. The lateral hypothalamus, nucleus accumbens, amygdala, periaqueductal gray, and ventral tegmental area all support morphine self-administration. Animals will perform an operant task, such as lever pressing, to have morphine delivered directly into these brain regions.

Further studies of the neurocircuitry involved in opioid reward revealed a dopamine-independent role for the nucleus accumbens and a dopamine-dependent role. Researchers found that dopamine receptor blockade with dopamine antagonists and dopamine denervation in the nucleus accumbens eliminated cocaine and amphetamine self-administration but spared heroin and morphine self-administration. The initiation of heroin self-administration was unaltered by administration of large doses of the dopamine antagonist haloperidol into the midbrain dopamine system, including the nucleus accumbens, prefrontal cortex, caudate putamen,

μ Opioid Receptors

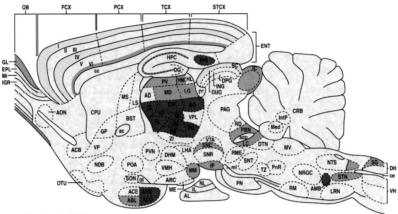

δ Opioid Receptors

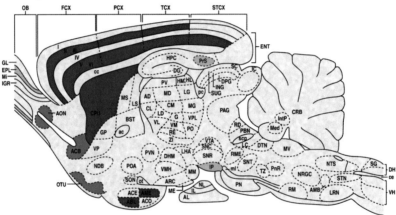

κ Opioid Receptors

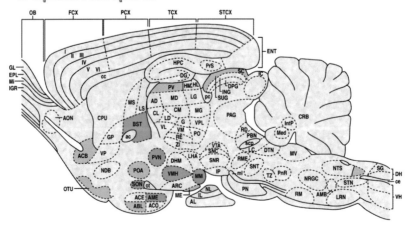

FIGURE 5.9 **Schematic representation of μ, δ, and κ₁ receptor mRNA expression and binding in the rat central nervous system.** The receptor densities, shown as different color hues, are within a receptor type and do not represent absolute receptor capacity. Therefore, dense binding of one receptor type is not equivalent in terms of receptor number to dense binding of another receptor type. This is particularly true for the κ₁ receptor binding sites, which represent only 10% of the total opioid receptor binding sites in the rat brain. These rat parasagittal sections are designed, however, to transmit qualitatively the correspondence between receptor mRNA expression and receptor binding distribution. This figure demonstrates that each opioid receptor mRNA has a unique distribution which correlates well with the known μ, δ, and κ₁ receptor binding distributions. μ *Receptor Distribution.* A high correlation between μ receptor mRNA expression and binding is observed in the striatal clusters and patches of the nucleus accumbens and caudate putamen, diagonal band of Broca, globus pallidus and ventral pallidum, bed nucleus of the stria terminalis, most thalamic nuclei, medial and cortical amygdala, mammillary nuclei, presubiculum, interpeduncular nucleus, median raphe, raphe magnus, parabrachial nucleus, locus coeruleus, nucleus ambiguus, and nucleus of the solitary tract. Differences in μ receptor mRNA and binding distributions are observed in regions such as the neocortex, olfactory bulb, superior colliculus, spinal trigeminal nucleus, and spinal cord which might be a consequence of receptor transport to presynaptic terminals. δ *Receptor Distribution.* A high correlation between δ receptor mRNA expression and binding is observed in such regions as the anterior olfactory nucleus, neocortex, caudate putamen, nucleus accumbens, olfactory tubercle, diagonal band of Broca, globus pallidus and ventral pallidum, septal nuclei, amygdala, and pontine nuclei, suggesting local receptor synthesis. Regions of high δ receptor mRNA expression and comparatively low receptor binding include the internal granular layer of the olfactory bulb and ventromedial nucleus of the hypothalamus. The apparent discrepancy between δ receptor mRNA expression and δ receptor binding in several brainstem nuclei and in the cerebellum is, in part, due to the increased sensitivity of *in situ* hybridization methods and high levels of nonspecific binding observed with δ-selective ligands. Differences in distributions indicative of receptor transport are observed in the substantia gelatinosa of the spinal cord, external plexiform layer of the olfactory bulb, and the superficial layer of the superior colliculus. κ *Receptor Distribution.* A high degree of correlation between κ₁ receptor mRNA expression and binding is observed in regions such as the nucleus accumbens, caudate putamen, olfactory tubercle, bed nucleus of the stria terminalis, medial preoptic area, paraventricular nucleus, supraoptic nucleus, dorsomedial and ventromedial hypothalamus, amygdala, midline thalamic nuclei, periaqueductal gray, raphe nuclei, parabrachial nucleus, locus coeruleus, spinal trigeminal nucleus, and the nucleus of the solitary tract. Differences in κ₁ receptor binding and mRNA distribution in the substantia nigra pars compacta, ventral tegmental area, and neural lobe of the pituitary might be due to receptor transport.

Abbreviations: **ABL** basolateral amygdaloid nucleus; **ac** anterior commissure; **ACB** nucleus accumbens; **ACE** central amygdaloid nucleus; **ACO** cortical amygdaloid nucleus; **AD** anteriodorsal thalamus; **AL** anterior lobe, pituitary; **AMB** nucleus ambiguus; **AME** medial amygdaloid nucleus; **AON** anterior olfactory nucleus; **ARC** arcuate nucleus, hypothalamus; **BST** bed nucleus of the stria terminalis; **cc** corpus callosum; **ce** central canal; **CL** centrolateral thalamus; **CM** centromedial thalamus; **CPU** caudate putamen; **CRB** cerebellum; **DG** dentate gyrus; **DH** dorsal horn, spinal cord; **DMH** dorsomedial hypothalamus; **DPG** deep gray layer, superior colliculus; **DTN** dorsal tegmental nucleus; **ENT** entorhinal cortex; **EPL** external plexiform layer, olfactory bulb; **FCX** frontal cortex; **G** nucleus gelatinosus thalamus; **GL** glomerular layer, olfactory bulb; **GP** globus pallidus; **HL** lateral habenula; **HM** medial habenula; **HPC** hippocampus; **IC** inferior colliculus; **IGR** intermediate granular layer, olfactory bulb; **IL** intermediate lobe, pituitary; **ING** intermediate gray layer, superior colliculus; **IntP** interposed cerebellar nucleus; **IP** interpeduncular nucleus; **LC** locus coeruleus; **LD** laterodorsal thalamus; **LG** lateral geniculate thalamus; **LHA** lateral hypothalamic area; **LRN** lateral reticular nucleus; **LS** lateral septum; **MD** dorsomedial thalamus; **ME** median eminence; **Med** medial cerebellar nucleus; **MG** medial geniculate; **Mi** mitral cell layer, olfactory bulb; **ml** medial leminscus; **MM** medial mammillary nucleus; **MS** medial septum; **MV** medial vestibular nucleus; **NDB** nucleus diagonal band; **NL** neural lobe, pituitary; **NRGC** nucleus reticularis gigantocellularis; **NTS** nucleus tractus solitarius; **OB** olfactory bulb; **ot** optic tract; **OTU** olfactory tubercle; **PaG** periaqueductal gray; **PBN** parabrachial nucleus; **pc** posterior commissure; **PCX** parietal cortex; **PN** pons; **PnR** pontine reticular; **PO** posterior nucleus thalamus; **POA** preoptic area; **PrS** presubiculum; **PV** paraventricular thalamus; **PVN** paraventricular hypothalamus; **RD** dorsal raphe; **RE** reuniens thalamus; **RM** raphe magnus; **RME** median raphe; **SC** superior colliculus; **scp** superior cerebellar peduncle; **SG** substantia gelatinosa; **SNC** substantia nigra pars compacta; **SNR** substantia nigra pars reticulata; **SNT** sensory nucleus trigeminal; **SON** supraoptic nucleus; **STCX** striate cortex; **STN** spinal trigeminal nucleus; **SUG** superficial gray layer, superior colliculus; **TCX** temporal cortex; **TZ** trapezoid nucleus; **VH** ventral horn, spinal cord; **VL** ventrolateral thalamus; **VM** ventromedial thalamus; **VMH** ventromedial hypothalamus; **VP** ventral pallidum; **VPL** ventroposteriolateral thalamus; **VTA** ventral tegmental area; **ZI** zona incerta *[Taken with permission from Mansour A, Fox CA, Akil H, Watson SJ. Opioid receptor mRNA expression in the rat CNS: anatomical and functional implications.* Trends in Neurosciences, *1995, (18), 22–29.]*

FIGURE 5.10 **Summary of responses to drugs and spontaneous behaviors in μ, δ, and κ opioid receptor knockout mice.** Responses to drugs are shown on the left with drugs indicated; behaviors in the absence of drugs are shown on the right. ↓, strongly reduced or abolished. ↑, increased. →, unchanged. ↓→, unchanged or decreased depending on the experimental conditions. Abbreviation: THC, Δ⁹-tetrahydrocannabinol. *[Modified with permission from Gaveriaux-Ruff C, Kieffer BL. Opioid receptor genes inactivated in mice: the highlights. Neuropeptides, 2002, (36), 62–71.]*

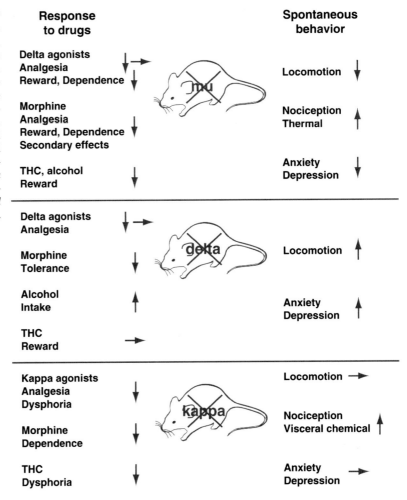

and amygdala. Both observations support the hypothesis that opioid reward is mediated by dopamine-dependent and -independent inputs to the nucleus accumbens (Figure 5.11).

A focal point for the involvement of the nucleus accumbens in opioid reward was the observation that selective destruction of the neurons themselves in the nucleus accumbens blocked cocaine, heroin, and morphine self-administration. Similarly, lesions of the ventral pallidum blocked both heroin and cocaine self-administration. Lesions of the pedunculopontine tegmental nucleus also blocked intravenous

heroin self-administration. These studies suggest that neurons in the nucleus accumbens mediate the acute reinforcing properties of opioids and involve the processing of a circuit that includes not only the nucleus accumbens but also the ventral pallidum and pedunculopontine nucleus.

Withdrawal/Negative Affect Stage

Pain

One contribution to the intoxication associated with opioids reflects their ability to block

Neurochemical Neurocircuits in Drug Reward
Opioids

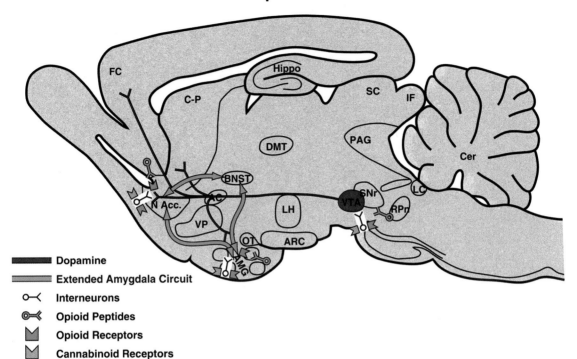

- ▬▬▬ **Dopamine**
- ▬▬▬ **Extended Amygdala Circuit**
- ⊶ **Interneurons**
- ⊶ **Opioid Peptides**
- ⋈ **Opioid Receptors**
- ⋈ **Cannabinoid Receptors**

FIGURE 5.11 **Sagittal section through a representative rodent brain illustrating the pathways and receptor systems implicated in the acute reinforcing actions of opioids.** Opioids activate opioid receptors in the ventral tegmental area, nucleus accumbens, and amygdala via direct actions or interneurons. Opioids facilitate the release of dopamine (red) in the nucleus accumbens via an action either in the ventral tegmental area or the nucleus accumbens, but also are hypothesized to activate elements independent of the dopamine system. Endogenous cannabinoids may interact with postsynaptic elements in the nucleus accumbens involving dopamine and/or opioid peptide systems. The blue arrows represent the interactions within the extended amygdala system hypothesized to have a key role in opioid reinforcement. AC, anterior commissure; AMG, amygdala; ARC, arcuate nucleus; BNST, bed nucleus of the stria terminalis; Cer, cerebellum; C-P, caudate putamen; DMT, dorsomedial thalamus; FC, frontal cortex; Hippo, hippocampus; IF, inferior colliculus; LC, locus coeruleus; LH, lateral hypothalamus; N Acc., nucleus accumbens; OT, olfactory tract; PAG, periaqueductal gray; RPn, reticular pontine nucleus; SC, superior colliculus; SNr, substantia nigra pars reticulata; VP, ventral pallidum; VTA, ventral tegmental area. *[Taken with permission from Koob GF, Le Moal M.* Neurobiology of Addiction. *Academic Press, London, 2006.]*

the affective dimension of pain. The analgesic effects of opioids are caused by direct inhibition of nociceptive activity that ascends from the dorsal horn of the spinal cord to the brain circuitry associated with pain and also by activation of pain control circuits that descend from the midbrain via the rostral ventromedial medulla to the dorsal horn of the spinal cord. Endogenous opioid peptides and their receptors are highly localized to both the ascending and descending pain control circuits (Figure 5.12; for further reading, see Shurman et al., 2010).

Tolerance

At the receptor level, two mechanisms have been implicated in the within-system changes

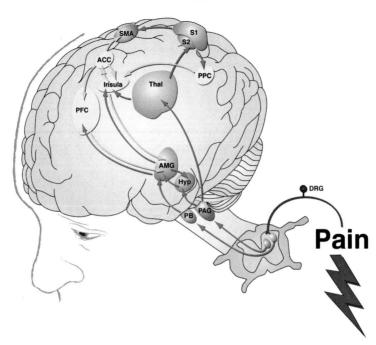

FIGURE 5.12   **Pathways for the supraspinal processing of pain superimposed on key elements of addiction circuitry implicated in negative emotional states.** Blue structures are involved in the "fast" processing of pain via the spinothalamic tract, and pain signals arrive indirectly in the amygdala. Pink structures are involved in the "fast" processing of pain via the spinal–parabrachial–amygdala pathway, and pain signals arrive directly in the amygdala. Yellow structures are involved in the "slower" cognitive processing of pain. Notice significant overlap of the supraspinal processing of pain and addiction in the amygdala. ACC, anterior cingulate cortex; AMG, amygdala; BNST, bed nucleus of the stria terminalis; DRG, dorsal root ganglion; DS, dorsal striatum; GP, globus pallidus; Hippo, hippocampus; Hyp, hypothalamus; Insula, insular cortex; OFC, orbitofrontal cortex; PAG, periaqueductal gray; PB, parabrachial nucleus; PPC, posterior parietal cortex; S1, S2, somatosensory cortex; SMA, supplementary motor area; Thal, thalamus; VS, ventral striatum. *[Modified with permission from Blackburn-Munro G,Blackburn-Monro R. Pain in the brain: are hormones to blame?* Trends in Endocrinology and Metabolism *2003, (14), 20–27.*

that may contribute to acute tolerance: receptor desensitization and receptor internalization. The role of desensitization in opioid tolerance remains controversial because tolerance develops at doses that do not produce desensitization. Opioid receptors are coupled to second messenger systems, and they may be involved in acute tolerance. μ and δ receptors but not κ receptors can also undergo rapid agonist-mediated internalization via endocytosis, in which cells absorb these proteins by surrounding them. Endogenous ligands (opioid peptides) cause rapid internalization, and others, such as morphine and oxycodone, do not, indicating that different intracellular events may

play a role in the relative efficacy of opioids. A significant proportion of tolerance to opioids may involve recruitment of between-system neuroadaptations as outlined below for opioid withdrawal (see also Chapter 1).

Withdrawal

As described above, opioid dependence is associated with a characteristic withdrawal syndrome that appears with the abrupt termination of opioid administration or administration of competitive opioid receptor antagonists, such as naloxone (termed "precipitated withdrawal"). The neural substrates for the physical and affective signs of opioid withdrawal can be dissociated. In rats, physical dependence has been characterized by an abstinence syndrome that includes the appearance of ptosis, teeth chattering, wet dog shakes (which are exactly what the phrase suggests), and diarrhea. This syndrome can be precipitated in dependent animals by systemic injections of opioid antagonists. Motivational withdrawal includes changes in brain reward thresholds, the disruption of trained operant behavior for food reward, and conditioned place aversions. Precipitated opioid withdrawal is associated with increased brain reward thresholds at doses of naloxone that do not elicit physical signs of withdrawal, which, as mentioned above, indicates that the mechanisms of the physical and motivational components of opioid withdrawal are different (Figure 5.13).

Opioid dependence and tolerance can begin with a single administration of the drug. Single opioid injections can induce a state of acute opioid dependence in both humans and animals. Acute dependence is particularly evident when evaluating motivational measures of withdrawal, such as the suppression of operant responding for food, place aversion, and brain stimulation reward (Figure 5.14). Repeated morphine administration results in a progressive increase in the potency of naloxone to elicit precipitated withdrawal. Greater shifts in potency were observed when naloxone was administered on all treatment days but only in the testing situation and not in the home cage where the rat had received no drug injections, suggesting an important conditioning component of acute dependence. An hypothetical, parallel human example is that of an individual with opioid use disorder who undergoes withdrawal in a particular environment and experiences conditioned withdrawal when exposed again to that environment. A lasting association between a specific environment and the aversive stimulus effects of opioid withdrawal can persist for a long time after the acute withdrawal state has dissipated.

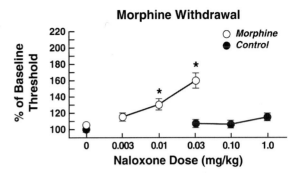

FIGURE 5.13 **Naloxone dose-dependently elevated intracranial self-stimulation reward thresholds in rats (reflecting a decrease in reward function) in the morphine group but not in the placebo group.** The minimum dose of naloxone that elevated ICSS thresholds in the morphine group was 0.01 mg/kg (*$p < 0.05$, compared with vehicle). *These results show that low doses of naloxone can "precipitate" a dysphoric-like effect (increased reward thresholds) in morphine-dependent rats at doses that do not cause any change in nondependent control rats. [Taken with permission from Schulteis G, Markou A, Gold LH, Stinus L, Koob GF. Relative sensitivity to naloxone of multiple indices of opiate withdrawal: a quantitative dose-response analysis.* Journal of Pharmacology and Experimental Therapeutics, *1994, (271), 1391–1398.]*

Animal studies have observed hyperalgesia during spontaneous (in which drug administration is simply ceased) or precipitated (in which an antagonist is administered) opioid withdrawal following acute or chronic opioid exposure (for further reading, see Simonnet and Rivat, 2003). Some studies have even suggested that pain sensitization might develop while the subjects are still exposed to the opioid. Moreover, heroin effectively facilitated pain in rats after just one exposure to the drug (Figure 5.15). This phenomenon may indicate the actual sensitization of pain systems because both the magnitude and duration of hyperalgesia increased as a function of opioid administration. For example, the first heroin administration may induce moderate hyperalgesia for 2 days, whereas the fifth injection of the same dose may induce hyperalgesia for 6 days. When the opioid is administered repeatedly, for example once daily for 2 weeks, a gradual and dose-dependent decrease in nociceptive

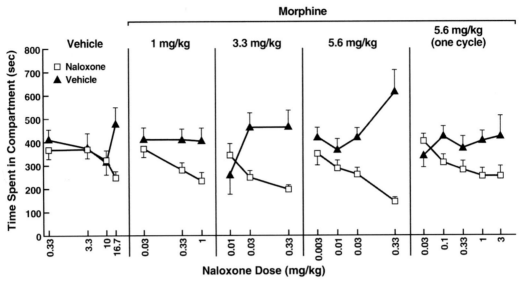

FIGURE 5.14 **Mean time spent by rats in each of three compartments of a place conditioning apparatus.** All morphine/naloxone treatment conditions represent two conditioning cycles, except where noted. As time spent in the naloxone-paired compartment declines as a function of naloxone dose, this extra time appears to be randomly spent in either the vehicle-paired or neutral compartment. *These data show that low doses of naloxone can "precipitate" an aversive-like effect in rats, even following an acute administration of morphine, suggesting that the opponent process (b process; see Chapter 1) produced by opioids begins with the first opioid injection.* [Taken with permission from Azar MR, Jones BC, Schulteis G. Conditioned place aversion is a highly sensitive index of acute opioid dependence and withdrawal. Psychopharmacology, 2003, (170), 42–50.]

threshold is observed that lasts for several weeks after drug administration (Figure 5.15). A small dose of heroin that was otherwise ineffective at triggering delayed hyperalgesia in non-heroin-treated rats enhanced pain sensitivity for several days after a series of heroin injections, suggesting the occurrence of pain sensitization. The effectiveness of naloxone in precipitating hyperalgesia in rats that had recovered their pre-drug nociceptive thresholds after single or repeated heroin injections indicates that heroin-deprived rats were in a new biological state associated with a functional balance between opioid-dependent analgesic systems and pronociceptive systems. Such a finding may also be another explanation of tolerance, in which a prolonged increase occurs in the excitability of nociceptive pathways that increasingly opposes analgesia induced by repeated opioid administration. Thus, a neuronal memory, characterized by a vulnerable state, may remain long after the complete wash-out of the drug and when apparent equilibrium near the pre-drug state has been re-established. These long-term effects may include the expression of other allostatic changes, such as negative emotional states, long after withdrawal from the drug (see Chapter 1).

The mechanism for such hyperalgesia may involve activation of glutamatergic systems. A noncompetitive glutamate receptor antagonist prevented both the long-lasting heroin-induced enhancement in pain sensitivity and naloxone-precipitated hyperalgesia. A parallel has been found between the development of thermal hyperalgesia in rats and tolerance to the analgesic effects of morphine administered for eight consecutive days. The concurrent development of tolerance was prevented by co-administration of morphine with a glutamate receptor antagonist and protein kinase C inhibitor.

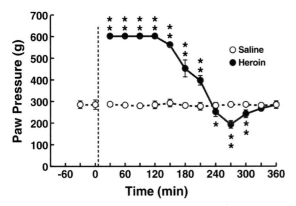

FIGURE 5.15 **Effects of heroin on vocalization threshold to paw pressure in rats.** (A) Rats received a subcutaneous injection of 2.5 mg/kg heroin or saline after the determination of basal paw pressure-inducing vocalization, and then the values were determined every 30 min for 6 h. Each point represents the mean paw pressure ± SEM of 8–10 animals. *p < 0.05, **p < 0.01. *These data show an opponent process-like effect on pain thresholds following a single dose of heroin in the rat. Initially, for 3 hours, heroin produced analgesia (an increase in pain thresholds). However, after the analgesia disappeared, hyperalgesia (a decrease in pain thresholds) developed (see text for a definition of hyperalgesia). [Taken with permission from Laulin JP, Larcher A, Celerier E, Le Moal M, Simonnet G. Long-lasting increased pain sensitivity in rat following exposure to heroin for the first time.* European Journal of Neuroscience, 1998, (10), 782–785.]

Studies of the neurobiological substrates of physical dependence have revealed multiple sites of action, including the periaqueductal gray, dorsal thalamus, and locus coeruleus. However, the brain sites responsible for the motivational and emotional changes associated with opioid withdrawal have been localized to the nucleus accumbens and amygdala. The aversive stimulus effects of opioid withdrawal that form the basis for its motivational effects can readily be measured in rats using conditioned place aversion or the suppression of operant responding for a food reward. Thus, during chronic morphine exposure, neural elements in the nucleus accumbens and amygdala may become sensitized to opioid antagonists and may be partially responsible for the negative stimulus effects of opioid withdrawal (Figure 5.16).

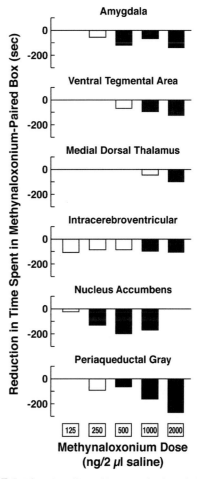

FIGURE 5.16 **The effect of intracerebral methylnaloxonium paired with a particular environment on the amount of time spent by rats in that environment during an injection-free test session.** Values represent the median difference between the postconditioning score and the preconditioning score. Darkened bars represent those doses where the conditioning scores were significantly different from the preconditioniong scores. Significance was set at p < 0.02 to control for multiple comparisons. *These results show that a naloxone derivative (methylnaloxium, an opioid antagonist) when injected directly into the brain can produce an aversive-like effect in opioid-dependent animals, with the lowest doses producing an aversive effect, particularly in the nucleus accumbens and central nucleus of the amygdala. [Taken with permission from Stinus L, Le Moal M, Koob GF. Nucleus accumbens and amygdala are possible substrates for the aversive stimulus effects of opiate withdrawal.* Neuroscience, 1990, (37), 767–773.]

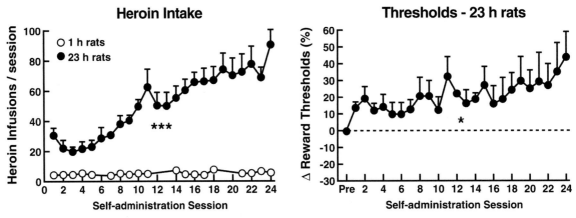

FIGURE 5.17 **Unlimited daily access to heroin escalated heroin intake and decreased the excitability of brain reward systems.** (Left) Heroin intake (20 μg per infusion) in rats during limited (1 h) or unlimited (23 h) self-administration sessions. ***$p < 0.001$, effect of access (1 or 23 h). (Right) Percentage change from baseline ICSS thresholds in 23 h rats. Reward thresholds, assessed immediately after each daily 23 h self-administration session, became progressively more elevated as exposure to self-administered heroin increased across sessions. *$p < 0.05$, effect of heroin on reward thresholds. *These data show that the overall increase in thresholds over days associated with extended access to heroin paralleled the overall increase in drug taking over days (termed escalation; see* Chapter 3*) associated with extended access. [Taken with permission from Kenny PJ, Chen SA, Kitamura O, Markou A, Koob GF. Conditioned withdrawal drives heroin consumption and decreases reward sensitivity.* Journal of Neuroscience, 2006, (26), 5894–5900.]

Data from conditioned place aversion studies and unlimited access to intravenous heroin self-administration provide a neuropharmacological framework for the neurocircuitry associated with opioid addiction. Studies of lesions of the extended amygdala while measuring precipitated withdrawal-induced place aversions support a role for the extended amygdala in the aversive stimulus effects of opioid withdrawal. Lesions of the central nucleus of the amygdala, one part of the extended amygdala, block the development of morphine withdrawal-induced place aversion but have less of an effect on the somatic signs of withdrawal.

Neurochemical elements within the extended amygdala involved in the aversive stimulus effects of opioid withdrawal include corticotropin-releasing factor (CRF) and norepinephrine. Blockade of CRF receptors in the central nucleus of the amygdala blocked conditioned place aversion produced by opioid withdrawal. Inactivation of noradrenergic (norepinephrine) function in the bed nucleus of the stria terminalis, another

region of the extended amygdala, blocked the aversive motivational effects of opioid withdrawal. Injections of a β-adrenergic receptor antagonist or α_2 receptor agonist into the lateral bed nucleus of the stria terminalis blocked precipitated opioid withdrawal-induced place aversion. Norepinephrine concentrations in the bed nucleus of the stria terminalis represent 10% of the brain's norepinephrine. Blockade of norepinephrine receptors in the central nucleus of the amygdala with β-adrenergic antagonists attenuated morphine withdrawal-induced conditioned place aversion.

Using the intravenous self-administration model of extended access, rats will steadily increase heroin intake, showing a pattern of responding not unlike humans with opioid addiction (Figure 5.17). The daily pattern of intake shifts, with decreases in food and water intake and the development of motivational signs of dependence (for further reading, see Chen et al., 2006). The same neuropharmacological systems implicated in the negative emotional effects of opioid withdrawal have been shown to be important for the compulsive drug taking and seeking associated with extended-access intravenous self-administration in animal models. Both CRF antagonists and α_1 noradrenergic antagonists dose-dependently decrease the compulsive drug intake observed in opioid-dependent rats.

Neuronal plasticity occurs in the nucleus accumbens and amygdala with the development of morphine dependence. Dopamine neuron firing and extracellular dopamine levels are decreased during opioid withdrawal. Chronic morphine administration is also associated with a decrease in the size of ventral tegmental area dopamine neurons and an increase in the sensitivity to dopamine antagonists. The cellular changes that occur during opioid withdrawal are accompanied by increased GABA activity and increased metabotropic glutamate receptor sensitivity, which both decrease glutamate release in the ventral tegmental area and lead to decreased dopamine cell firing. Chronic opioid administration, therefore, has multiple effects on the neuropharmacological systems that interface with the ventral tegmental area and extended amygdala (see Chapter 2), which may provide the cellular basis for the neuroadaptations associated with the development of dependence. Opioids act indirectly via GABA and glutamate systems to activate reward pathways, and these same systems show neuroadaptations with chronic opioid exposure.

Acute opioid receptor activation leads to the inhibition of adenylyl cyclase (Figure 5.18), the cyclic adenosine monophosphate (cAMP) protein phosphorylation cascade via the recruitment of G_i and related G proteins, activation of voltage-gated Ca^{2+} channels, and activation of K^+ channels. More K^+ flows out of the cell, and less Ca^{2+} flows into the cell. Reductions in cellular Ca^{2+} levels alter Ca^{2+}-dependent protein phosphorylation cascades. Alterations in the activity of these protein phosphorylation cascades, which can vary among different cell

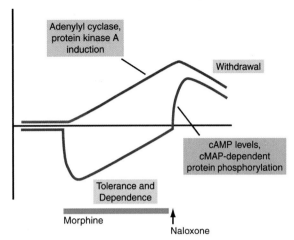

FIGURE 5.18 **Upregulation of the cyclic adenosine monophosphate (cAMP) pathway as a mechanism of opioid tolerance and dependence.** Opioids acutely inhibit the functional activity of the cAMP pathway (indicated by cellular levels of cAMP and cAMP-dependent protein phosphorylation). With continued opioid exposure, functional activity of the cAMP pathway gradually recovers and then increases far above control levels following removal of the opioid (e.g., by administration of the opioid receptor antagonist naloxone). These changes in the functional state of the cAMP pathway are mediated by the induction of adenylyl cyclase and protein kinase A in response to chronic administration of opioids. The induction of these enzymes accounts for the gradual recovery in the functional activity of the cAMP pathway that occurs during chronic opioid exposure (tolerance and dependence) and activation of the cAMP pathway observed upon removal of opioid (withdrawal). *[Taken with permission from Nestler EJ. Historical review: molecular and cellular mechanisms of opiate and cocaine addiction.* Trends in Pharmacological Sciences. *2004. (25), 210–218.]*

types, lead to the regulation of still other ion channels, which further contributes to the acute effects of the drug.

Chronic exposure to opioids increases adenylyl cyclase, leading to other perturbations in intracellular messenger pathways, such as in protein phosphorylation mechanisms. These perturbations eventually elicit long-term adaptations that can lead to changes in many other neural processes within target neurons. These target neurons include those that trigger the long-term effects of the drugs, eventually leading to tolerance, dependence, withdrawal, sensitization, and addiction (Figure 5.18). Opioid withdrawal increases the expression of the transcription factor Fos, a marker of neural activation, with particular sensitivity in the extended amygdala. Such Fos changes correlate with the motivational effects (place aversion) rather than somatic effects of opioid withdrawal (for further reading, see Nestler, 2001).

Preoccupation/Anticipation Stage

Animal models of the *preoccupation/anticipation* stage of the addiction cycle include models of drug-, cue-, and stress-induced reinstatement (see Chapter 3). The reinstatement of heroin self-administration induced by a priming injection of heroin after extinction depends on the activation of μ opioid receptors. μ Opioid receptor agonists reinstate responding when injected systemically or directly into the ventral tegmental area, and these effects are blocked by naloxone. In contrast, cue-induced reinstatement is not blocked by opioid antagonists. A runway model of cue-induced reinstatement with heroin-trained rats found evidence of resistance to dopamine and opioid blockade of olfactory cue-induced reinstatement. Similarly, the dopamine antagonist haloperidol does not block conditioned place preference produced by heroin cues. However, the blockade of glutamate activity attenuates the cue-induced reinstatement of heroin seeking.

The stress of an intermittent footshock reinstates heroin self-administration in nondependent rats after extinction and reactivates opioid-induced place preference after drug-free periods without extinction. These effects are also not readily blocked by opioid or dopamine receptor antagonists. However, CRF can reinstate heroin seeking, and stress-induced reinstatement can be blocked with combination CRF_1/CRF_2 receptor antagonists and selective CRF_1 receptor antagonists. A CRF_2 antagonist, however, was ineffective, indicating that the CRF_1 subtype is most likely more important for this type of reinstatement. The brain sites critical for the role of CRF in footshock-induced reinstatement include the bed nucleus of the stria terminalis and central nucleus of the amygdala. Reversible functional inactivation of these structures also blocked the footshock-induced reinstatement of heroin seeking.

Similarly, a role for norepinephrine projections that originate in the ventral noradrenergic pathway and project to the bed nucleus of the stria terminalis and central nucleus of the amygdala has also been shown in studies that evaluate footshock-induced reinstatement of opioid seeking. α_2 Adrenergic agonists, which are known to inhibit norepinephrine release, block the footshock-induced reinstatement of heroin seeking. The brain sites for these effects appear to be the ventral noradrenergic bundle from the lateral tegmental nucleus that projects to the ventral portion of the forebrain, such as the bed nucleus of the stria terminalis. Lesions of this pathway attenuated the footshock-induced reinstatement of heroin seeking.

Humans with opioid addiction are well known to have a dysregulated hypothalamic-pituitary-adrenal (HPA) stress axis (see Chapter 2) that persists during cycles of addiction. These persistent physiological abnormalities stabilize during methadone maintenance. In an experiment that blocked cortisol synthesis, the reduced HPA axis reserve in individuals with heroin addiction returned to normal and then stabilized during methadone maintenance. Conversely, reactivation of a hyperactive HPA axis occurred during opioid withdrawal. During protracted abstinence, hyper-responsiveness of the cortisol negative feedback system regulates the HPA axis. Cycles of heroin addiction were associated with hyporesponsivity of the temporary shutoff of the negative feedback on the HPA axis produced by the blockade of cortisol synthesis, but this hypoactivity may be paralleled by an ongoing sensitization of CRF systems in the amygdala (see Chapter 2).

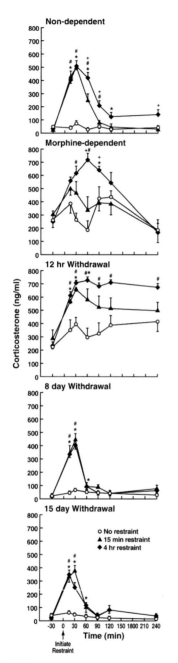

In morphine-dependent rats during opioid dependence and acute withdrawal, a marked increase in basal corticosterone concentrations and exaggerated response to stressors are found (Figure 5.19). Rats that had undergone 12 h withdrawal displayed increased basal corticosterone and a potentiated and prolonged corticosterone response to restraint stress. After eight and 16 day withdrawals, they recovered normal baseline HPA activity and showed a blunted response to a stressor. This reduced response to a stressor was suggested to be attributable to the increased sensitivity of the negative feedback systems to glucocorticoids and reduced CRF function, similar to what is seen in individuals with heroin addiction. Thus, chronic stress exposure and chronic morphine exposure have similar effects in rats, and hormonal stress responses may play a role in the maintenance and relapse to opioid use long after acute withdrawal from opioids.

The protracted abstinence component of the *preoccupation/anticipation* stage of drug addiction is also accompanied by an attentional bias to drugs and drug-related stimuli that helps to channel an individual's behavior toward drug seeking. In electrophysiological studies, heroin-dependent subjects had larger slow-wave components of event-related potentials in response to heroin-related stimuli during abstinence, and these observations correlated with post-experiment craving. In animal studies, hippocampal long-term potentiation (in which neurons are

FIGURE 5.19 **Plasma corticosterone responses to 15 min and 4 h restraint stress in vehicle- and morphine-treated rats.** The arrow indicates the time of the initiation of restraint. The data are expressed as mean ± SEM (n = 5–9). *$p < 0.05$, 15 min restraint vs. no restraint groups; #$p < 0.05$, 4 h restraint vs. no restraint groups; +$p < 0.05$, 15 min restraint vs. 4 h restraint groups. *These results show that rodents made dependent on opioids have an increased glucocorticoid response to acute opioid withdrawal in unrestrained animals but a blunted glucocorticoid response to restraint stress in protracted abstinence, suggesting dysregulation of the hypothalamic–pituitary–adrenal axis in opioid dependence, similar to the dysregulation observed with chronic administration of other drugs of abuse.* [Taken with permission from Houshyar H, Cooper ZD, Woods JH. Paradoxical effects of chronic morphine treatment on the temperature and pituitary-adrenal responses to acute restraint stress: a chronic stress paradigm. Journal of Neuroendocrinology, 2001, (13), 862–874.]

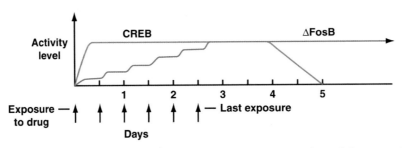

FIGURE 5.20   **Whether a user is tolerant to a drug or, conversely, sensitized to it, depends in part on the levels of active cyclic adenosine monophosphate response element binding protein (CREB) and ΔFosB in nucleus accumbens cells.** Initially, CREB dominates, leading to tolerance and, in the drug's absence, discomfort that only more drug can alleviate. But CREB activity decreases within days when not boosted by repeated administrations of opioids. In contrast, ΔFosB concentrations stay elevated for weeks after the last drug exposure. As CREB activity declines, the dangerous long-term sensitizing effects of ΔFosB come to dominate. [*Adapted with permission from Nestler EJ, Malenka RC. The addicted brain. Scientific American, 2004, (290), 78–85. © Terese Winslow.*]

turned on and take longer than usual to turn off) was reduced by chronic opioid treatment, and the chronically treated animals showed partial learning deficits in a water maze in which they had to locate a platform hidden beneath the water's surface. These studies suggest that opioids can impair executive function, and this may contribute to the phenomenon of craving.

The studies of the opioid regulation of second messenger systems in the nucleus accumbens has led to the identification of long-term changes in molecular elements of the brain motivational circuits associated the protracted abstinence of the *preoccupation/anticipation* stage. As noted above (see Figure 5.18), heroin exposure increases protein kinase A activity in the nucleus accumbens, and cyclic adenosine monophosphate (cAMP) response element binding protein (CREB) in the nucleus accumbens is decreased during chronic morphine exposure, whereas upregulation of cAMP response element (CRE) transcription has been observed in the nucleus accumbens during opioid withdrawal.

Another transcription factor activated by the chronic administration of opioids is ΔFosB. This transcription factor is responsible for persistently high levels of activator protein-1 (AP-1) complexes, which are transcriptionally active dimers of Fos and related Jun-family proteins. ΔFosB overexpression increases an individual's sensitivity to the rewarding effects of morphine, and expression of the "dominant negative" form of ΔFosB decreases the sensitivity to morphine. Because the effects of drugs of abuse on ΔFosB are stable for weeks to months after the last drug exposure, it may help to initiate and maintain the allostatic state of addiction and may be a common long-term molecular motivational change across drug classes (Figure 5.20).

SUMMARY

Opioids are defined as all drugs, both natural and synthetic, with morphine-like action. Opium contains morphine and other opioid alkaloids, such as thebaine and codeine. Opioids are the most powerful pain relievers known to man. Similarly to other drugs of abuse, the self-limited, controlled use of opioids is accompanied by a lack of withdrawal symptoms and limited pathology. However, opioid addiction remains a serious problem worldwide, and the diversion of opioid pain medications from their prescribed use to abuse has reached epidemic-like levels. Opioids have very powerful psychotropic effects. They relieve not only physical pain but also emotional pain, thus forming their main behavioral mechanism of action. Opioid intoxication from intravenous or smoked use is characterized by different stages that include the rush, nod, high, and being straight. Opioid withdrawal is characterized by very severe motivational and physical symptoms. Motivational signs can begin with a single administration. Protracted abstinence is characterized by powerful craving that derives from both conditioned positive and negative reinforcement and a hypersensitivity to pain and stress. Much is known about the neurobiological substrates for the acute reinforcing effects of opioids. At the neurocircuitry level, neural elements in the region of the ventral tegmental area and nucleus accumbens are important. At the cellular level, evidence exists for a disinhibitory effect of opioids via glutamatergic or GABAergic interneurons, both in the nucleus accumbens and ventral tegmental area. At the molecular level, the μ opioid receptor is the subtype most critical for the acute reinforcing effects of opioids. μ Opioid receptor knockout mice do not show opioid dependence or withdrawal. During the development of dependence on opioids, major between-system changes occur at the level of the ventral tegmental area and nucleus accumbens that contribute to the motivational effects of withdrawal. Chronic morphine produces a sensitized aversive response to opioid antagonists in the extended amygdala, with recruitment of norepinephrine and CRF activity. A decrease in the neuronal firing of dopamine neurons in the ventral tegmental area occurs during withdrawal that may be mediated by the increased release of GABA and decreased release of glutamate. Opioid and dopaminergic mechanisms are involved in opioid-induced (primed) reinstatement, glutamate is involved in cue-induced reinstatement, and the brain stress systems (CRF and norepinephrine) are involved in stress-induced reinstatement. All of these changes may contribute to the decreased reward system activity and increased stress system activity associated with opioid dependence and the allostatic molecular changes that drive craving during protracted abstinence associated with opioid dependence.

Suggested Reading

Chen, S.A., O'Dell, L., Hoefer, M., Greenwell, T.N., Zorrilla, E.P., Koob, G.F., 2006. Unlimited access to heroin self-administration: independent motivational markers of opiate dependence. Neuropsychopharmacology 3 (1), 2692–2707. [corrigedum: 3(1), 2802].

Gutstein, H.B., Akil, H., 2001. Opioid analgesics. In: Hardman, J.G., Limbird, L.E., Goodman-Gilman, A. (Eds.), Goodman and Gilman's The Pharmacological Basis of Therapeutics, tenth ed. McGraw-Hill, New York, pp. 569–619.

Himmelsbach, C.K., 1942. Clinical studies of drug addiction: physical dependence, withdrawal and recovery. Arch. Intern. Med. 69, 766–772.

Jansson, L.M., Velez, M., Harrow, C., 2009. The opioid-exposed newborn: assessment and pharmacologic management. J. Opioid Manag. 5, 47–55.

Nestler, E.J., 2001. Molecular basis of long-term plasticity underlying addiction. Nat. Rev. Neurosci. 2, 119–128.

Shurman, J., Koob, G.F., Gutstein, H.B., 2010. Opioids, pain, the brain, and hyperkatifeia: a framework for the rational use of opioids for pain. Panminerva. Med. 11, 1092–1098.

Simonnet, G., Rivat, C., 2003. Opioid-induced hyperalgesia: abnormal or normal pain? Neuroreport 14, 1–7.

DEFINITIONS

"Alcohol is the king of liquids. It excites the taste to the highest degree, its various preparations have opened up to mankind new sources of enjoyment. It supplies to certain medicines an energy which they could not have without it." *(Brillat-Savarin JA. Physiologie du Goût. Feydeau, Paris, 1826).*

The word "alcohol," according to Merriam-Webster's dictionary, finds its roots in the Arabic *al-kuhul* (or *kohl, cohol,* or *kohol*) to mean a powder of antimony or galena used by women to darken the eyebrows. The name *alcohol* was derived through Medieval Latin from Arabic. Because of the fineness of this powder, it was later applied to highly rectified spirits, a signification unknown in Arabia. Alcohol generically represents a wide range of compounds (Figure 6.1), but the alcohol suitable for drinking is ethanol (or ethyl alcohol or ethanol; Box 6.1). Alcohol is found in all substances that contain glucose. It is the product of the "saccharine principle," which is the term used in distillation for the conversion of any carbohydrate to glucose that can then be subjected to fermentation. Fermentation is the conversion of glucose and water in the presence of yeast to ethanol and carbon dioxide, and this is a common biological reaction in nature. Five agents are required for alcoholic fermentation: sugar (or starch to form glucose), water, heat, ferment (usually the yeast *Saccharomyces cerevisiae*), and air. Yeast converts glucose to alcohol up to a level of approximately 12%. Above this level, the alcohol becomes toxic to the yeast, which then dies. Such a process occurs in nature in seed germination and fruit ripening. Any source of glucose is sufficient to produce alcohol through the process of fermentation, and a wide range of glucose sources is used as the basis of numerous alcoholic beverages worldwide (Table 6.1). To raise alcohol (ethanol)

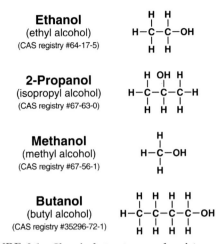

FIGURE 6.1 **Chemical structures and registry numbers for various alcohols from the Chemical Abstracts database.** Notice that each structure has a chain of four carbons or less. *[Taken with permission from Koob GF, Le Moal M. Neurobiology of Addiction. Academic Press, London, 2006.]*

BOX 6.1
_____

SYNOPSIS OF THE NEUROPHARMACOLOGICAL TARGET FOR ALCOHOL

All alcoholic products contain ethyl alcohol (ethanol), which is the main psychoactive ingredient in alcoholic beverages. Alcohol does not bind as a direct agonist at receptors in the brain but rather appears to be sequestered in transmembrane water pockets and modulates receptors (termed ethanol-receptive elements) to produce its behavioral effects. Alcohol is considered a sedative-hypnotic, but it can also produce psychostimulant-like effects that are attributable to disinhibition. Alcohol-receptive elements have been hypothesized to be located on ion-gated receptors, such as γ-aminobutyric acid-A (GABA$_A$), glycine, and glutamate receptors. The intoxicating effects of alcohol are mediated by the activation of multiple neurotransmitter systems (predominantly GABA, opioid peptides, and dopamine) in the origin areas (ventral tegmental area) and terminal areas (nucleus accumbens) of the mesocorticolimbic dopamine system and extended amygdala (central nucleus of the amygdala, bed nucleus of the stria terminalis, and a transition zone in the shell of the nucleus accumbens). The addiction potential of alcohol largely derives from powerful within-system neuroadaptations (signal transduction mechanisms) and between-system neuroadaptations (neurocircuitry changes) in the brain motivational and stress systems.

TABLE 6.1   Common Alcoholic Beverages

Beverage	Source of Glucose	Fermentation	Distillation	Alcohol by Volume
Beer (ale, lager)	barley, hops	×		3–6%
Beer (wheat)	wheat, hops	×		3–6%
Cider (alcohol)	apples	×		3–6%
Gin	juniper berries		×	40%
Vodka	rye, wheat, potatoes	×	×	35–60%
Schnapps	potatoes (flavored with various fruit juices)		×	20–45%
Rum	sugar cane molasses	×	×	35–40%
Tequila	agave cactus, corn, sugar cane	×	×	40–70%
Mead	honey	×		11–17%
White wine	white grapes and other grapes without skins	×		13%
Red wine	red or black grapes with skins	×		12.5%
Rose wine	red or black grapes with skins for short time	×		13%
Port wine	grapes (fermentation halted by addition of distilled grape spirits)	×	×	20%
Champagne	grapes	×		12%
Sherry	grapes (fortified with neutral spirits)	×		14–20%
Sake	rice	×		10–20%
Brandy (cognac, armagnac)	grapes, plums		×	40–60%
Liqueur	grapes (flavored with fruit, herbs, spices, flowers, wood)		×	14–40%
Drambuie	scotch, heather honey (flavored with herbs)		×	40%
Whiskey	corn, rye, barley		×	40–60%
Scotch	barley, wheat, maize (flavored with peat)		×	40–60%

For more information, visit http://en.wikipedia.org/wiki/Alcoholic_beverage#Types_of_alcoholic_beverages.

concentrations above 12%, the yeast-converted fermentation mixture must be distilled. The fermentation mixture is heated, and the ethanol vaporizes at a lower temperature than water. When cooled in some form of a condensation device (often a cool metal or glass container), the ethanol can again be captured as a liquid.

HISTORY OF ALCOHOL USE

Alcohol is a ubiquitous substance in our society and is widely used in alcoholic beverages for its beneficial effects; both social and medicinal. Alcoholic beverages are considered to have both nutritional and drug effects. As such, alcohol is unique among drug preparations.

Alcohol ingestion per capita has been steady in the United States since 1850, with the exception of the "Prohibition" period from 1919 to 1933 when the 18th Amendment to the US Constitution was ratified, prohibiting the sale of alcohol (the only two states that voted against the amendment were Rhode Island and Connecticut).

Alcohol is a well known "social lubricant" used to produce disinhibition in social situations, but at the same time excessive use produces the most harm to society of all drugs of abuse. The following address to the legislature by Mississippi State Senator Judge Noah S. Sweat in 1952 represents the dilemma faced by society in addressing the various aspects of the impact of alcohol on society:

> "You have asked me how I feel about whisky. All right, here is just how I stand on this question: If when you say whisky, you mean the devil's brew, the poison scourge; the bloody monster that defiles innocence, yea, literally takes the bread from the mouths of little children; if you mean the evil drink that topples the Christian man and woman from the pinnacles of righteous, gracious living into the bottomless pit of degradation and despair, shame and helplessness and hopelessness, then certainly I am against it with all of my power ... But if when you say whisky, you mean the oil of conversation, the philosophic wine, the stuff that is consumed when good fellows get together, that puts a song in their hearts and laughter on their lips and the warm glow of contentment in their eyes, if you mean holiday cheer; if you mean the stimulating drink that puts the spring in the old gentlemen's step on a frosty morning; if you mean the drink that enables a man to magnify his joy, and his happiness and to forget, if only for a little while, life's great tragedies and heartbreaks and sorrows, if you mean that drink, the sale of which pours into our treasuries untold millions of dollars, which are used to provide tender care for our little crippled children, our blind, our deaf, our dumb, our pitiful aged and infirmed, to build highways, hospitals and schools, then certainly I am in favor of it. This is my stand. I will not retreat from it; I will not compromise." (*Associated Press. Ex-judge Sweat, of "Whisky Speech" fame, dies.* The Commercial Appeal, *Memphis TN. Feb 24, 1996: A4.*)

An overwhelming majority of persons in the United States have used alcohol at least once in their lives. The 2011 United States *National Survey on Drug Use and Health* from the Substance Abuse and Mental Health Services Administration estimated that 211.7 million people aged 12 and older (82.1%) had ever engaged in alcohol use, and 170.4 million people aged 12 and older were last-year users of alcohol (65.9%). Notable statistics from this survey included the following. In 2011, of those people aged 12 or older who ever consumed alcohol in the last year, 16.7 million (6.5%) showed alcohol abuse or dependence (Substance Use Disorder based on the *Diagnostic and Statistical Manual of Mental Disorders*, 5th edition [DSM-5], criteria), and 7.8 million (4.6%) of those who ever consumed alcohol in the last year showed alcohol dependence (DSM-IV criteria; see Chapter 1).

Alcohol abuse and alcoholism can lead to numerous medical conditions, ranging from cirrhosis of the liver and heart disease to pancreatitis, Korsakoff's dementia, and fetal alcohol syndrome. According to the *State Trends in Alcohol-Related Mortality, 1979–92* by the National Institute on Alcohol Abuse and Alcoholism, alcohol was implicated in 32% of all deaths in the United States, including fatal automobile crashes, other accidents, liver disease, heart disease, neurological diseases, and cancer. Although the number has steadily declined since the early 1980s, alcohol was involved in 37% of all traffic deaths in the United States in 2008 among persons aged 16 to 20. In 2006, the Centers for Disease Control and Prevention reported that the cost of alcohol to US society was over $223 billion, including losses in workplace productivity (72% of the total cost), healthcare expenses (11%), criminal justice expenses (9%), and motor vehicle crashes (6%).

TABLE 6.2   Representative Listing by the World Health Organization of per Capita Alcohol Consumption (in Liters) in 2000

Country	Total	Beer	Wine	Spirits
France	11.7**	2.0**	7.1**	2.6**
Spain	11.17	3.76	4.61	2.79
United Kingdom*	10.39	4.86	2.10	1.50
Greece	9.16	2.10	4.82	2.24
Italy	9.16	1.47	7.11	0.58
United States	9.08	5.11	1.67	2.29
Venezuela	7.28	4.86	0.07	2.34
Sweden*	6.86	2.77	1.86	1.00
Japan	6.26	2.30	0.41	2.81
Chile	6.05	1.18	4.25	0.63
China	5.17	1.03	0.09	4.04
Brazil	4.79	2.40	0.36	2.03
South Korea	4.13	0.25	0	3.88
Mexico	4.01	2.92	0.30	0.79
Israel	2.06	0.93	0.25	0.87
India	1.01	0.03	0	0.98

These values estimate the level of alcohol consumption per adult (15 years of age or older) of pure alcohol during a calendar year as calculated from official statistics on production, sales, import, and export, taking into account stocks whenever possible. Conversion factors used to estimate the amount of pure alcohol in (barley) beer is 5%, wine 12%, and spirits 40% of alcohol (other conversion factors were used for some types of beer and other beverages). Data were collected and calculations were made mainly using three sources: FAOSTAT – United Nations Food and Agriculture Organization's Statistical Database, World Drink Trends, regularly published by Produktschap voor Gedistilleerde Dranken (Netherlands), and in some cases direct government data. Data are available from the World Health Organization "Adult Per Capita Alcohol Consumption" database for most countries of the world since 1961 onward. Data are presented for the groups of total, and also beer, wine, and spirits separately. The category *Beer* includes data on barley, maize, millet, and sorghum beer combined. The amounts from beer, wine, and spirits do not necessarily add up to the presented total, as in some cases the total includes other beverage categories, including palm wine, vermouths, cider, fruit wines, and so on. It is important to note that these figures comprise in most cases the recorded alcohol consumption only and have some inherent problems. Factors which influence the accuracy of per capita data are: informal production, tourists, overseas consumption, stockpiling, waste, spillage, smuggling, duty-free sales, variation in beverage strength, and the quality of the data upon which this table is based. In some countries there exists a significant unrecorded alcohol consumption that should be added for a comprehensive picture of total alcohol consumption.

* *Data from 2001.*
** *Data from* World Drink Trends: International Beverage Alcohol Consumption and Production Trends. *Produktschap voor Gedistilleerde Dranken, Henley-on-Thames, Oxfordshire, 2002.*

Patterns of alcohol use vary between cultures (Table 6.2, Box 6.2). Per capita alcohol consumption also varies between countries, from a low of 1 liter per person in India to a high of over 11 liters per person in France. France, Spain, Greece, and Italy have the highest per capita consumption, corresponding to a pattern of high wine drinking that pervades nearly all facets of daily life.

BOX 6.2

CULTURAL DIFFERENCES IN PATTERNS OF ALCOHOL CONSUMPTION

France. France has the highest per capita alcohol consumption (approximately 12 liters per person per year) of any country. Two-thirds of this total consumption is in the form of wine drinking. For men, and to a lesser extent women, wine is drunk at meals as part of the diet. This has declined, however, in the last 50 years. Wine also is consumed as part of social and festive occasions, and as part of an entirely aesthetic experience (i.e., for oenological reasons). There has existed a purported popular French belief that "wine is not alcohol" (which stems from the mid-1800s when Pasteur deemed wine as beneficial and "hygienic" because it could kill microbes) and the word *alcohol* had two meanings, one in the singular referring to a chemical element in fermented beverages, and the other referring to distilled drinks. The majority of habitual or excessive drinkers are men – although drinking has increased in women – and alcohol consumption remains an expression of the masculine identity (Nahoum-Grappe, 1995).

Italy. Similar to France, wine pervades most public and private sectors of life in Italy, with wine drinking being the most prevalent. Italians rank 5th in alcohol consumption. Abstainers are viewed with curiosity, as "odd persons" who should explain why they do not drink. In young people, males drink more than females, more wine in northeastern Italy, and in the home, and more beer in southern Italy and outside the home. Although Italians do not stigmatize heavy consumption, they do tend to blame problem drinkers who lose control. Italian physicians are known to suggest moderate wine consumption to prevent cardiovascular disease, an approach that has recently received scientific justification, but both media and medical lobbies of late are

increasingly emphasizing the breadth of alcohol-related problems, particularly drunk driving and cirrhosis of the liver (Cottino, 1995).

Sweden. Sweden has half the alcohol consumption of France, but Swedes often are characterized as binge-drinkers, being one of the countries of the so-called "vodka belt" across northeastern Europe, a long-standing drinking pattern that has ancient cultural roots. The most prevalent beverage is beer that is drunk on rare occasions, usually weekends; therefore, a small part of the population is responsible for a large part of total consumption. For men, getting deliberately intoxicated is a sign of masculinity, but for women, the act can bring condemnation. Swedes also look down on those with persistent alcohol problems, with blame directed toward the individual rather than the family or workplace. Even though the Swedes are labeled as binge-drinkers, they have a relatively low incidence of alcohol-related problems compared with other Western countries and a significantly lower overall consumption (Nyberg, 1995).

China. China ranks low on total alcohol consumption, with per capita consumption that is significantly less than half that of France, with the majority in the form of spirits (liquors). The Chinese stress the role of alcohol in all aspects of life, affecting structures of belief, behavior, values, attitudes, and religion. It is an important adjunct to hospitality, with both the host and guest honoring each other with drink as a combined expression of welcome and appreciation. Everyone toasts for the Chinese New Year, for good health, and for long-lasting prosperity for their elders. Alcohol still plays a role in Chinese medicine (in fact, the Chinese written characters for "alcohol" and "medicine" share the same root). The majority of men (64%) are moderate drinkers, while the majority of women (51%) abstain. A very low percentage of the population (10%, all male), however, are heavy drinkers. Overall, approximately 30% abstain. There is a high proportion of individuals (50%) with the inactive allele for acetaldehyde dehydrogenase which produces a flushing reaction which is hypothesized to form a protective factor against excessive drinking and subsequent alcoholism. However, socially, the Chinese people seem generally unaware of the flushing reaction, and if they are, it has little or no impact on their attitudes in relation to alcohol despite the high abstinence rate and very low heavy drinking (Xiao, 1995).

BEHAVIORAL EFFECTS

Alcohol has a wide range of behavioral effects and for centuries has been widely regarded as both a sedative and stimulant. To quote Shakespeare from *Macbeth*, Act II, Scene III:

Porter. Faith, sir, we were carousing till the second cock; and drink, sir, is a great provoker of three things.
Macduff. What three things does drink especially provoke?
Porter. Merry, sir, nose-painting, sleep, and urine. Lechery, sir, it provokes, and unprovokes; it provokes the desire, but it takes away the performance; therefore, much drink may be said to be an equivocator with lechery; it makes him, and it mars him; it sets him on, and it takes him off; it persuades him, and disheartens him; makes him stand to, and not stand to; in conclusion, equivocates him in a sleep, and, giving him the lie, leaves him.

Alcohol, a sedative hypnotic, produces dose-dependent behavioral effects in humans, including sedation (decreases in activity) and hypnosis (sleep induction). At low doses (blood alcohol levels of 0.01–0.05 g%), alcohol produces personality changes, including increased sociability, increased talkativeness, and a more expansive personality (Figure 6.2, Table 6.3, Box 6.3). Such blood alcohol levels are associated with mild euphoria, improved mood, good feelings, increased confidence, and increased assertiveness. Some release of inhibitions also occurs, with tension reduction and increased responsiveness (and sometimes combativeness) in conflict situations. As the dose increases from 0.08 to 0.10 g%, mood swings become more pronounced, with euphoria, emotional outbursts, and a greater release of inhibitions. Blood alcohol levels of 0.08 g% produce distinct impairment in judgment, and motor dysfunction is apparent. Blood alcohol levels of 0.15 to 0.20 g% are associated with marked ataxia, major motor impairment, staggering, slurred speech, muscular incoordination, and impairment in reaction time. Sensory responses are also impaired, including a loss of vestibular sense and decreased pain sensation. Such blood levels also dull concentration and insight, impair discrimination and memory, significantly impair judgment, cause greater emotional instability, and profoundly release inhibitions. At this level, "blackouts" can occur, in which a person will have no later memory of the events that transpired while the person was intoxicated. At blood levels of 0.30 g%, people become stuporous but are still conscious. This is an anesthetic level of intoxication, with marked decreases in responsivity to environmental stimuli, severely impaired motor function, and rapid and dramatic changes in mood. Vomiting can occur at this level. The lethal dose in 50% of individuals (referred to as the LD_{50})

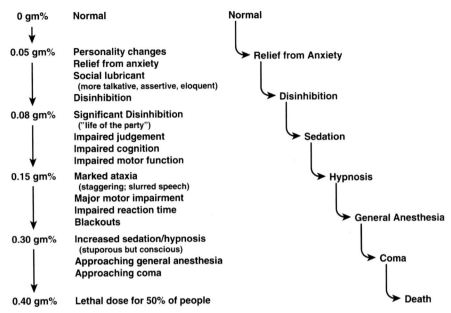

FIGURE 6.2   **Progression of subjective and physiological changes that correspond to increased blood alcohol levels.**

is approximately 0.50 g% in nondependent individuals (alcohol-dependent individuals may have a significantly higher LD_{50}; see section on tolerance below; Box 6.4).

PHARMACOKINETICS

Alcohol has been described as the "universal solvent." It is readily miscible in water (meaning that it forms a homogeneous solution) and has significant lipid solubility. Therefore, alcohol readily crosses cell membranes. Alcohol is absorbed in the stomach (20%) and small intestine (80%). In normal adults, 80–90% of absorption occurs within 30–60 min. The absorption of alcohol is delayed by up to 4–6h if food is present in the stomach, and the total amount of alcohol absorbed is reduced (Figure 6.3). The "absorption" of a drug means the movement of the drug into the blood stream. Blood alcohol levels have become the standard by which to assess the absorption of alcohol and make comparisons between animals and

humans, and between experimental conditions (Table 6.3).

Alcohol is largely eliminated through catabolism in the liver by three enzymatic pathways. Only 5–10% of alcohol is excreted unchanged from the lungs or urine. A factor of 2100 will convert breath alcohol concentration to arterial blood concentration, which is the basis of the "Breathalyzer" test. Alcohol is broken down to acetaldehyde in the liver by the enzyme alcohol dehydrogenase, which is responsible for a large part of its oxidation (Figure 6.4). Acetaldehyde is then broken down to acetic acid by acetaldehyde dehydrogenase and then further broken down to water and carbon dioxide in some organs. Allelic (genetic) variations in this pathway are responsible for the differential alcohol elimination rates in the human population. Inactivation of acetaldehyde dehydrogenase-2 (ALDH2) provides the basis for the alcohol-induced flush reaction seen in many individuals with Asian heritage. The flush reaction is characterized by facial flushing, tachycardia (increased

TABLE 6.3 Blood Alcohol Level (gm%) Estimations for Men and Women

BAL for Men

Drinks	Body Weight (lb)							
	100	120	140	160	180	200	220	240
1	0.04	0.03	0.03	0.02	0.02	0.02	0.02	0.02
2	0.08	0.06	0.05	0.05	0.03	0.03	0.03	0.03
3	0.11	0.09	0.08	0.07	0.06	0.06	0.05	0.05
4	0.15	0.12	0.11	0.09	0.08	0.08	0.07	0.06
5	0.19	0.16	0.13	0.12	0.11	0.09	0.09	0.08
6	0.23	0.19	0.16	0.14	0.13	0.11	0.10	0.09
7	0.26	0.22	0.19	0.16	0.15	0.13	0.12	0.11
8	0.30	0.25	0.21	0.19	0.17	0.15	0.14	0.13
9	0.38	0.31	0.27	0.23	0.21	0.19	0.17	0.16

BAL for Women

Drinks	Body Weight (lb)							
	100	120	140	160	180	200	220	240
1	0.05	0.04	0.03	0.03	0.03	0.02	0.02	0.02
2	0.09	0.08	0.07	0.06	0.05	0.05	0.04	0.04
3	0.14	0.11	0.10	0.09	0.08	0.07	0.06	0.06
4	0.18	0.15	0.13	0.11	0.10	0.09	0.08	0.08
5	0.23	0.19	0.16	0.14	0.13	0.11	0.10	0.09
6	0.27	0.23	0.19	0.17	0.15	0.14	0.12	0.11
7	0.32	0.27	0.23	0.20	0.18	0.16	0.14	0.13
8	0.36	0.30	0.26	0.23	0.20	0.18	0.17	0.15
9	0.41	0.34	0.29	0.26	0.23	0.20	0.19	0.17
10	0.45	0.38	0.32	0.28	0.25	0.23	0.21	0.19

Subtract 0.01 gm% for each 40 min of drinking.
1 drink = 1.25 ounce 80 Proof liquor, 12 ounce beer, or 5 ounce wine.
[http://www.alcohol.vt.edu/Students/alcoholEffects/estimatingBAC/]

heart rate), hypotension, elevated skin temperature, increased body sway, and nystagmus and is attributable to the buildup of acetaldehyde caused by a lack of acetaldehyde dehydrogenase activity. Initially, the surge in acetaldehyde produces more intense feelings of intoxication, but with increased drinking, the flush reaction produces nausea, vomiting, and an aversive reaction. Disulfiram (Antabuse) inhibits acetaldehyde dehydrogenase and produces an identical flush reaction. This is extremely aversive and forms the basis of its use in the treatment of alcoholism (see Chapter 9).

In certain ethnic groups, a mutation in two nucleotides of the ALDH2 gene produces complete inactivation of acetaldehyde dehydrogenase if a person is homozygous for both alleles and partial inactivation in heterozygous individuals. Forty to 50% of the Japanese, Chinese, and Vietnamese populations are heterozygous for the ALDH2 gene mutation, and the Japanese are approximately 7% homozygous for the mutation. Europeans show virtually 0% of the population with the mutation, Koreans are 30% heterozygous and 3% homozygous for the mutation, and Native North Americans also show a very low incidence of the ALDH2 mutation (Table 6.4).

In a 150 lb person, the average rate of metabolism of pure alcohol is approximately 7–9 ml/h (0.3 ounces/h). This converts to approximately 0.01–0.015 g% per hour or approximately half of a standard drink per hour. Individuals with alcoholism can double this rate of metabolism through the mechanism of metabolic tolerance, which has been theorized to be largely attributable to the induction of the liver enzyme cytochrome P4502E1 (although some have argued for increased activity of alcohol dehydrogenase as well). P4502E1 was found to be increased by four to 10-fold in liver biopsies of recently drinking humans and can contribute to the production of highly toxic metabolites in the liver in individuals with alcoholism. Importantly, this type of tolerance results in lower blood alcohol levels for the tolerant individual than the nontolerant individual for the same dosing at the same body weight. Pharmacodynamic tolerance results from changes in the response to the drug when the blood alcohol levels are the same (see Chapter 2).

BOX 6.3

BLOOD ALCOHOL MEASURES

Blood alcohol levels are measured in gram%. The degree of intoxication throughout the United States is measured by a blood alcohol level, and the legal limit is 0.08 gram%. For example, *0.08 grams alcohol/100 ml = 0.08 gram% = 17 mM.* Generally, for a male who weighs 150 lbs, 4 ounces of spirits (100 proof = 50% alcohol), four glasses of wine, or four beers will result in a blood alcohol level of approximately 0.10 gram%.

For a female who weighs 150 lbs, these same amounts of alcohol will result in a blood alcohol level of 0.12 gram%. The difference in blood alcohol levels in males and females has been attributed to differences in the distribution of body fat, with more fat per kilogram (thus less water) for females, and lower gastric levels of the alcohol-metabolizing enzyme alcohol dehydrogenase in females.

BOX 6.4

GIRL DOWNS QUART OF LIQUOR ON DARE, DIES

ORLAND PARK, Ill. – A high school cheerleader who downed a quart of 107-proof liquor on a dare passed out and died after she was dropped off at a friend's house to sleep it off.

Authorities said 16-year-old Elizabeth Wakulich might have been saved if someone had taken her to a hospital sooner.

Wakulich was out with friends early Monday when she answered a challenge to drink a bottle of schnapps with an alcohol content of more than 53 percent.

Wakulich was pronounced dead with a blood alcohol level of .38 percent, nearly four times the legal limit for driving in Illinois. The medical examiner estimated her level was closer to .60 shortly after the binge. A level of .40 to .50 can kill.

Associated Press

From: San Diego Union Tribune, *Thursday, June 19, 1997.* © *The Associated Press, 2013.*

A third pathway for alcohol metabolism is a non-oxidative pathway catalyzed by fatty acid ethyl ester (FAEE) synthase, which leads to the formation of fatty acid esters, which in turn produce mono-, di-, and triglycerides. FAEEs are found in the highest concentrations in the liver, adipose tissue, and the heart and are hypothesized to contribute to the toxic effects of alcohol.

USE, ABUSE, AND ADDICTION

Alcoholism

Alcoholism is equivalent to Substance Dependence on Alcohol as defined by the *Diagnostic and Statistical Manual of Mental Disorders*, 4th edition, and Dependence as defined by the ICD-10, both of which are equivalent to alcohol addiction.

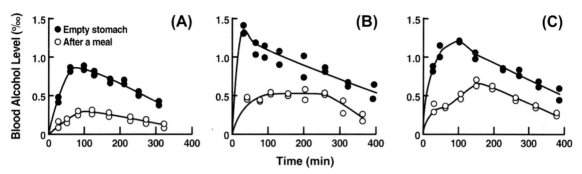

FIGURE 6.3 Influence of a meal, taken with alcohol, on blood alcohol levels, showing three different patterns of responses (A, B, and C) in a function that relates blood alcohol levels over time. Closed circles correspond to the blood alcohol level when the alcohol was taken on an empty stomach, and open circles correspond to the alcohol level after consuming the same quantity of alcohol with a meal. Each subject was tested with and without food. Units are expressed as ‰, which refers to Δ/baseline per mil. In an example of such annotation, 1.5‰ would be equivalent to 150 mg% (0.15 g%). (A) This "food curve" shows a large depression in relation to the fasting curve with a low maximum and a slowly descending limb. This finding is interpreted as the result of a great delay in absorption, both with regard to rate and time, with absorption continuing for 4–6 h. (B) A plateau was maintained for the 2–3 h interval after a delayed absorption period. The horizontal course was followed by a rather rapid fall, implying that absorption, distribution, and combustion balance each other. When absorption is completed, distribution is maintained which caused the rapid fall of the post-absorptive phase. (C) The post-absorptive period had a parallel course to that of the fasting curve. Absorption in this case was delayed to such an extent that the maximum appeared later, and the normal over-shooting of alcohol was prevented. The distribution phase was not reflected in the blood alcohol level as under fasting conditions, and the rate of disappearance of alcohol from the blood stream during the post-absorptive period was the same as in fasting. *These data show that the ingestion of a meal delays the absorption of alcohol ingested with the meal in three different patterns (A, B, and C). However, in no case did the level of the "food" blood alcohol curve reach the values of the "fasting" curve. [Taken with permission from Goldberg L. Quantitative studies on alcohol tolerance in man. Acta Physiologica Scandinavica Supplementum, 1943, (5), 1–128.]*

Substance Use Disorders as defined by the *Diagnostic and Statistical Manual of Mental Disorders*, 5th edition, grades the disorder as mild, moderate, and severe, and future studies will link these gradations to the commonly used terms of "addiction" and "alcoholism" (see Chapter 1). The stages of alcoholism vary significantly and can be manifested at any time of life and take on many forms (Box 6.5). A sample time course of alcoholism in a person's work life is shown in Table 6.5.

A strong genetic component is well established in alcoholism. Twin and adoption studies have shown that the hereditability of alcoholism may be as high as 50–60%. The phenotype of individuals with a positive family history for alcoholism is unique and suggests characteristics that can be linked to patterns of behavior that lead to excessive drinking and ultimately alcoholism. Family history-positive

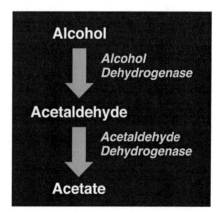

FIGURE 6.4 Alcohol metabolism. The liver has three metabolic systems that are able to oxidize alcohol. Alcohol dehydrogenase oxidizes alcohol into acetaldehyde, and acetaldehyde dehydrogenase then oxidizes acetaldehyde into carbon dioxide and water, which is then secreted in the urine. The anti-relapse medication disulfiram (Antabuse) blocks acetaldehyde dehydrogenase at therapeutic doses. Females have less of the alcohol dehydrogenase enzyme than males and a larger amount of body fat for a given weight.

TABLE 6.4   Frequency of Acetaldehyde Dehydrogenase Isozyme Deficiency in American Indians, Asian Mongoloids, and Other Populations

Population	Sample Size	% Deficient
South American Indians		
Atacameños (Chile)	133	43
Mapuche (Chile)	64	41
Shuara (Ecuador)	99	42
North American Indians		
Sioux (North Dakota)	90	5
Navajo (New Mexico)	56	2
Mexican Indians		
Mestizo (Mexico City)	43	4
Asian Mongoloids		
Japanese	184	44
Chinese Mongolian	198	30
Chinese Zhuang	106	45
Chinese Han	120	50
Korean (Mandschu)	209	25
Chinese (living abroad)	196	35
South Korean	75	27
Vietnamese	138	53
Indonesian	30	39
Thai (North)	110	8
Filipino	110	13
Ainu	80	20
Other populations		
German	300	0
Egyptian	260	0
Sudanese	40	0
Kenyan	23	0
Liberian	184	0
Turk	65	0
Fang	37	0
Israeli	77	0
Asian Indian	50	0

[Taken with permission from Goedde HW, Agarwal DP, Harada S, Rothhammer F, Whittaker JO, Lisker R. Aldehyde dehydrogenase polymorphism in North American, South American, and Mexican Indian populations. American Journal of Humam Genetics, *1986, (38), 395–399.]*

individuals show a low level of responsiveness to alcohol, perhaps reflecting a low sensitivity to the drug. The low response to alcohol can be seen relatively early in life and carries a similar heritability to alcoholism. This phenotypic characteristic predicts later heavy drinking and alcohol dependence but is not associated with heavy use or problems associated with substance use disorders with other drugs. The low response to alcohol as an endophenotype can enhance the risk of heavier drinking and drinking problems through environmental influences, such as associations with heavier-drinking peers, alterations in the expectations of the likely effects of drinking, and the enhanced probability of using alcohol to cope with stressors.

Alcohol Withdrawal

Alcohol withdrawal is characterized by a latent state of hyperexcitability, representing a "rebound" phenomenon from the previously chronically depressed central nervous system caused by alcohol. In humans, alcohol withdrawal after ingesting 10–15 drinks per day for 10 days leads to time-dependent effects that begin within a few hours of abstinence, depending on the blood alcohol levels obtained (Table 6.6). Early stages of withdrawal, up to 36 h, are characterized by tremor and elevated sympathetic nervous system responses, including increased heart rate, blood pressure, and body temperature. Such physical signs are accompanied by insomnia, anxiety, anorexia, and dysphoria. Later stages of withdrawal, if left untreated (which is rare today), can include more severe tremor, sympathetic responses, anxiety, and delirium tremens. Delirium tremens is characterized by vivid hallucinations and psychotic behavior. High fever can also occur and be life-threatening, but, again, this is rare in modern medicine because of the availability of benzodiazepines for treatment.

BOX 6.5

I am David. I am an alcoholic. I have always been an alcoholic. I will always be an alcoholic. I cannot touch alcohol. It will destroy me. It is like an allergy – not a real allergy – but *like* an allergy.

I had my first drink at sixteen. I got drunk. For several years I drank every week or so with the boys. I didn't always get drunk, but I know now that alcohol affected me differently than other people. I looked forward to the times I knew I could drink. I drank for the glow, the feeling of confidence it gave me. But maybe that's why my friends drank too. They didn't become alcoholics. Alcohol seemed to satisfy some specific need I had, which I can't describe. True, it made me feel good, helped me forget my troubles, but that wasn't it. What was it? I don't know, but I know I liked it, and after a time, I more than liked it, I needed it. Of course, I didn't realize it. It was maybe ten or fifteen years before I realized it, *let* myself realize it.

My need was easy to hide from myself and others (maybe I'm kidding myself about the others). I only associated with people who drank. I married a woman who drank. There were always reasons to drink. I was low, tense, tired, mad, happy. I probably drank as often because I was happy as for any other reason. And occasions for drinking – when drinking was appropriate, expected – were endless. Football games, fishing trips, parties, holidays, birthdays, Christmas, or merely Saturday night. Drinking became interwoven with everything pleasurable – food, sex, social life. When I stopped drinking, these things, for a time, lost all interest for me, they were so tied to drinking. I don't think I will ever enjoy them as much as I did when drinking. But if I had kept drinking, I wouldn't be here to enjoy them. I would be dead.

So, drinking came to dominate my life. By the time I was 25 I was drinking every day, usually before dinner, but sometimes after dinner (if there was a "reason"), and more on weekends, starting in the afternoon. By 30, I drank all weekend, starting with a beer or Bloody Mary in the morning, and drinking off and on, throughout the day, beer or wine or vodka, indiscriminately. The goal, always, was to maintain a glow, not enough, I hoped, that people would notice, but a glow. When five o'clock came. I thought, well, now it's cocktail hour and I would have my two of three scotches or martinis before dinner as I did on non-weekend nights. After dinner I might nap, but just as often felt a kind of wakeful calm and power and happiness that I've never experienced any other time. These were the dangerous moments. I called friends, boring them with drunken talk; arranged parties; decided impulsively to drive to a bar. In one year, at the age of 33. I had three accidents, all on Saturday night, and was charged with drunken driving once (I kept my licence, but barely). My friends became fewer, reduced to other heavy drinkers and barflies. I fought with my wife, blaming her for her drinking, and once or twice hit her (or so she said – like many things I did while drinking, there was no memory afterward).

And by now I was drinking at noontime, with the lunch hour stretching longer and longer. I began taking off whole afternoons, going home potted. I missed mornings at work because of drinking the night before, particularly Monday mornings. And I began drinking weekday mornings to get going. Vodka and orange juice. I thought vodka wouldn't smell (it did). It usually lasted until an early martini luncheon, and I then suffered through until cocktail hour, which came earlier and earlier.

By now I was hooked and knew it, but desperately did not want others to know it. I had been sneaking drinks for years – slipping out to the kitchen during parties and such – but now I began hiding alcohol, in my desk, bedroom, car glove compartment, so it would never be far away, ever. I grew panicky even thinking I might

Continued

BOX 6.5   *(cont'd)*

not have alcohol when I needed it, which was just about always.

For years, I drank and had very little hangover, but now the hangovers were gruesome. I felt physically bad – headachy, nauseous, weak – but the mental part was the hardest. I loathed myself. I was waking early and thinking what a mess I was, how I had hurt so many others and myself. The words "guilty" and "depression" sound superficial in trying to describe how I felt. The loathing was almost physical – a dead weight that could be lifted in only one way, and that was by having a drink, so I drank, morning after morning. After two or three, my hands were steady, I could hold some breakfast down, and the guilt was gone, or almost.

Despite everything, others knew. There was the odor, the rheumy eyes, and flushed face. There was missing work and not working well when there. Fights with wife, increasingly physical. She kept threatening to leave and finally did. My boss gave me a leave of absence after an embarrassed remark about my "personal problems." At some point I was without

wife, home, or job. I had nothing to do but drink. The drinking was now steady, days on end. I lost appetite and missed meals (besides, money was short). I awoke at night, sweating and shaking, and had a drink. I awoke in the morning vomiting and had a drink. It couldn't last. My ex-wife found me in my apartment shaking and seeing things, and got me in the hospital. I dried out, left, and went back to drinking. I was hospitalized again, and this time stayed dry for six months. I was nervous and couldn't sleep, but got some of my confidence back and found a part-time job. Then my ex-boss offered my job back and I celebrated by having a drink. The next night I had two drinks. In a month I was drinking as much as ever and again unemployed. That was three years ago. I've had two big drunks since then but don't drink other times. I think about alcohol and miss it. Life is gray and monotonous. The joy and gaiety are gone. But drinking will kill me. I know this and have stopped – for now.

From: anonymous

Such a description is reasonably accurate with regard to the physical signs of alcohol withdrawal, but it does not address the *motivational* effects of alcohol withdrawal. Individuals with alcoholism also show dramatic evidence of dysphoric states during acute withdrawal that persist into protracted abstinence, including symptoms of anxiety, dysphoria, and depression. In a number of inpatient studies, acute withdrawal (i.e., the first week post-alcohol) is characterized by Beck Depression Inventory scores and Hamilton Depression Scores in the range of moderate depression. In these inpatient studies, depression scores decline during subsequent weeks of treatment but remain at an intermediate elevated level for up to 4 weeks after withdrawal. Similar results were found for anxiety measures, even in subjects without comorbid anxiety or depression. Independent of comorbidity status, individuals who relapsed had higher trait anxiety scores than those who abstained. Although individuals with alcoholism show significant decreases in measures of depression and anxiety during withdrawal, there is a measurable level of depression/anxiety symptoms that persist long after acute withdrawal into protracted abstinence that may be relevant for the treatment of alcoholism.

TABLE 6.5 Progressively Worsening Alcoholic Employee Behavior Patterns

| Employee Behavior Pattern | Observable Signs | | Performance on the Job |
	Absenteeism	General Behavior	
Early stage drinking to relieve tension increase in tolerance memory lapses	tardiness at lunchtime early departure	overreacts to real or imagined criticism complains of not feeling well	misses deadlines lowered job efficiency
Middle stage sneaking drinks feeling guilty tremors loss of interest	frequent days off for vague ailments or implausible reasons	marked changes (e.g., statements are not dependable, begins avoiding associates, repeated minor injuries on and off job)	spasmodic work pace lapses of attention cannot concentrate
Late Middle stage unable to discuss problems efforts for control fail neglect of food drinking alone	frequent time off (perhaps several days) does not return from lunch	domestic problems interfere with work financial problems more frequent hospitalization will not discuss problems	far below what is expected
Terminal stage now thinks, "My job interferes with my drinking"	prolonged unpredictable absences	completely undependable repeated hospitalization physical deterioration visible serious financial problems serious family problems	uneven generally incompetent

Source: Cline S. Alcohol and Drugs at Work. *Drug Abuse Council, Washington DC, 1975.*

Alcohol Tolerance

Multiple forms of tolerance develop to the effects of alcohol, but they can generally be divided into two major types: dispositional tolerance and functional tolerance. With dispositional tolerance, chronic alcohol use can lead to an increased ability to metabolize alcohol through the induction of alcohol dehydrogenase and other metabolic enzymes. Such metabolism can double, reaching 30–40 mg/dl/h compared with a nontolerant adult who metabolizes alcohol at about 15–20 mg/dl/h. This dispositional tolerance requires 3–14 days of drinking and can take several weeks of abstinence to return to normal.

Functional tolerance requires a higher blood alcohol level to achieve intoxication and is mediated by neuroadaptational changes in the central nervous system. It can be divided into three categories: acute, chronic, and behavioral. Acute functional tolerance was originally defined as the "Mellanby effect," in which a greater degree of impairment was observed at a given concentration of alcohol on the ascending limb of the blood alcohol curve than at the same concentration on the descending limb. Similarly to other drugs of abuse, rapid initial tolerance occurs within one drinking session. The subjective sense of intoxication follows the ascending limb of the blood alcohol curve but not the descending limb (Figure 6.5). Importantly, such tolerance to the *intoxicating* effects of alcohol is not necessarily accompanied by any marked increase in the lethal dose.

Chronic functional tolerance in humans is reflected by an increase in intake needed to produce intoxication (that is, a shift to the right of the concentration-response function).

TABLE 6.6   Stages of Alcohol Withdrawal in Humans Following Ingestion of 10–15 Drinks per Day over a Ten Day Period

Stage	Period of Withdrawal	Signs	Comments
Early Stage	from a few hours to 36–48 hours	Anxiety	
		Anorexia	
		Insomnia	
		Tremor	This tremulous phase (shakes) often is observed on admission and can be severe enough to prevent a patient from feeding himself.
		Mild disorientation	
		Convulsions	Between 24 and 48 h; similar to tonic-clonic seizures of grand mal epilepsy.
		Sympathetic response	Elevated blood pressure and body temperature; increased heart rate (heart rate is a useful index of continuing toxicity and may warn of impending delirium tremens).
Late Stage	begins after 2–4 days and can last 2–3 days	Delirium tremens	The most severe withdrawal state: • marked tremor, anxiety, and insomnia • marked paranoia and disorientation • severe autonomic overactivity, including sweating, nausea, vomiting, diarrhea, and fever • agitation • vivid hallucinations • reality testing fails, and patient must be protected from self-harm during outbursts of irrational behavior • seizures are rare in this stage • high fever, in which prognosis is poor and can be life-threatening • death usually occurs secondary to complicating illness, infection, or injury • shock and hyperthermia can be fatal • fatality rate used to be upward of 15% but now has decreased to 1–2%

Source: Goldstein DB. Pharmacology of Alcohol. Oxford University Press, New York, 1983.

Heavy drinkers were shown to be less sensitive to alcohol than moderate drinkers or abstainers in the "finger-finger" motor coordination test (Figure 6.6). Behavioral tolerance can be defined as learning to compensate for the effects of the drug. One example of behavioral tolerance is someone who practices performing a task (like walking) while intoxicated.

ALCOHOL TOXICITY

Behavioral Toxicity

Different patterns of drinking predominate in society and can be categorized as social drinking, binge drinking, and heavy drinking according to the National Institute on Alcohol

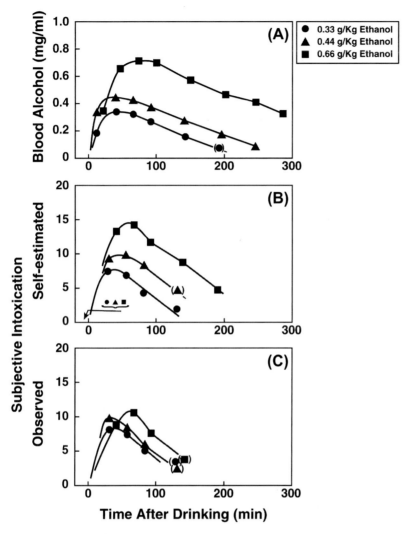

FIGURE 6.5 **Comparison of effects of 0.33, 0.44, and 0.66 g/kg ethanol on (A) blood alcohol levels, (B) self-estimated subjective intoxication, and (C) observed degree of intoxication.** Alcohol was taken in the form of whisky on an empty stomach, and the time allowed for drinking was 10–15 min. Means (data points) within parentheses include one zero and thus may be too high. *These data show what is called "within-session tolerance" or "acute tolerance." The degree of intoxication parallels the ascending limb of the function that relates intoxication and blood alcohol levels, but the degree of intoxication does not parallel the descending limb of the function that relates intoxication and blood alcohol levels. Blood alcohol levels remain high long after the intoxication disappears.* [Modified with permission from Ekman G, Frankenhaeuser M, Goldberg L, Hagdahl R, Myrsten AL. Subjective and objective effects of alcohol as functions of dosage and time. Psychopharmacologia, 1964, (6), 399–409.]

Abuse and Alcoholism (Table 6.7). Binge drinking remains a major problem among college students. Although there has been a 16% decrease in college binge drinking in the U.S. over the past 20 years, absolute numbers remain high, with 36% of college students reporting binge drinking in the 2 weeks prior to the survey (five or more drinks in a row) as outlined by the 2012 Monitoring the Future national survey results. Such binge drinking is associated with serious consequences, ranging from serious injury to death. The health and psychosocial consequences range from motor vehicle accidents, legal problems, blackouts, and missing classes to date rape, other types of violence, and unwanted or unprotected sex, with resulting problems such as sexually transmitted diseases. Binge drinking between the ages of 10 and 21 is more likely to progress to alcohol abuse or dependence, with earlier excessive drinking increasing the probability of later problems (Table 6.8; see Chapter 1).

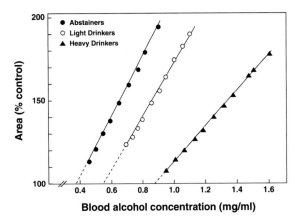

FIGURE 6.6   Performance on the "finger-finger" test (in which subjects must touch the tip of the left index finger to the tip of the right index finger at arm's length) as a function of blood alcohol concentration in abstainers, light drinkers, and heavy drinkers. The non-overlapping lines were described as evidence of tolerance to the motor-incoordinating effects of alcohol. *These data show dose-dependent chronic tolerance to a motor measure of intoxication in humans. For the heavy drinkers, it takes over twice the blood alcohol level to produce the same amount of impairment as observed in abstainers. [Taken with permission from Goldberg L. Quantitative studies on alcohol tolerance in man.* Acta Physiologica Scandinavica Supplementum, *1943, (5), 1–128.]*

TABLE 6.7   Alcohol Use Definitions

Term	Definition
Current use	At least one drink in the past 30 days (includes binge and heavy use).
Binge use	Five or more drinks on the same occasion at least once in the past 30 days. A pattern of drinking that brings blood alcohol concentration to 0.08 gm% or above. For the typical adult, this pattern corresponds to consuming five or more drinks (male), or four or more drinks (female), in about two hours.
Heavy use	Five or more drinks on the same occasion on at least five different days in the past 30 days.
Drink	A 12 ounce can or bottle of beer or wine cooler, a 5 ounce glass of wine, or 1.5 ounces of 80 proof (40% alcohol) distilled spirits.

Source: Substance Abuse and Mental Health Services Administration. Results from the 2002 National Survey on Drug Use and Health: National Findings (Office of Applied Statistics, NHSDA Series H-22, DHHS publication no. SMA 03–3836). Rockville MD, 2003; National Institute on Alcohol Abuse and Alcoholism. State of the Science Report on the Effects of Moderate Drinking. National Institute on Alcohol Abuse and Alcoholism, Bethesda, 2004.

Alcohol can also be extremely toxic when high doses are consumed acutely or chronically or when ingested during pregnancy. Overdoses occur under situations of binge drinking or simply by accident, fostered by ignorance of its potential toxicity. Numerous examples can be given of young people who overdose at parties, especially when engaging in challenges or games that involve drinking excessively (see Box 6.4). In 2009, nearly 32% (over 650,000) of all drug-related emergency room visits involved alcohol. The US Drug Abuse Warning Network reported that nearly 200,000 of these alcohol-related emergency room visits were made by people under the age of 21. Others have estimated that over 1,400 students aged 18–24 and enrolled in 2- to 4-year colleges died due to alcohol-related unintentional injuries. Of the 8 million college students in the US, 25% drove under the influence of alcohol, and

remarkably, 37% rode with a drinking driver. Alcohol misuse-related damage is not limited to deaths and emergency room visits; it also extends to a wide range of individual and social consequences (Table 6.8). Half a million college students were unintentionally injured under the influence of alcohol, and an additional 100,000 were assaulted by another student who had been drinking.

Alcohol also facilitates sexual desire and sexual behavior by lessening a person's inhibitions, but alcohol at higher doses also impairs sexual performance. In males, taking small amounts of alcohol acutely has been associated with an increase in self-reported sexual arousal and a slight increase or decrease in sexual response measured by penile vasocongestion. However, higher doses of alcohol lead to substantial reductions in sexual arousal, measured by both self-report and penile vasocongestion, and an

TABLE 6.8   Potential Negative Consequences of College Student Drinking

Damage to self	academic impairment
	blackouts
	personal injury or death
	short-term and long-term physical illness
	unintended and unprotected sexual activity
	suicide
	sexual coercion/rape victimization
	impaired driving
	legal repercussions
	impaired athletic performance
Damage to other people	property damage and vandalism
	fights and interpersonal violence
	sexual violence
	hate-related incidents
	noise disturbances
Institutional costs	property damage
	student attrition
	loss of perceived academic rigor
	poor town relations
	added time demands and emotional strain on staff
	legal costs

From: Perkins HW. *Surveying the damage: a review of research on consequences of alcohol misuse in college populations.* Journal of Studies on Alcohol Supplement, *2002, (14), 91–100.*

impaired ability to ejaculate. Similar results for acute alcohol administration in females have been reported. Although many women reported that low-dose alcohol increases sexual pleasure, sexual arousal and the ability to achieve orgasm dose-dependently decreased with increases in blood alcohol levels. All of these effects reverse when the alcohol is cleared from the body.

Chronic alcohol use and alcoholism in males is associated with a higher frequency of sexual dysfunction. Individuals with alcoholism in outpatient treatment reported a three-fold higher prevalence of serious erectile dysfunction compared with individuals without alcoholism. Chronic alcohol use is associated with low testosterone and sperm count, smaller testes, feminization, and gynecomastia (increase in the size of the mammary glands in the breast).

Some of these effects can persist even with prolonged abstinence but ultimately are reversible. Alcoholism in women is associated with numerous sexual dysfunctions, including low sexual desire, lack of orgasm, contractions of the vagina that interfere with intercourse, and painful intercourse. They also said that alcohol relieved their sexual problems by relieving sexual inhibitions. Expectations of disinhibiting sexuality may serve as a motivation for drinking. Women with alcoholism also reported more guilt surrounding sexual behavior and sexuality than women without alcoholism. Thus, sexual dysfunction may be both the cause and result of high alcohol use in women.

Heavy alcohol consumption in women is also associated with menstrual dysfunction, including anovulation (a menstrual cycle occurs without ovulation), recurrent amenorrhea (the absence of a menstrual period), early menopause, and a higher incidence of spontaneous abortions. All of these effects may be related to hormonal changes in females that are caused by acute and chronic alcohol intake. Acute alcohol intoxication increased estradiol levels in both pre- and post-menopausal women. These alcohol-induced increases in estradiol and testosterone levels may be related to a decrease in the body's ability to catabolize steroids.

Contribution of Alcohol to Medical Diseases

Alcohol contributes to many major medical diseases, including liver damage, heart disease, and neurological disorders. Alcohol abuse and alcoholism account for 4.5% of worldwide disability-adjusted life years (DALYs), the number of years one loses from a working life expectancy, and these values increase to 6.7% in high-income countries (Box 6.6).

Chronic, high-dose alcohol can lead to fatty liver, alcoholic hepatitis, and ultimately cirrhosis of the liver. In such a diseased condition,

---

BOX 6.6

DISABILITY-ADJUSTED LIFE YEARS (DALYs)

The World Health Organization (WHO) provides a comprehensive framework for studying health risks that was developed for *The World Health Report 2002*, which presented estimates for the year 2000. An update for the year 2004 for 24 global risk factors has been provided. It uses updated information from WHO programs and scientific studies for both exposure data and the causal associations between risk exposure and disease and injury outcomes. The burden of disease attributable to risk factors is measured in terms of lost years of healthy life using the metric "disability-adjusted life year" (DALY). The DALY combines years of life lost due to premature death and years of healthy life lost due to illness and disability. Although there are many possible definitions of "health risk," it is defined in the report as "a factor that raises the probability of adverse health outcomes." The report focuses on selected risk factors that have global spread, for which data are available to estimate population exposures or distributions, and for which the means to reduce them are known. Five leading risk factors were identified in this report: childhood underweight, unsafe sex, alcohol use, unsafe water and sanitation, and high blood pressure. These were responsible for 25% of all deaths in the world and 20% of all DALYs. Reducing exposure to these risk factors would increase global life expectancy by nearly 5 years.

World Health Organization. Global Health Risks: Mortality and Burden of Disease Attributable to Selected Major Risks. World Health Organization, *Geneva, 2009.*

---

alcohol is used preferentially for fuel in the liver, displacing up to 90% of the liver's normal metabolic substrates. Acetaldehyde accumulates, alcohol-oxidizing activity increases, and alcohol dehydrogenase-mediated nicotinamide adenine dinucleotide reductase (NADH) accumulates. All of these metabolic effects can lead to hepatotoxicity. Alcoholic cirrhosis usually develops after more than a decade of heavy drinking. The amount of alcohol that can injure the liver varies greatly from person to person. In women, as few as two to three drinks per day have been linked with cirrhosis. In men, as few as three to four drinks per day are needed. The US National Institute on Alcohol Abuse and Alcoholism reported that liver cirrhosis was the 12th leading cause of death in 2009 (a total of 31,522 deaths). Of these cirrhosis deaths, 48% were directly attributable to alcohol.

Heavy drinking is also associated with increased mortality from heart disease. Alcohol can cause cardiomyopathy, which is decreased function of the heart muscle. Moderate drinking, in contrast, has been associated with beneficial effects on the cardiovascular system caused by increases in high-density lipoproteins (that is, "good cholesterol"). Heavy alcohol intake is also associated with cancers of the mouth, tongue, esophagus, liver, pancreas, pharynx, larynx, stomach, lung, colon, and rectum.

Alcohol and cancer vulnerability involve a powerful interaction with smoking, which is historically high among individuals with alcoholism. Over decades, the association between alcohol drinking and smoking has been high, as has the negative association between alcohol consumption and the likelihood to quit smoking. In 2000, the National Institute on Alcohol Abuse and Alcoholism reanalyzed data from its 1992 National Longitudinal Alcohol Epidemiology Survey. The total sample size was 42,862. The prevalence of smoking was 28% among lifetime abstainers from alcohol, 49% among light drinkers, and 73%

among heavy drinkers. According to this same survey, of the people with a lifetime history of alcohol abuse or dependence, 68% smoked, compared with 46% of people without these disorders.

Wernicke–Korsakoff Syndrome

Heavy drinking in people who also have thiamine deficiency, usually caused by poor nutrition, can lead to two neuropsychiatric disorders, one of which is reversible (Wernicke's encephalopathy) and the other is not (Korsakoff's psychosis). These syndromes are now considered a unitary disorder called Wernicke–Korsakoff syndrome. Wernicke's encephalopathy is characterized by a confusional state, ataxia, abnormal eye movements, blurred vision, double vision, nystagmus, and tremor. It is associated with a prolonged history of alcoholism with steady drinking and an inadequate nutritional state. The neurological syndrome (ataxia, opthalmoplegia, and nystagmus) can be reversed in its early stages by thiamine supplementation in the diet, but the learning and memory impairments respond more slowly and incompletely. Untreated Wernicke's encephalopathy leads to death in up to 20% of cases, and a large percentage (85%) of people who survive Wernicke's encephalopathy go on to develop Korsakoff's psychosis.

Korsakoff's psychosis is characterized by severe anterograde amnesia with intact retrograde memory (that is, memories prior to the onset of Korsakoff's remain intact). Other cognitive functions may be spared, but the amnesia is irreversible and is associated with actual loss of neurons in the brain, such as anterior portions of the diencephalon, including the paratenial nucleus, mesial temporal lobe structures, orbitofrontal cortices, nucleus basalis, basal forebrain structures, and the hippocampus.

Fetal Alcohol Syndrome

Alcohol has significant adverse effects on the developing embryo when mothers drink during pregnancy, and fetal alcohol exposure is the leading cause of mental retardation in the Western world. Originally described as fetal alcohol syndrome, this teratogenic syndrome is now recognized as part of a spectrum of detrimental effects due to alcohol, termed fetal alcohol spectrum disorder, which affects approximately 1% of live births in the United States. Fetal alcohol syndrome is diagnosed when the following are present: characteristic facial dysmorphology, growth restriction, and central nervous system/neurodevelopmental abnormalities. The effects on growth include prenatal growth deficiency, postnatal growth deficiency, and a low weight-to-height ratio. The characteristic facial features include short palpebral tissues between the upper and lower eyelids, maxillary hypoplasia (underdevelopment of the upper jaw), epicanthal folds from the nose to inner side of the eyebrow, a thin upper lip, and a flattened philtrum (the cleft from the nose to upper lip; Figure 6.7). Central nervous system anomalies include microcephaly (a smaller head compared with children of the same age and gender), developmental delays, intellectual disability, and neonatal problems. Fetal alcohol spectrum disorder describes a continuum of permanent birth defects caused by the maternal consumption of alcohol and refers to a complex pattern of behavioral or cognitive dysfunction, including learning difficulties, poor school performance, poor impulse control, problems relating to others, and deficits in language, abstract thinking, memory, attention, and judgment. Other disorders within this spectrum include alcohol-related neurodevelopmental disorders with only central nervous system abnormalities and alcohol-related birth defects with physical abnormalities (Box 6.7).

Factors such as the pattern and quantity of maternal drinking, stage of fetal development at the time of alcohol exposure, the use of other drugs, and sociobehavioral risk factors strongly

Fetal Alcohol Syndrome

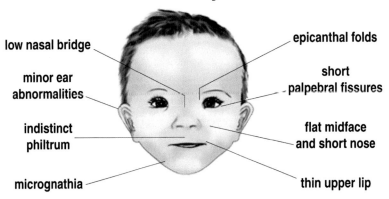

low nasal bridge

minor ear abnormalities

indistinct philtrum

micrognathia

epicanthal folds

short palpebral fissures

flat midface and short nose

thin upper lip

FIGURE 6.7 **Facial characteristics that are associated with fetal alcohol exposure.** *[Taken with permission from Warren KR, Hewitt BG, Thomas JD. Fetal alcohol spectrum disorders: research challenges and opportunities.* Alcohol Research and Health, *2011, (34), 4–14.]*

BOX 6.7

FETAL ALCOHOL SPECTRUM DISORDERS

This is an umbrella term that describes a range of effects that can occur in an individual whose mother drank alcohol during pregnancy. These effects may include physical, mental, behavioral, and/or learning disabilities with possible life-long implications. The term FASD is not intended for use as a clinical diagnosis (for further reading, see Warren KR, Hewitt BG, Thomas JD. Fetal alcohol spectrum disorders: research challenges and opportunities. *Alcohol Research and Health*, 2011, 34: 4–14).

Fetal Alcohol Syndrome

A diagnosis of full Fetal Alcohol Syndrome is made if the following three primary defining features are present:

- Documentation of characteristic facial abnormalities (smooth philtrum, thin vermillion border, and short palpebral fissures; see Figure 6.11)
- Documentation of prenatal and postnatal growth deficits
- Documentation of central nervous system abnormalities (i.e., structural, neurological, or behavioral, or a combination thereof).

---

influence the probability of developing fetal alcohol effects. The current recommendation of the Surgeon General of the United States is to drink no alcohol at all during pregnancy, because even small amounts of alcohol can lead to fetal alcohol spectrum disorder. According to the Institute of Medicine, 0.5 to 2.0 cases of fetal alcohol syndrome occur with every 1,000 live births in the United States. An epidemiological study conducted in

2000 found that the prevalence of fetal alcohol syndrome was 39.2 per 1,000 live births in the Western Cape Province of South Africa.

Low-Risk Drinking

Many would argue that no significant harm occurs with social drinking, sometimes referred to as "acceptable low-risk drinking"

BOX 6.8

ACCEPTABLE LOW-RISK DRINKING

Two different federal government definitions of acceptable low-risk drinking have been formulated:

1. US Dietary Guidelines, based on health and nutrition factors

   "No more than two drinks per day for a man, and no more than 14 drinks in a week (no saving drinks for another day), and for a female one drink per day/and no more than seven drinks per week." A drink is defined here as containing 14 grams of ethanol.

2. National Institute on Alcohol Abuse and Alcoholism (NIAAA) guidelines, based on longitudinal data from NIAAA's National Epidemiologic Study on Alcohol-Related Conditions (NESARC)

   "These guidelines suggest thresholds for the probability of transitioning to DSM-defined alcohol abuse or alcohol dependence. The NESARC data showed that the risk is minimal for men when they do not drink more than four drinks per day coupled with no more than 14 per week; and for women, no more than three drinks per day and seven drinks per week. Exceeding either of these daily or weekly limits increases the risk of transitioning to alcohol abuse or dependence (together now defined as Alcohol Use Disorder), especially when both the daily and weekly limits are exceeded."

(Box 6.8) with the exception of drinking during pregnancy. Indeed, significant evidence suggests beneficial effects from moderate amounts of alcohol, particularly in the form of red wine to reduce the risk of heart disease (for further reading, see Movva and Figueredo, 2013).

BEHAVIORAL MECHANISM OF ACTION

Sedative-hypnotic drugs in general and alcohol in particular produce a common behavioral action – disinhibition – that can explain many of their behavioral effects, from "social lubrication" to paradoxical rage reactions. At low to moderate doses (blood alcohol levels of 0.05–0.10 g%), alcohol disinhibits behavior (that is, individuals show a release of inhibitions in situations where they normally might be socially constrained). Alcohol is widely used at social events to promote conversation and social interaction; the "social lubricant" effect. This disinhibition is often mistaken for a psychostimulant effect. As a result, alcohol at lower doses is often mislabeled as a stimulant. To understand alcohol's well-documented aggression-promoting actions, one can look to benzodiazepines.

Benzodiazepines (tranquilizers) are sedative-hypnotic drugs that are commonly used to treat anxiety. They have long been known to produce a paradoxical rage reaction, reflected by aggression and impulsive behavior, presumably because of the disinhibited release of long-suppressed anger that only surfaces when the repression is lifted by the drug treatment. The disinhibition produced by alcohol is part of the classic continuum of behavioral effects of sedative-hypnotic drugs that relates behavioral effects to dose. Such disinhibition may also contribute to the use of alcohol as a form of self-medication.

The suffering of individuals with alcoholism has been hypothesized to be deeply rooted in disordered emotions characterized by unbearable and painful affect, a painful sense of emptiness, and an inability to express personal feelings that result in self-humiliation and frustration in interpersonal relationships (Box 6.9). Individuals who are cut off from their emotions will welcome repeated moderate doses of alcohol or depressants as medications to allow them to express feelings that they are usually unable to communicate (referred to as alexithymia). Such individuals are thus intrinsically vulnerable and exhibit deficits in how they care for themselves. They cannot control their behaviors and cannot contain what is repeatedly endangering their well-being, family, social relationships, and survival. Fundamentally, these individuals cannot adequately evaluate the consequences of dangers of the situation either rationally or emotionally, and they often exhibit fear, worry, and apprehension. In some cases, the individual seeks to relieve painful feelings or control his feelings. The paradox is that using alcohol to self-medicate emotional pain or a life out of control can perpetuate a life that revolves exclusively around alcohol, which, in turn, causes emotional pain caused by physiological consequences (withdrawal) and social consequences (neglect of responsibilities to family and work).

NEUROBIOLOGICAL EFFECTS

Molecular Site of Action for Alcohol: Ethanol-Receptive Elements

Alcohol does not bind to any given receptor in a classic steric or allosteric manner, in contrast to other drugs of abuse. It has, however, been shown to interact at the molecular level with specific neuronal elements, termed ethanol-receptive elements, to produce changes in specific synaptic targets at the cellular and system levels, resulting in its pharmacological effects (for further reading, see Harris et al., 2008). Low to moderate doses of alcohol (10–50 mM, which reflect blood alcohol levels of 0.04 to 0.2 g% from *in vivo* administration) have wide-ranging effects on the nervous system, acting directly on the GABA receptor complex, serotonin 5-HT$_3$ receptors, and glycine receptors and inhibiting glutamate receptors, potassium channels, G-proteins, and protein kinases (Figure 6.8). Alcohol is a small molecule with low binding energy compared with other drugs of abuse. This is reflected in the requirement for much higher doses of alcohol to produce intoxication (millimolar levels compared with nanomolar levels for other drugs, such as opioids and psychostimulants). These pharmacological characteristics of alcohol suggest that multiple alcohol-receptive sites in the brain are required to influence the structure and function of proteins, possibly via water-filled membrane pockets.

The way that alcohol affects specific protein-receptive pockets was first modeled using the LUSH protein in the *Drosophila* fruit fly. LUSH is an odorant binding protein that is used by the fly to sense alcohols and was purposefully named for its role in alcohol's effects. Short carbon-chain alcohols, such as ethanol, bind at only a single site in the LUSH protein, and this binding dramatically stabilizes the protein. In a separate study, pharmacologically relevant concentrations of ethanol stabilized the opening of a ligand-gated ion channel of a bacterial variant homolog of GABA and glycine receptors. Crystal structures of the alcohol-sensitized variant showed that alcohol binds to a transmembrane hydrophilic cavity between channel subunits and may stabilize the open form of the channel (Figure 6.9). This type of cavity may be preserved in human alcohol-sensitive glycine and GABA$_A$ receptors, suggesting a structural basis for what have previously been termed ethanol-receptive elements.

BOX 6.9

I DRANK

I drank Fumé Blanc at the Ritz-Carlton Hotel, and I drank double shots of Johnnie Walker Black on the rocks at a dingy Chinese restaurant across the street from my office, and I drank at home. For a long time I drank expensive red wine, and I learned to appreciate the subtle differences between a silky Merlot and a tart Cabernet Sauvignon and a soft, earthy Beaucastel from the south of France, but I never really cared about those nuances because, honestly, they were beside the point. Toward the end I kept two bottles of Cognac in my house: the bottle for show, which I kept on the counter, and the real bottle, which I kept in the back of a cupboard beside an old toaster. The level of liquid in the show bottle was fairly consistent, decreasing by an inch or so, perhaps less, each week. The liquid in the real bottle disappeared quickly, sometimes within days. I was living alone at the time when I did this, but I did it anyway and it didn't occur to me not to: it was always important to maintain appearances.

I drank when I was happy and I drank when I was anxious and I drank when I was bored and I drank when I was depressed, which was often. I started to raid my parents' liquor cabinet the year my father was dying. He'd be in the back of their house in Cambridge, lying in the hospital bed in their bedroom, and I'd steal into the front hall bathroom and pull out a bottle of Old Grand-dad that I'd hidden behind the toilet. It tasted vile – the bottle must have been fifteen years old – but my father was dying, dying very slowly and gradually from a brain tumor, so I drank it anyway and it helped.

A love story. Yes: this is a love story.

It's about passion, sensual pleasure, deep pulls, lust, fears, yearning hungers. It's about needs so strong they're crippling. It's about saying good-bye to something you can't fathom living without.

I loved the way drink made me feel, and I loved its special power of deflection, its ability to shift my focus away from my own awareness of self and onto something else, something less painful than my own feelings. I loved the sounds of drink: the slide of a cork as it eased out of a wine bottle, the distinct glug-glug of booze pouring into a glass, the clatter of ice cubes in a tumbler. I loved the rituals, the camaraderie of drinking with others, the warming, melting feelings of ease and courage it gave me.

Our introduction was not dramatic; it wasn't love at first sight, I don't even remember my first taste of alcohol. The relationship developed gradually, over many years, time punctuated by separations and reunions. Anyone who's ever shifted from general affection and enthusiasm for a lover to outright obsession knows what I mean: the relationship is just there, occupying a small corner of your heart, and then you wake up one morning and some indefinable tide has turned forever and you can't go back – You need it; it's a central part of who you are.

Still, I look in the mirror sometimes and think, "What happened?" I have the CV of a model citizen or a gifted child, not a common drunk. Hometown: Cambridge, Massachusetts, backyard of Harvard University. Education: Brown University, class of '81, magna cum laude. Parents: esteemed psychoanalyst (dad) and artist (mom), both devoted and insightful and keenly intelligent.

In other words, nice person, from a good, upper-middle-class family. I look and I think, "What *happened?*"

Of course, there is no simple answer. Trying to describe the process of becoming an alcoholic

Continued

BOX 6.9 *(cont'd)*

is like trying to describe air. It's too big and mysterious and pervasive to be defined. Alcohol is everywhere in your life, omnipresent, and you're both aware and unaware of it almost all the time; all you know is you'd die without it, and there is no simple reason why this happens, no single moment, no physiological event that pushes a heavy drinker across a concrete line into alcoholism. It's a slow, gradual, insidious, elusive *becoming.*

When you love somebody, or something, it's amazing how willing you are to overlook the flaws. Around that same time, in my thirties, I started to notice that tiny blood vessels had burst all along my nose and cheeks. I started to dry-heave in the mornings, driving to work in my car. A tremor in my hands developed, then grew worse, then persisted for longer periods, all day sometimes.

I did my best to ignore all this. I struggled to ignore it, the way a woman hears coldness in a lover's voice and struggles, mightily and knowingly, to misread it.

The phrase is *high-functioning alcoholic.* Smooth and ordered on the outside; roiling and chaotic and desperately secretive underneath, but not noticeably so, never noticeably so. I remember sitting down in my cubicle that morning, my leg propped up on a chair, and thinking: *I wonder if she knows. I wonder if anyone can tell by looking at me that something is wrong.* I used to wonder that a lot, that last year or two of drinking –*Something is different about me,* I'd think, sitting in an editorial meeting and looking around at everyone else, at their clear eyes and well-rested expressions. *Can anybody see it?* The wondering itself made me anxious, chipping away at the edges of denial.

Perception versus reality. Outside versus inside. I never missed a day of work because of

drinking, never called in sick, never called it quits and went home early because of a hangover. But inside I was falling apart. The discrepancy was huge.

Beneath my own witty, professional façade were oceans of fear, whole rivers of self-doubt. I once heard alcoholism described in an AA meeting, with eminent simplicity, as "fear of life." and that seemed to sum up the condition quite nicely. I, for example, had spent half my professional life as a reporter who lived in secret terror of the most basic aspects of the job, of picking up the phone and calling up strangers to ask questions. Inside, I harbored a long list of qualities that made my own skin crawl: a basic fragility; a feeling of hypersensitivity to other peoples' reactions, as though some piece of my soul might crumble if you looked at me the wrong way; a sense of being essentially inferior and unprotected and scared. Feelings of fraudulence are familiar to scores of people in and out of the working world – the highly effective, well-defended exterior cloaking the small, insecure person inside – but they're epidemic among alcoholics. You hide behind the professional persona all day; then you leave the office and hide behind the drink.

Sometimes, in small flashes, I'd be aware of this. One night after work, on my way to a bar to meet a friend for drinks, a sentence popped into my head. I thought: *This is the real me, this person driving in the car.* I was anxious. My teeth were clenched, partly from spending a long day hunched over the computer and partly from the physical sensation of wanting a drink badly, and I was aware of an undercurrent of fear deep in my gut, a barely definable sensation that the ground beneath my feet wasn't solid or real. I think I understood in that instant that I'd created two versions of myself: the working version, who sat at the desk and pounded away at

---

BOX 6.9 *(cont'd)*

---

the keyboard, and the restaurant version, who sat at a table and pounded away at white wine. In between, for five or ten minutes at a stretch, the real version would emerge: the fearful version, tense and dishonest and uncertain. I rarely allowed her to emerge for long. Work – all that productive, effective, focused work – kept her distracted and submerged during the day. And drink – anesthetizing and constant – kept her too numb to feel at night.

My reflection in the mirror looked awful: my skin was pale and my face was drawn and I had large dark circles under my eyes. I had on a scoop-necked sweater and I could see little burst blood vessels all over my chest, red marks that looked like the beginnings of a rash. My twin sister Becca, a doctor, would see those periodically and tell me she thought they were alcohol related, and I always thought. *Nonsense: they're from too much sun, back when I was younger.* In any event, I looked like hell, and somewhere inside I understood that if I kept this up, kept drinking and working and flailing around like this, I'd die, slowly, but literally kill myself.

Around the time that Wicky died, I started taking those little quizzes about drug and alcohol abuse that you sometimes find in women's magazines or pamphlets at the doctor's office, and I started answering a lot of the questions positively. Do you find yourself having a drink or two before you go to a party where you know alcohol will be served, just to "get yourself in the mood?" Yes. Do you find yourself gulping drinks? Um … check. Do you drink more when you're under stress? Sure. But some of the questions seemed a little obvious, even kind of stupid. Do you drink alone? Well, of course I drink alone; I *live* alone. What kind of a question is that?

The knowledge that some people can have enough while you never can is the single most compelling piece of evidence for a drinker to suggest that alcoholism is, in fact, a disease, that it has powerful physiological roots, that the alcoholic's body simply responds differently to liquor than a nonalcoholic's. Once I started to drink, I simply did not know how or when to stop: the feeling of need kicked in, so pervasively that stopping didn't feel like an option. My friend Bill explains it this way to his mother, who has a hard time wrapping her mind around the disease concept of alcoholism and who holds fast to the belief that he could have controlled his drinking if only he'd exerted enough will. He says, "Mom, next time you have diarrhea, try controlling *that*." Crude, perhaps, but he gets the point across.

The need is more than merely physical: it's psychic and visceral and multilayered. There's a dark fear to the feeling of wanting that wine, that vodka, that bourbon: a hungry, abiding fear of being without, being exposed, without your armor. In meetings you often hear people say that, by definition, an addict is someone who seeks physical solutions to emotional or spiritual problems. I suppose that's an intellectual way of describing that brand of fear, and the instinctive response that accompanies it: there's a sense of deep need, and the response is a grabbiness, a compulsion to latch on to something outside yourself in order to assuage some deep discomfort.

And there it was again, the connection: Repression + Drink = Openness. At heart, alcoholism feels like the accumulation of dozens of such connections, dozens of tiny fears and hungers and rages, dozens of experiences and memories that collect in the bottom of your soul, coalescing over many many many drinks into a single liquid solution.

Continued

You drink long and hard enough and your life gets messy. Your relationships (with nondrinkers, with yourself) become strained. Your work suffers. You run into financial trouble, or legal trouble, or trouble with the police. Rack up enough pain and the old math – Discomfort + Drink = No Discomfort – ceases to suffice; feeling "comfortable" isn't good enough anymore.

You're after something deeper than a respite from shyness, or a break from private fears and anger. So after a while you alter the equation, make it stronger and more complete. Pain + Drink = Self-Obliteration.

From: Knapp C, Drinking: A Love Story, Dial Press, New York, 1996.

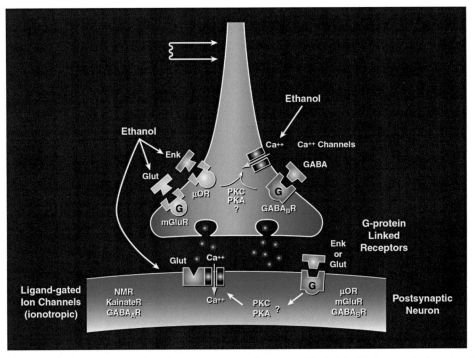

FIGURE 6.8   **Probable synaptic sites of alcohol action in central neurons.** Alcohol facilitates γ-aminobutyric acid (GABA) release in the nucleus accumbens, ventral tegmental area, and central nucleus of the amygdala, and these actions may be mediated in some cases by presynaptic $GABA_B$ receptors. In chronic alcohol-treated animals, GABA release increases at some of these sites. Alcohol acutely inhibits the release of glutamate in both the nucleus accumbens and central nucleus of the amygdala, possibly through metabotropic glutamate (Glut) receptors (mGluR), μ opioid receptors (μOR), or calcium (Ca^{2+}) channels. In chronic alcohol-treated animals, an increase in release is observed. Enk, enkephalin; PKA, protein kinase A; PKC, protein kinase C.

One classic action of alcohol is that it potentiates GABA-gated currents by activating GABA-mediated chloride ion uptake by the GABA-benzodiazepine ionophore complex. Some researchers have argued that the actions of alcohol on the GABA-benzodiazepine ionophore complex are GABA receptor subunit-dependent. Alcohol may require the presence of the α4β1δ, α4β3δ, α6β3δ, and δ subunits. Other extra-synaptic GABA receptors that are composed of α4β3δ subunits in some cells have been hypothesized to be the primary targets for alcohol in the GABA receptor systems that facilitate alcohol's effects on sleep, anxiety, memory, and cognition. However, total knockout of any of these specific GABA receptor subunits does not dramatically change alcohol sensitivity.

Another mechanism by which receptors and ion channels are modulated by alcohol occurs via changes in protein kinase phosphorylation (that is, turning the functions of proteins on and off). Alcohol facilitates protein kinase Cγ (PKCγ)-mediated phosphorylation and inhibits PKCε-mediated phosphorylation. PKCγ knockout mice are less sensitive to alcohol's effects on $GABA_A$ receptors, while PKCε knockout mice are more sensitive to alcohol's effects on $GABA_A$ receptors (for further reading, see Ron and Messing, 2013). Alcohol also inhibits adenosine reuptake by inhibiting equilibrative nucleoside transporter-1, which increases extracellular adenosine levels and activates adenosine A_2 receptors. This activation, in turn, activates the cyclic adenosine monophosphate (cAMP) response element binding protein (CREB) system via the cAMP-PKA second-messenger system. Thus, alcohol has two notable direct and sensitive molecular effects: to change ion channel function and to modify signal transduction pathways to alter neurotransmitter function, again presumably via water-filled membrane pockets that change protein function. How such molecular actions actually translate to the release of endogenous transmitters that are

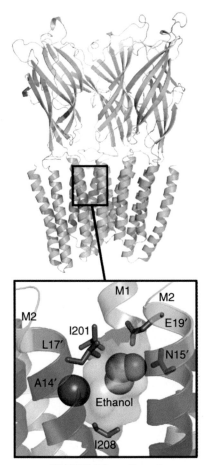

GLIC F14'A + ethanol

FIGURE 6.9 **X-ray structures of wildtype and alcohol-sensitized GLIC, in which GLIC F140A mutant co-crystallized with alcohol (Protein Data Bank ID 4HFE).** The GLIC receptor is a bacterial (*Gloeobacter violaceus*) Ligand-gated Ion Channel, homologous to brain ligand-gated ion channels, such as γ-aminobutyric acid-A ($GABA_A$) receptors and nicotinic acetylcholine receptors. GLIC is a protein-gated, cation-selective channel. Like nicotinic acetylcholine receptors, it is a functional pentameric oligomer. The blow-up of the small box shows the binding cavity in the protein that contains ethanol (orange and red spheres). The complete GLIC pentameric protein complex is shown above the box. GLIC was mutated by changing one amino acid, F (phenylalanine), to A (alanine), at the 14' position in the protein. The other letters and numbers represent the amino acids at specific positions. M indicates a membrane-spanning section of the protein. [*Taken with permission from Sauguet L, Howard RJ, Malherbe L, Lee US, Corringer PJ, Harris RA, Delarue M. Structural basis for potentiation by alcohols and anesthetics in a ligand-gated ion channel.* Nature Communications, *2013, (4), 1697.*]

known to cause intoxication remains an area to be explored in the alcohol research field.

Binge/Intoxication Stage

Neurocircuitry Mechanisms

Alcohol-induced disinhibition in humans can be modeled in animals by evaluating the anti-stress or anti-anxiety (anxiolytic) effects of alcohol. The anti-anxiety and tension-reducing-like properties of alcohol have been demonstrated in various behavioral situations in animals. An early observation in 1946 illustrated the effects of alcohol on "neurotic"-like behavior induced in cats in a conflict situation. The cats were trained to run down an alley and open a box to obtain food when signaled by a bell-light conditioned stimulus. The "conflict" arose when a blast of air accompanied the food delivery at irregular intervals. The animals subsequently developed bizarre, neurotic-like behaviors, such as inhibition of feeding, startle reflexes, phobic responses, and aversive behavior in response to stimuli associated with the food/air blast conditioned stimuli. Alcohol significantly reduced this neurotic-like behavior. The cats showed a restoration of simpler responses and an attenuation of phobias, motor disturbances, and other abnormal behaviors. Nonetheless, alcohol also disrupted the timing, spatial orientation, sequence, and efficiency of normal goal-oriented responses. This early study elaborated many of the features of alcohol's effect on conflict behavior, notably the ability of alcohol to block or reduce the suppression of behavior induced by punishment and decrease unpunished behavior, often at the same time or at the same doses.

Similarly to benzodiazepines and barbiturates, alcohol dose-dependently increases punished responding in the Geller–Seifter conflict test, in which the animals learn to press a lever for food or some other reward. After they are trained, each reward delivery is accompanied by an aversive stimulus, such as a mild footshock

or puff of air (see Chapter 3). Alcohol increases the number and/or intensity of aversive stimuli that the animal will endure. Alcohol exerts anxiolytic-like effects in several animal models of anxiety, including the lick suppression test, social interaction test, elevated plus maze, and behavioral contrast test (see Chapter 3).

In animals, alcohol has similar reinforcing effects to that in humans. Early paradigms that assessed the reinforcing effects of alcohol typically used an oral preference paradigm, in which animals were allowed to drink alcohol or water. A later approach was the development of a training procedure that involved access to a sweetened solution and subsequent fading in of alcohol to temper alcohol's naturally aversive taste. When the sweetness was finally faded out of the solution, the rats readily self-administered alcohol, resulting in blood alcohol levels of 0.04–0.08 g% (see Chapter 3). In both procedures, rodents appear to readily learn to associate the ingestion of alcohol with psychotropic effects and to negate the aversive taste effects.

The use of animal models of the acute reinforcing effects of alcohol and selective receptor antagonists for specific neurochemical systems has shown that alcohol at intoxicating doses has wide but selective actions on neurotransmitter systems in the brain reward systems. Neuropharmacological studies have implicated multiple neurochemical systems in the acute reinforcing effects of alcohol, including GABA, opioid peptides, dopamine, serotonin, and glutamate (Figure 6.10). Systemic injections of $GABA_A$ receptor antagonists reversed the motor-impairing effects of alcohol, anxiolytic-like effects of alcohol, and alcohol drinking. The opioid antagonist naltrexone decreased alcohol self-administration in various animal models, suggesting a role for endogenous opioid peptide systems in the reinforcing effects of alcohol. Such studies led to the clinical use of naltrexone for reducing alcohol consumption and preventing relapse (Figure 6.11).

Neurochemical Neurocircuits in Drug Reward
Alcohol

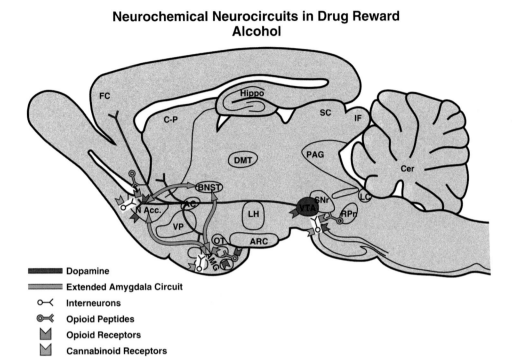

Dopamine

Extended Amygdala Circuit

o—< **Interneurons**

⊙—< **Opioid Peptides**

⋈ **Opioid Receptors**

⋈ **Cannabinoid Receptors**

⋈ **GABA_A Receptors**

FIGURE 6.10 **Sagittal section through a representative rodent brain that illustrates the pathways and receptor systems implicated in the acute reinforcing actions of alcohol.** Alcohol activates γ-aminobutyric acid-A (GABA_A) receptors in the ventral tegmental area, nucleus accumbens, and amygdala via either direct actions at the GABA_A receptor or through the indirect release of GABA. Alcohol is hypothesized to facilitate the release of opioid peptides in the ventral tegmental area, nucleus accumbens, and central nucleus of the amygdala. Alcohol facilitates the release of dopamine (*red*) in the nucleus accumbens via an action either in the ventral tegmental area or nucleus accumbens. Endogenous cannabinoids and adenosine may interact with postsynaptic elements in the nucleus accumbens, involving dopamine and/or opioid peptide systems. The blue arrows represent the interactions within the extended amygdala system hypothesized to play a key role in alcohol reinforcement. AC, anterior commissure; AMG, amygdala; ARC, arcuate nucleus; BNST, bed nucleus of the stria terminalis; Cer, cerebellum; C-P, caudate-putamen; DMT, dorsomedial thalamus; FC, frontal cortex; Hippo, hippocampus; IF, inferior colliculus; LC, locus coeruleus; LH, lateral hypothalamus; N Acc., nucleus accumbens; OT, olfactory tract; PAG, periaqueductal gray; RPn, reticular pontine nucleus; SC, superior colliculus; SNr, substantia nigra pars reticulata; VP, ventral pallidum; VTA, ventral tegmental area. *[Taken with permission from Koob GF, Le Moal M. Neurobiology of Addiction. Academic Press, London, 2006.]*

The mesocorticolimbic dopamine system also participates in the reinforcing properties of alcohol. Systemic injections of dopamine receptor antagonists decrease responding for alcohol. Alcohol self-administration increases extracellular levels of dopamine in the nucleus accumbens in nondependent rats (Figure 6.12). Such increases not only occur during the actual self-administration session but also precede the self-administration session, possibly reflecting the incentive motivational properties of environmental cues associated with alcohol. Mesocorticolimbic dopamine, however, does not appear to be critical for the acute reinforcing effects of alcohol. Lesions of the mesocorticolimbic dopamine system in rats failed to block operant alcohol self-administration. The modulation of various other aspects of monoamine

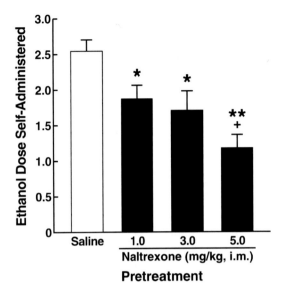

FIGURE 6.11 **Effects of saline (0.9% NaCl, 1.0 ml, i.m.) or naltrexone (1.0, 3.0, or 5.0 mg/kg, i.m.) on intravenous alcohol self-administration over a 4 h session in rhesus monkeys.** Each bar represents the mean alcohol intake for all animals and all days of pretreatment with a given naltrexone dose or saline. All doses of naltrexone were associated with alcohol intake below saline levels (*$p < 0.05$, compared with saline; **$p < 0.01$, compared with saline). The differences between the effects of 1.0 and 3.0 mg/kg naltrexone were not significant, but the effects of 5.0 mg/kg differed significantly from the 1.0 and 3.0 mg/kg doses (+$p < 0.05$). *These data show that naltrexone injected intramuscularly in rhesus monkeys dose-dependently decreased intravenous alcohol self-administration. Such early studies ultimately led to the use of naltrexone as a medication to treat alcoholism (see Chapter 9).* [Taken with permission from Altshuler HL, Phillips PE, Feinhandler DA. Alteration of ethanol self-administration by naltrexone. Life Sciences, 1980, (26), 679–688.]

transmission can also decrease alcohol intake, including increases in the synaptic availability of serotonin with precursor loading, the blockade of serotonin reuptake, and the antagonism of serotonin 5-HT$_3$ and 5-HT$_2$ receptors (for further reading, see Koob, 2003).

The neuroanatomical substrates for the reinforcing actions of alcohol involve the same ventral striatal neurocircuitry and extended amygdala circuitry as elaborated for psychostimulants and opioids. Very low doses of the dopamine receptor antagonist fluphenazine injected directly into the nucleus accumbens block alcohol self-administration at low doses (Figure 6.13). A potent GABA$_A$ receptor antagonist, SR 95531, when microinjected into the nucleus accumbens, bed nucleus of the stria terminalis, and central nucleus of the amygdala, reduced alcohol intake, with the most sensitive site being the central nucleus of the amygdala (Figure 6.14). Injections of an opioid receptor antagonist into the nucleus accumbens, ventral tegmental area, and central nucleus of the amygdala also reduced alcohol consumption, suggesting a role for opioid peptides in both the ventral striatum and extended amygdala in the acute reinforcing actions of alcohol (Figure 6.15).

Cellular Mechanisms of Intoxication

The action of alcohol at the cellular level is based on the premise that alcohol has a specific action on synaptic transmission, and the synapse is hypothesized to be one of the most sensitive sites for alcohol's action. This hypothesis originated in part from early electrophysiological studies that showed a greater effect of alcohol in multisynaptic pathways than in monosynaptic pathways. Cellular studies of brain slices of the ventral striatum and extended amygdala supported this hypothesis. The neurotransmitter systems that have been the most studied at the cellular level are GABA and glutamate. For example, in the extended amygdala, alcohol has been shown to directly facilitate GABA function by enhancing GABA release in rats and mice. In contrast, alcohol has powerful glutamate antagonist effects.

Alcohol at intoxicating doses also activates neurons in the ventral tegmental area. At least part of this activation was shown to occur via a direct action on dopaminergic neurons in the ventral tegmental area. Acetaldehyde, a product of alcohol metabolism, also activates dopamine neuronal activity in the ventral tegmental area and may contribute to the reinforcing effects of

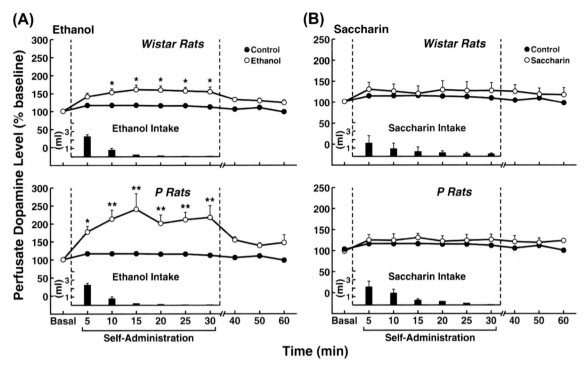

FIGURE 6.12   (A) Effects of oral alcohol self-administration on dopamine release in the nucleus accumbens in genetically heterogeneous Wistar rats ($n = 11$) and alcohol-preferring (P) rats ($n = 9$). Data from both strains are contrasted against the same control group ($n = 9$), consisting of alcohol-naive Wistar and P rats trained to respond for water only. Alcohol significantly increased dopamine release in both groups of rats (Wistar rats: *$p < 0.01$; P rats: *$p < 0.05$, **$p < 0.01$). The insets show the mean $\pm$ SEM alcohol intake per 5 min interval. (B) Dopamine release in the nucleus accumbens in Wistar rats ($n = 4$) and P rats ($n = 4$) that responded to saccharin reinforcement. The data for both strains are contrasted against the same control group that consisted of saccharin-naive Wistar and P rats trained to respond for water. Saccharin produced only negligible increases in dopamine efflux compared with alcohol. *These data show that alcohol self-adminstration in rats can increase the release of dopamine in the nucleus accumbens, an effect produced by its pharmacological effects. Notice, however, that the increase in the release of dopamine was greater in the alcohol-preferring rats than in the outbred Wistar strain of rats. Saccharin produced similar amounts of self-administration and had no significant effect on dopamine release in the nucleus accumbens.* [Taken with permission from Weiss F, Lorang MT, Bloom FE, Koob GF. Oral alcohol self-administration stimulates dopamine release in the rat nucleus accumbens: genetic and motivational determinants. Journal of Pharmacology and Experimental Therapeutics, 1993, (267), 250–258.].

alcohol. Other studies have identified non-dopaminergic, alcohol-sensitive neurons in the ventral tegmental area, including GABA neurons. Acute alcohol administration at doses within the intoxicating range decreased the spontaneous activity of ventral tegmental area GABAergic neurons, suggesting the possibility of both disinhibitory mechanisms and direct effects on dopaminergic neurons.

Molecular Genetic Approaches Using Knockout Models

Many molecular genetic knockouts have been studied. Alcohol-drinking mouse models have been identified using two-bottle choice drinking and operant responding for alcohol (see Chapter 3). The knockout of several different neurotransmitters, modulators, receptors, and other molecules decreases drinking behavior

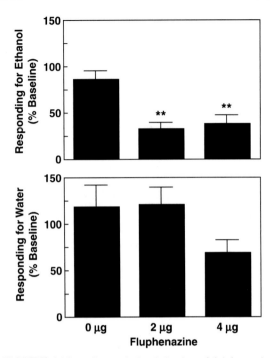

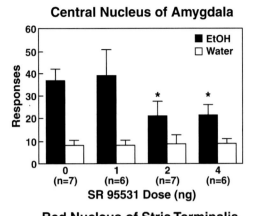

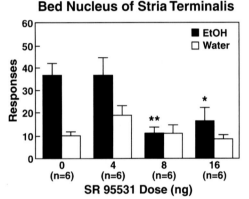

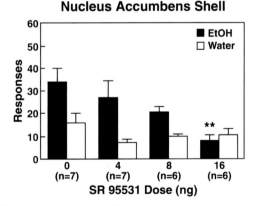

FIGURE 6.13 **Effects of microinjection of the dopamine antagonist fluphenazine into the nucleus accumbens in rats on responding for alcohol (10% w/v) and water.** The data are expressed as the mean percentage of baseline responding and are plotted as a function of fluphenazine dose. Asterisks (**) indicate a significant difference in responding compared with responding after vehicle injection ($p < 0.01$). *These data show that a dopamine D_2 receptor antagonist injected into the nucleus accumbens dose-dependently decreased alcohol self-administration, suggesting a key role for dopamine release in the nucleus accumbens in the rewarding effects of alcohol. [Taken with permission from Rassnick S, Pulvirenti L, Koob GF. Oral ethanol self-administration in rats is reduced by the administration of dopamine and glutamate receptor antagonists into the nucleus accumbens.* Psychopharmacology, *1992, (109), 92–98.]*

and the preference for alcohol, contributing to a detailed symphony of brain systems that contribute to the acute reinforcing effects of alcohol. For example, μ opioid receptor knockout mice do not self-administer alcohol. The knockout of cannabinoid CB_1 and δ opioid receptors, neuropeptide Y (NPY) and NPY_1 receptors, and PKA, among others, increases alcohol drinking. This complex interplay provides clues to the systems

FIGURE 6.14 **The effect of γ-aminobutyric acid-A receptor antagonist SR 95531 injections into the central nucleus of the amygdala, bed nucleus of the stria terminalis, and shell of the nucleus accumbens on responding for alcohol and water in rats.** The data are expressed as the mean number of responses for alcohol and water during 30 min sessions for each injection site. Notice the change

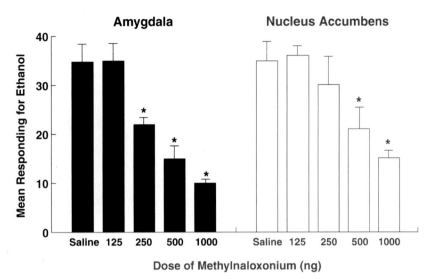

FIGURE 6.15 **The effects of intracerebral administration of the opioid receptor antagonist methylnaloxonium into the amygdala and nucleus accumbens on responding for alcohol in rats.** The data are expressed as the mean total responses. Asterisks (*) indicate significant differences from saline injections ($p < 0.05$). *These data show that the opioid receptor antagonist methylnaloxonium injected into the central nucleus of the amygdala and nucleus accumbens dose-dependently decreased alcohol self-administration. Notice that the most potent effects were observed with the injections into the central nucleus of the amygdala (250 ng was a significant dose), suggesting a key role for opioid peptide activity in the central nucleus of the amygdala in the rewarding effects of alcohol. [Modified with permission from Heyser CJ, Roberts AJ, Schulteis G, Koob GF. Central administration of an opiate antagonist decreases oral ethanol self-administration in rats.* Alcoholism: Clinical and Experimental Research, *1999, (23), 1468–1476.]*

in which inhibition may contribute to the reinforcing effects of alcohol (for further reading, see Crabbe et al., 2006).

in the abscissa scale for injections into the bed nucleus of the stria terminalis and nucleus accumbens shell. Significant differences from corresponding saline control values: *$p < 0.05$, **$p < 0.01$, for ethanol responses; #$p < 0.05$, for water responses. *These data show that a highly potent GABA$_A$ receptor antagonist injected into the central nucleus of the amygdala, bed nucleus of the stria terminalis, and nucleus accumbens dose-dependently decreased alcohol self-administration. Notice that the most potent effects were observed with the injections into the central nucleus of the amygdala (2 ng was a significant dose), suggesting a key role for GABA activity in the central nucleus of the amygdala in the rewarding effects of alcohol. [Taken with permission from Hyytia P, Koob GF. GABA$_A$ receptor antagonism in the extended amygdala decreases ethanol self-administration in rats.* European Journal of Pharmacology, *1995, (283), 151–159.]*

Withdrawal/Negative Affect Stage

Alcohol Tolerance

Metabolic tolerance can account for some of the resistance of the brain to alcohol, as noted above. Early animal studies, however, also showed that rats treated chronically with alcohol had higher brain levels of alcohol than control animals at the time of recovery from overt intoxication, arguing for pharmacodynamic tolerance (see Chapter 1). In rodents, chronic functional tolerance has been measured by changes in the sedative effects of alcohol, usually reflected by the ability of the animal to perform a motor task, such as run on a treadmill or balance on a rotating rod. Behavioral factors, including learning, play a prominent role in the development of tolerance. Animals and humans can learn to counteract the effects of alcohol through Pavlovian or operant conditioning. For example, rats that were allowed to experience a treadmill task while intoxicated showed much more rapid and complete tolerance to alcohol than rats that were not allowed to experience the task while intoxicated but received alcohol after completion of the task.

Numerous neuropharmacological substrates are involved in behavioral tolerance as a model of the neuroadaptive processes associated with the development of pharmacodynamic tolerance. These include serotonin, glutamate, and vasopressin. Blockade of the activity of any of these systems blocks acute and chronic tolerance. A neural circuit that involves these neurotransmitters and connections between the septum and hippocampus has been proposed to play an essential role in the development and retention of tolerance (for further reading, see Kalant, 1998).

Alcohol Withdrawal and Dependence

In rodents, alcohol withdrawal is characterized by irritability, hyper-responsiveness, abnormal motor responses, anxiety-like responses, and decreased reward, all similar to the human condition. Seizures can also occur at high doses. At high doses, alcohol withdrawal signs in rats become maximal after 3–4 days. The anxiety-like responses and seizures can be "kindled" (that is, they increase with repeated withdrawal; Figure 6.16).

The neurobiological basis for the motivational effects of alcohol withdrawal, in which individuals engage in alcohol-seeking behavior during withdrawal, extends the neuroadaptive concept described above for tolerance to include counteradaptive neurochemical events within the brain's emotional systems that are normally used to maintain emotional homeostasis (see Chapter 1). Acute alcohol withdrawal compromises brain reward systems, reflected by an elevation in brain reward thresholds (that is, more electrical current is needed for the animal to perceive the stimulation as rewarding),

which is opposite to the threshold-lowering effect of acute alcohol exposure. Rats that are made dependent on alcohol using alcohol vapor or a liquid diet, resulting in blood alcohol levels greater than $0.1\,g\%$, exhibit elevations in reward thresholds during withdrawal from alcohol. This effect has been shown to persist up to 72 h after alcohol exposure (Figure 6.17).

Decreases in neurotransmitter function in the ventral striatum and extended amygdala (e.g., GABA, enkephalins, endorphins, dopamine, and serotonin) associated with the acute reinforcing effects of alcohol and increases in glutamatergic responses represent some of the neurochemical counteradaptations that are motivationally important in the development of alcohol dependence. Rats and mice will drink more and work more for alcohol during withdrawal after becoming dependent (see Chapter 3). Neuropharmacological studies have shown that the increase in alcohol self-administration during acute withdrawal can be dose-dependently reduced by intracerebral injections of $GABA_A$ receptor agonists. Acamprosate, a hypothesized partial agonist or antagonist of brain glutamate systems, also decreases excessive drinking associated with dependence and abstinence in rats (for further reading, see Koob et al., 2009).

Dopaminergic function is also compromised during acute alcohol withdrawal. Dependent animals have decreased extracellular dopamine levels in the nucleus accumbens (Figure 6.18). In contrast to the activation of dopaminergic systems during acute intoxication, dopaminergic activity decreases in the ventral tegmental area during withdrawal. This has been linked to the dysphoria associated with acute and protracted withdrawal. The decrease in dopaminergic activity in the ventral tegmental area is consistent with studies that found decreased dopamine release in the nucleus accumbens during alcohol withdrawal. The reduction of dopaminergic neurotransmission is prolonged, outlasting the physical signs of withdrawal. Similar effects have been observed

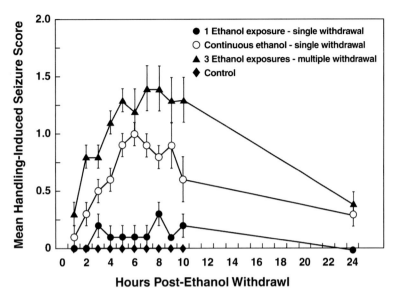

FIGURE 6.16 **The progressive development of handling-induced seizures during alcohol withdrawal in male C3H mice.** The multiple withdrawal group received three cycles of 16h alcohol vapor separated by 8h periods of abstinence. A single withdrawal group received a single bout of alcohol exposure (16h). A second group experienced a single withdrawal episode after receiving the equivalent amount of alcohol intoxication as the multiple withdrawal group (16 × 3 = 48h) but received it continuously (uninterrupted). The control group did not receive ethanol. The severity of handling-induced seizures was greatest in the multiple withdrawal group, intermediate for the continuous alcohol-single withdrawal group, and minimal for the single ethanol exposure-single withdrawal group. The incidence of spontaneous handling-induced seizures was virtually negligible in the control group. Peak seizure intensity was reached approximately 6–8h after withdrawal for all alcohol-exposed groups and generally subsided by 24h, although withdrawal signs were still evident in the multiple withdrawal and continuous ethanol-single withdrawal groups at this time. *These results show that multiple withdrawals from alcohol in mice can produce a "kindling" of seizures (a sensitization of seizures such that seizures are more likely to occur with each successive withdrawal). A similar kindling of anxiety-like responses has been observed in animals. A kindling of both seizures and anxiety has been observed in humans with repeated withdrawal. [Taken with permission from Becker HC, Hale RL. Repeated episodes of ethanol withdrawal potentiate the severity of subsequent withdrawal seizures: an animal model of alcohol withdrawal "kindling." Alcoholism: Clinical and Experimental Research, 1993, (17), 94–98.]*

for virtually all major drugs of abuse. Remarkably, when animals were allowed to self-administer alcohol during acute withdrawal, they self-administered just enough alcohol to return extracellular dopamine levels in the nucleus accumbens back to normal, pre-dependence baseline levels (Figure 6.18). Overall, these findings indicate that the classic neurotransmitters that regulate the positive reinforcing properties of drugs of abuse, including alcohol, are compromised during withdrawal.

Alcohol is also a powerful modulator of stress systems. Dysregulation of the brain's stress systems has been hypothesized to be another neurochemical counteradaptation that is motivationally significant during the development of alcohol dependence, an effect that may be crucial for understanding dependence and relapse. Two other brain stress systems have prominent roles in mediating the stress-like effects of alcohol withdrawal and the compulsive-like drinking associated with alcohol dependence. Although less well-developed, evidence supports a role for norepinephrine systems in the extended amygdala in the negative motivational state and increased

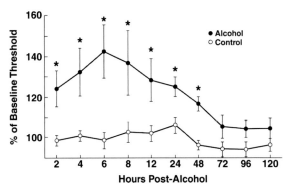

FIGURE 6.17 **Time-dependent elevation of intracranial self-stimulation thresholds in rats during alcohol withdrawal.** Mean blood alcohol levels were 197.29 mg%. The data are expressed as the mean percentage of baseline threshold. Asterisks (*) indicate thresholds that were significantly elevated above control levels at 2–48 h post-alcohol ($p < 0.05$). Open circles indicate the control condition. Closed circles indicate the ethanol withdrawal condition. *These data show that animals made dependent on alcohol using an alcohol vapor procedure and withdrawn from the alcohol show elevations in reward thresholds measured by intracranial self-stimulation (see Chapter 3 for details on intracranial self-stimulation and the alcohol withdrawal procedure). These increases can be interpreted as dysphoric-like effects.* [Taken with permission from Schulteis G, Markou A, Cole M, Koob G. Decreased brain reward produced by ethanol withdrawal. Proceedings of the National Academy of Sciences USA, 1995, (92), 5880–5884.]

self-administration associated with dependence. Substantial evidence has accumulated that suggests that in animals and humans, central noradrenergic systems are activated during acute withdrawal from alcohol and alcohol withdrawal in rats and humans by noradrenergic blockade. In dependent rats, the α_1 receptor antagonist prazosin selectively blocked the increased drinking associated with acute withdrawal. Dynorphin, an opioid peptide that binds to κ opioid receptors, is activated by chronic psychostimulant and opioid administration (see Chapters 2, 4, and 5), and κ opioid receptor agonists produce aversive effects in animals and humans. κ Opioid antagonists also block the excessive drinking associated with alcohol withdrawal and dependence, and this effect appears to be mediated by the shell of the nucleus accumbens.

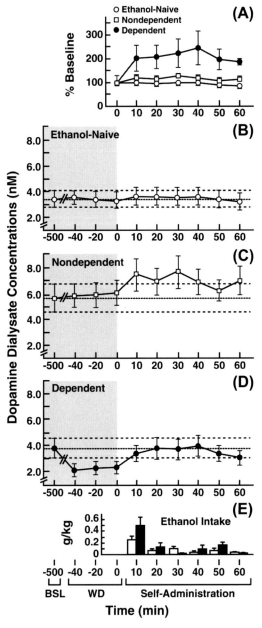

FIGURE 6.18 **Effects of operant alcohol self-administration in nondependent and dependent rats (alcohol liquid diet; see Chapter 3) that underwent alcohol withdrawal on dopamine efflux in the nucleus accumbens.** Dialysate neurotransmitter levels were compared with those in alcohol-naive rats trained to self-administer water. Average water intake in this group was negligible (<0.8 ml) and

Both acute and chronic alcohol activate the hypothalamic-pituitary-adrenal (HPA) axis (see Chapter 2), which appears to be the result of the release of corticotropin-releasing factor (CRF) in the hypothalamus that, in turn, activates the neuroendocrine stress response. However, abstinent individuals with alcoholism are well known to have persistently impaired HPA function, reflected by low basal cortisol levels and blunted adrenocorticotropic hormone and cortisol responses to CRF. Similar results have been observed in animal studies. Functional changes in the CRF system in the paraventricular nucleus may be a mechanism by which the HPA system becomes dysregulated in alcoholism. However, the acute and chronic activation of the HPA system sensitizes the extensive extra-hypothalamic, extra-neuroendocrine CRF system implicated in behavioral

◄ is not shown. (A) Changes in neurotransmitter output from levels recorded during the last hour of withdrawal. The data are expressed as a percentage of baseline values calculated as the average of three 20 min samples collected during hour 8 of withdrawal (shown in B–D). The corresponding dialysate neurotransmitter concentrations are shown in B (Ethanol-Naive), C (Nondependent), and D (Dependent). To illustrate the changes in neurotransmitter efflux over the various experimental phases, B–D also show pre-withdrawal (BSL) and withdrawal (WD) dialysate concentrations of dopamine during hour 8 of withdrawal. Dashed lines represent the mean pre-withdrawal dialysate dopamine concentrations. (E) Amounts of self-administered alcohol (10% w/v) during 10 min intervals in the dependent (solid bars) and nondependent (open bars) groups. Alcohol self-administration in dependent rats restored dopamine levels to pre-withdrawal values. *These data show that ethanol-dependent rats exhibit a decrease in the release of dopamine in the nucleus accumbens during withdrawal. However, if the rats are given access to alcohol self-administration during withdrawal, then they drink a sufficient amount to restore extracellular dopamine levels to pre-withdrawal levels. Notice that the nondependent rats exhibit an increase in dopamine release in the nucleus accumbens independent of withdrawal. This reflects extracellular dopamine efflux in the nucleus accumbens that parallels both positive and negative reinforcement (see Chapter 1). [Taken with permission from Weiss F, Parsons LH, Schulteis G, Hyytia P, Lorang MT, Bloom FE, Koob GF. Ethanol self-administration restores withdrawal-associated deficiencies in accumbal dopamine and 5-hydroxytryptamine release in dependent rats.* Journal of Neuroscience, *1996, (16), 3474–3485.].*

responses to stress. Chronic alcohol produces anxiogenic-like responses during acute and protracted withdrawal, which can be reversed by intracerebral administration of a CRF receptor antagonist directly into the central nucleus of the amygdala and systemic administration of CRF_1 antagonists. Increases in extracellular levels of CRF are observed in the amygdala and bed nucleus of the stria terminalis during alcohol withdrawal (Figure 6.19). Even more compelling, a competitive CRF receptor antagonist that normally has no effect on alcohol self-administration in nondependent rats eliminates excessive drinking in dependent rats when injected into the central nucleus of the amygdala (Figure 6.20; for further reading, see Koob, 2008).

Acute withdrawal from alcohol also decreases neuropeptide Y levels in the central and medial nuclei of the amygdala and piriform cortex (for further reading, see Koob, 2008). When administered intracerebroventricularly or directly into the central nucleus of the amygdala, neuropeptide Y decreases alcohol intake. Other neurochemical systems that are potentially involved in the anxiety-inducing effects of alcohol withdrawal that also can modulate excessive drinking are norepinephrine, vasopressin, dynorphin, nociceptin, and endocannabinoids (Table 6.9).

The facilitation of GABA interneuron neurotransmission in the central nucleus of the amygdala is enhanced in dependent animals, a physiological effect that has been confirmed by directly measuring GABA levels in awake, freely moving animals (Figure 6.21). However, both the acute alcohol and chronic alcohol effects do not occur in neurons in knockout mice that lack the CRF_1 receptor. Several selective CRF_1 receptor antagonists block the effects of alcohol in rats and mice. Such studies suggest that the GABA facilitation in the central nucleus of the amygdala observed during acute ethanol exposure may rely on an interaction with CRF neurons. Thus, CRF activity increases at the system level during alcohol withdrawal and thus may be an

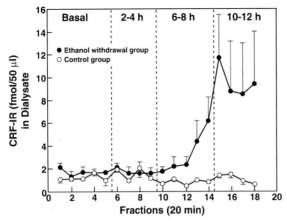

FIGURE 6.19 **Effects of alcohol withdrawal on corticotropin-releasing factor immunoreactivity (CRF-IR) levels in the rat amygdala as determined by microdialysis.** Dialysate was collected over four 2h periods that regularly alternated with nonsampling 2h periods. The four sampling periods corresponded to the basal collection (before removal of ethanol) and 2–4, 6–8, and 10–12h after withdrawal. Fractions were collected every 20min. The data are expressed as means ($n = 5$ per group). Significant differences were observed between groups over time ($p < 0.05$). *These data show that rats made dependent on alcohol using an alcohol liquid diet exhibit an increase in the release of corticotropin-releasing factor (CRF) in the central nucleus of the amygdala measured by in vivo microdialysis. Notice that this increase in CRF occurs during a period of withdrawal characterized by a decrease in the release of dopamine and serotonin in the nucleus accumbens and increases in reward thresholds. [Taken with permission from Merlo-Pich E, Lorang M, Yeganeh M, Rodriguez de Fonseca F, Raber J, Koob GF, Weiss F. Increase of extracellular corticotropin-releasing factor-like immunoreactivity levels in the amygdala of awake rats during restraint stress and ethanol withdrawal as measured by microdialysis.* Journal of Neuroscience, *1995, (15), 5439–5447.]*

early neuroadaptation of the brain to the effects of alcohol.

In summary, acute withdrawal from alcohol increases CRF in the central nucleus of the amygdala, which has motivational significance for the anxiety-like effects of acute withdrawal from alcohol and the increased drug intake associated with dependence. Acute withdrawal may also increase the release of norepinephrine in the bed nucleus of the stria terminalis and dynorphin in the nucleus accumbens, both of which may contribute to the negative emotional

state associated with dependence. Decreased activity of neuropeptide Y in the central nucleus of the amygdala may contribute to the anxiety-like state associated with ethanol dependence. Activation of brain stress systems (CRF, norepinephrine, dynorphin) combined with inactivation of brain anti-stress systems (neuropeptide Y) elicits powerful emotional dysregulation in the extended amygdala (Table 6.9). Such dysregulation of emotional processing may significantly contribute to between-system opponent processes that maintain dependence and set the stage for more prolonged state changes in emotionality, such as in protracted abstinence.

Preoccupation/Anticipation Stage

Protracted Abstinence

Prolonged abstinence from alcohol in humans involves a residual negative emotional state that can persist for weeks or months after acute withdrawal. To study protracted abstinence in animal models, one can define such a state as spanning a period when acute physical withdrawal has subsided, but behavioral changes persist. Increases in alcohol intake over the pre-dependence baseline and increases in stress responsivity persist for 2–8 weeks post-withdrawal from chronic alcohol. Rats tested 3–5 weeks post-withdrawal in the elevated plus maze, which is commonly used to evaluate anxiety-like behavior in rodents, did not show anxiogenic-like responses at baseline. However, angiogenic-like responses were induced by mild restraint stress only in rats with a history of alcohol dependence. This stress-induced anxiogenic-like response was reversed by a CRF receptor antagonist (Figure 6.22). The increase in alcohol self-administration during protracted abstinence was blocked by CRF antagonists. Similar effects on alcohol self-administration during protracted abstinence have been observed with administration of a glucocorticoid receptor antagonist. Thus, brain CRF systems appear to remain hyperactive during protracted abstinence, and

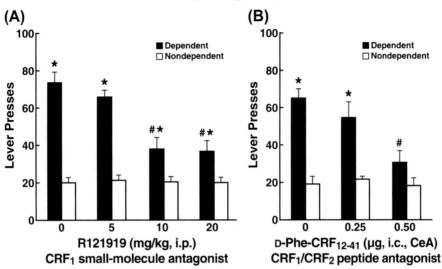

Ethanol Responding in Dependent Rats

FIGURE 6.20 (A) Effects of CRF$_1$ receptor small-molecule antagonist R121919 on ethanol self-administration in dependent and nondependent rats. Ethanol dependence was induced by intermittent exposure to ethanol vapors for 4 weeks. Animals were subsequently tested for ethanol and water self-administration following 2 hours of acute withdrawal. Withdrawn, ethanol-dependent animals displayed a significant increase in ethanol lever pressing compared with nondependent animals. R121919 significantly decreased ethanol self-administration in withdrawn, dependent but not nondependent animals. Neither ethanol vapor exposure nor R121919 altered water responding. *$p < 0.001$ compared with same drug dose in nondependent animals. #$p < 0.0001$ compared with vehicle treatment in dependent animals. (B) Effects of CRF$_1$/CRF$_2$ peptide antagonist D-Phe CRF$_{12-41}$ administered directly into the central nucleus of the amygdala on ethanol and water self-administration in ethanol-dependent and nondependent rats. Ethanol dependence was induced by intermittent exposure to ethanol vapors for 4 weeks. Animals were subsequently tested for ethanol and water self-administration after 2 hours of acute withdrawal. Withdrawn, ethanol-dependent animals displayed a significant increase in ethanol lever pressing compared with nondependent animals. D-Phe CRF$_{12-41}$ significantly decreased ethanol self-administration in withdrawn, dependent but not nondependent animals when administered directly into the central nucleus of the amygdala. Neither ethanol vapor exposure nor D-Phe CRF$_{12-41}$ altered water responding. *$p < 0.0001$, compared with same drug dose in nondependent animals. #$p < 0.0001$, compared with vehicle treatment in dependent animals. Error bars indicate SEM. *These data show that systemic administration of the small-molecule CRF$_1$ receptor antagonist or intracerebral injection of a mixed peptide CRF$_1$/CRF$_2$ antagonist into the central nucleus of the amygdala selectively blocked only the excessive drinking induced by withdrawal from alcohol in dependent rats using the alcohol vapor procedure (see Chapter 3 for details). Notice that the CRF antagonists had no effect in nondependent rats with limited access.* [Taken with permission from Funk CK, Zorrilla EP, Lee MJ, Rice KC, Koob GF. Corticotropin-releasing factor 1 antagonists selectively reduce ethanol self-administration in ethanol-dependent rats. Biological Psychiatry, 2007, (61), 78–86.] [Taken with permission from Funk CK, O'Dell LE, Crawford EF, Koob GF. Corticotropin-releasing factor within the central nucleus of the amygdala mediates enhanced ethanol self-administration in withdrawn, ethanol-dependent rats. Journal of Neuroscience, 2006, (26), 11324–11332.].

this hyperactivity is motivationally relevant to excessive alcohol drinking. Results such as these suggest that the emotional substrates of the brain that are dysregulated in the *binge/intoxication* and *withdrawal/negative affect* stages remain dysregulated and contribute to craving and relapse (see Chapters 1 and 2).

Reinstatement of Alcohol Reinforcement

Behavioral procedures have been developed to reinstate alcohol seeking after extinction. Previously neutral stimuli, such as a tone, light, or odor, that are paired with alcohol self-administration or predict alcohol self-administration can induce relapse. Rats can

TABLE 6.9 Stress and Anti-Stress Neurotransmitters Implicated in the Motivational Effects of Alcohol Dependence and Withdrawal

Increased Activity	Decreased Activity
↑ Corticotropin-releasing factor	↓ Neuropeptide Y
↑ Norepinephrine	↓ Nociceptin (orphanin FQ)
↑ Vasopressin	↓ Endocannabinoids
↑ Orexin (hypocretin)	
↑ Dynorphin	
↑ Substance P	

come to associate a specific olfactory stimulus with alcohol availability, and that olfactory stimulus can then reinstate responding in animals subjected to extinction. Consistent with the well-established conditioned cue reactivity in human individuals with alcoholism (see Chapter 9), the motivational effects of alcohol-related stimuli are highly resistant to extinction and retain their efficacy to elicit alcohol-seeking behavior over more than 1 month of repeated testing. Such reinstatement can be blocked by systemic administration of naltrexone and selective μ and δ opioid receptor antagonists. Dopamine D_1 and D_2 receptor antagonists also block cue-induced reinstatement. Stress exposure can reinstate responding for alcohol in previously extinguished rats, and this stress-induced reinstatement is blocked by CRF antagonists. CRF antagonists block stress-induced reinstatement but not cue-induced reinstatement, and naltrexone blocks cue-induced reinstatement but not stress-induced reinstatement, suggesting two independent neuropharmacological routes to reinstatement and relapse (for further reading, see Liu and Weiss, 2002; Table 6.10).

Molecular Genetics of Alcoholism

The precise molecular genetic basis for the hereditability of alcoholism is largely unknown, but several lines of evidence have provided some insights into possible genetic factors. Early studies on alcoholism found that individuals with alcoholism or certain subgroups of individuals with alcoholism have reduced cerebrospinal fluid levels of 5-hydroxyindoleacetic acid (5-HIAA), the major metabolite of the neurotransmitter serotonin. A series of studies highlighted the role of serotonin in impulse control, and low cerebrospinal 5-HIAA levels were associated with increased irritability and impaired impulse control in violent individuals with alcoholism with antisocial personality disorder. These characteristics are hallmarks of the young male with alcoholism. Studies of the association between single-nucleotide polymorphisms and alcohol dependence have revealed some possible polymorphisms in the genes that encode GABA, dopamine, opioid peptides, serotonin, and CRF. One of the associations is with a specific subunit of the $GABA_A$ receptor (the α2 subunit; for further reading, see Palmer et al., 2012).

Alcohol reinforcement has long been associated with the activation of opioid peptides. In animal studies, opioid receptor antagonists blocked alcohol self-administration, and opioid receptor antagonists have also been shown to have efficacy in treating alcoholism in humans (see Chapter 9). Some human genetic studies have identified an association between a functional polymorphism of the μ opioid receptor gene (A118G single-nucleotide polymorphism) and the therapeutic response to naltrexone in the treatment of alcoholism (see Chapter 9). Such studies point to a polymorphism that may contribute to the genetic vulnerability to alcoholism.

A parallel approach to the study of the neuropharmacological basis of excessive drinking involves the selective breeding of rodents for high alcohol consumption. Investigators capitalized on well-known within-species preference for alcohol drinking to develop lines of rats that voluntarily consume large amounts of alcohol (see Chapter 3). Extensive innate

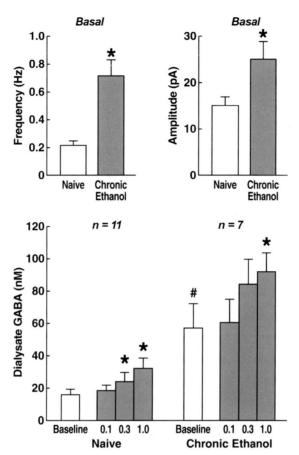

FIGURE 6.21 **Increased GABA release in the central nucleus of the amygdala in ethanol-dependent rats.** (Top) Chronic alcohol treatment increased the mean frequency and amplitude of spontaneous mini inhibitory postsynaptic currents (mIPSCs). The average frequency of mIPSCs in the central nucleus of the amygdala neurons in naive rats ($n = 9$) and chronic alcohol-treated rats ($n = 15$) is shown on the left (*$p < 0.001$). The same group of neurons showed an increase in the mean amplitude of mIPSCs in chronic alcohol-treated rats (*$p < 0.05$). (Bottom) Acute and chronic alcohol increased dialysate levels of GABA in the central nucleus of the amygdala. In both the naive and chronic alcohol-treated rats, alcohol administration into the central nucleus of the amygdala significantly (*$p < 0.05$) and dose-dependently increased mean dialysate GABA levels. The mean baseline dialysate GABA level was significantly (#$p < 0.001$) increased in chronic alcohol-treated rats compared with naive rats. *These data provide electrophysiological and neurochemical evidence of an increase in GABA release in the central nucleus of the amygdala in alcohol-dependent rats. Increases in the mean frequency and amplitude of spontaneous mini inhibitory postsynaptic currents (mIPSCs) indicate the presynaptic release of GABA. The microdialysis results provide neurochemical confirmation. The hypothesized change in GABA release in the central nucleus of the amygdala is driven by CRF and parallels the development of dependence in rats. [Taken with permission from Roberto M, Madamba SG, Stouffer DG, Parsons LH, Siggins GR. Increased GABA release in the central amygdala of ethanol-dependent rats. Journal of Neuroscience, 2004, (24), 10159–10166.]*

differences exist in the neurochemical systems implicated in the reinforcing effects of alcohol between selectively bred high- and low-drinking rodents. Alcohol-preferring rats have lower levels of serotonin and dopamine function, upregulation of the GABA system, and downregulation of the neuropeptide Y system (for further reading, see Murphy et al., 2002).

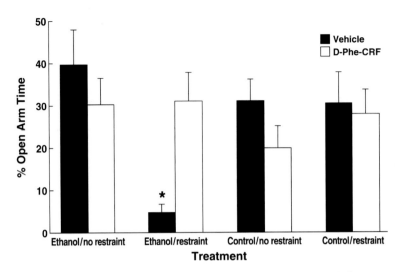

FIGURE 6.22 **Effect of restraint stress on exploratory behavior in rats in the elevated plus maze 6 weeks after exposure to an alcohol liquid diet over a 3 week period.** Control rats received a sucrose-containing liquid diet. The rats were injected intracerebroventricularly with $10\,\mu g$ of the corticotropin-releasing factor antagonist D-Phe-CRF$_{12-41}$ ($n = 8$–11/group) or vehicle ($n = 7$–8/group) and subsequently placed in restraint tubes or returned to their home cages for 15 min. The mean percentage of time spent in the open arms of the elevated plus maze was measured. *$p < 0.05$, compared with all other groups. *These data show that rats with a history of dependence present no overt anxiety-like effects during protracted abstinence but present an exaggerated stress response when challenged with mild restraint stress. The exaggerated stress response in the animals with a history of dependence is blocked by intracerebroventricular administration of a peptide CRF$_1$/CRF$_2$ receptor antagonist. These results suggest residual long-term "sensitization"of the extrahypothalamic CRF systems in animals with a history of alcohol dependence. [Taken with permission from Valdez GR, Zorrilla EP, Roberts AJ, Koob GF. Antagonism of corticotropin-releasing factor attenuates the enhanced responsiveness to stress observed during protracted ethanol abstinence. Alcohol, 2003, (29), 55–60.]*

TABLE 6.10 Effects of Drugs on Animal Models of Cue- and Stress-Induced Reinstatement of Alcohol Drinking

	Naltrexone	Acamprosate	CRF Antagonist	κ Opioid Antagonist	Vasopressin Antagonist
Baseline drinking	↓	–	–	–	–
Dependence-induced drinking	↓	↓	↓	↓	↓
Cue-induced reinstatement	↓	↓	–		
Stress-induced reinstatement	–		↓	↓	↓
Alcohol deprivation effect/ Protracted abstinence	↓	↓	↓		

Given that alcoholism is heritable, genetic differences may also be relevant to the role of brain stress systems in driving compulsive alcohol seeking. Animal models support the hypothesis that gene variants of CRF system molecules may promote compulsive-like alcohol intake.

For example, many msP alcohol-preferring rats carry two G-to-A polymorphisms in allelic identity with one another in the distal promoter region of the CRF$_1$ receptor *Crhr1* gene. These mutations are not seen in other alcohol-preferring lines or outbred rats. This msP line exhibits increased CRF$_1$ receptor expression in several stress-related brain regions, increased anxiety-like behavior, and increased sensitivity to the ability of CRF$_1$ receptor antagonists to reduce alcohol self-administration and stress-induced reinstatement of alcohol seeking. Similarly, rhesus monkeys that carry a C-to-T single-nucleotide polymorphism in the promoter region of the *Crh* gene (the gene for CRF) do not show normal glucocorticoid feedback inhibition of CRF peptide expression, and this gene variant is associated with two-fold greater alcohol consumption in monkeys exposed to early life stress, without altering the basal drinking of unstressed monkeys. Several polymorphisms in human CRF system molecules have also been associated with alcohol use phenotypes, often in an interaction with stress history. *Crhr1* single-nucleotide polymorphisms predicted greater alcohol consumption in already-dependent individuals and interacted with stress history. Converging evidence suggests that some individuals may be more vulnerable to the transition to dependence via negative reinforcement mechanisms that involve the activation of brain stress systems.

SUMMARY

Alcohol is widely used in society for both its social and medicinal benefits. It is readily derived in nature from fermentation. Early in human history, individuals learned to exploit the fermentation process to produce beverages and tonics. Alcohol is a sedative hypnotic that has euphoric and disinhibitory effects, explaining why some see it as a "social lubricant." Many of the alleged stimulant effects of alcohol probably result from such disinhibitory effects, which define its behavioral mechanism of action. As the dose of alcohol increases to levels associated with binge drinking, however, disinhibition gives way to motor impairment, muscular incoordination, impairments in reaction

time, impairments in judgment, impairments in sensory processing, and impairments in cognitive function – all behavioral effects that contribute to its behavioral toxicity. Binge drinking is defined as four drinks (in females) or five drinks (in males) over a 2 hour period. The chronic use of alcohol can lead to alcoholism or Dependence on Alcohol as defined by the ICD-10 and Substance Use Disorder on Alcohol as defined by the DSM-5. Numerous other medical diseases can also result from chronic alcohol use, ranging from cirrhosis of the liver to heart disease and pancreatitis to Wernicke–Korsakoff syndrome. All-to-frequent serious pathologies produced by drinking during pregnancy include fetal alcohol syndrome and fetal alcohol spectrum disorder. During the *binge/intoxication* stage, the neurobiological mechanism of action for the acute reinforcing effects of alcohol involves prominent actions on the GABAergic system and activation of some of the same reward neurotransmitters implicated in the actions of psychostimulants and opioids, including dopamine and opioid peptides. For a colorful representation of the symphony of alcohol's effects, see Figure 6.23. At the cellular level, alcohol has been shown to have specific synaptic effects, with very low doses of alcohol enhancing GABAergic neurotransmission and inhibiting glutamate neurotransmission, actions that show neuroadaptations during abstinence. Alcohol also interacts with second-messenger systems, notably the actions of protein kinases that can change the sensitivity of ligand-gated receptors or enhance gene transcription. Molecular genetic and knockout studies have confirmed some of the more powerful neuropharmacological effects that involve actions at μ opioid and neuropeptide Y systems but also have identified specific genes that are implicated in alcohol preference and excessive drinking. During the *withdrawal/negative affect* stage, abstinence from chronic alcohol, similar to other drugs of abuse, disrupts reward neurotransmitter function, such as dopamine,

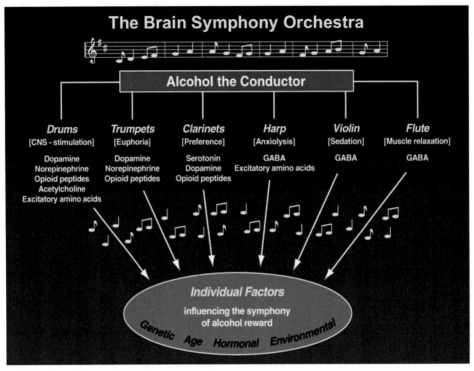

FIGURE 6.23 Schematic figure of the involvement of various neurotransmitters and individually related factors in the reward profile of alcohol. [*Modified with permission from Engel JA, Fahlke C, Hård E, Johannessen K, Svensson L, Söderpalm B. Serotonergic and dopaminergic involvement in ethanol intake. Clinical Neuropharmacology, 1992, 15(Suppl. 1 Pt A): 64A–65A.*]

opioid peptides, and GABA, and recruits the brain stress CRF system and dysregulates the brain anti-stress neuropeptide Y system, all of which appear to contribute to motivational withdrawal and excessive drinking during dependence. These effects have been localized to the ventral striatum and extended amygdala, providing support for the role of the extended amygdala in the acute and chronic motivational effects of alcohol in the development of dependence. During the *preoccupation/anticipation* stage, disruptions in reward function and the sensitization of brain stress systems persist into protracted abstinence. Animal models of relapse have provided evidence of a role for opioid peptides, dopamine, and glutamate in cue-induced reinstatement and CRF in stress-induced reinstatement. The challenge for future research is to identify how receptor proteins, neurons, and circuits convey the vulnerability to excessive and compulsive drinking associated with substance use disorders on alcohol.

Suggested Reading

Cottino A., 1995. Italy. In: Heath, D.B. (Ed.), International Handbook on Alcohol and Culture. Greenwood Press, Westport, CT, pp. 156–167.

Crabbe, J.C., Phillips, T.J., Harris, R.A., Arends, M.A., Koob, G.F., 2006. Alcohol-related genes: contributions from studies with genetically engineered mice. Add. Biol. 11, 195–269.

Harris, R.A., Trudell, J.R., Mihic, S.J., 2008. Ethanol's molecular targets. Sci. Signal. 1 (28). re7.

Kalant, H., 1998. Research on tolerance: what can we learn from history? Alcohol. Clin. Exp. Res. 22, 67–76.

Koob, G.F., 2003. Alcoholism: allostasis and beyond. Alcohol. Clin. Exp. Res. (27), 232–243.

Koob, G.F., 2008. A role for brain stress systems in addiction. Neuron 59, 11–34.

Koob, G.F., Lloyd, G.K., Mason, B.J., 2009. Development of pharmacotherapies for drug addiction: a Rosetta Stone approach. Nat. Rev. Drug Discov. 8, 500–515.

Liu, X., Weiss, F., 2002. Additive effect of stress and drug cues on reinstatement of ethanol seeking: exacerbation by history of dependence and role of concurrent activation of corticotropin-releasing factor and opioid mechanisms. J. Neurosci. 22, 7856–7861.

Movva, R., Figueredo, V.M., 2013. Alcohol and the heart: to abstain or not to abstain? Int. J. Cardiol 164, 267–276.

Murphy, J.M., Stewart, R.B., Bell, R.L., Badia-Elder, N.E., Carr, L.G., McBride, W.J., Lumeng, L., Li, T.K., 2002. Phenotypic and genotypic characterization of the Indiana University rat lines selectively bred for high and low alcohol preference. Behavior Genetics 32, 363–388.

Nahoum-Grappe, V., 1995. France. In: Heath, D.B. (Ed.), International Handbook on Alcohol and Culture. Greenwood Press, Westport, CT, pp. 75–87.

Nyberg, K., Allebeck, P., 1995. Sweden. In: Heath, D.B. (Ed.), International Handbook on Alcohol and Culture. Greenwood Press, Westport, CT, pp. 156–167.

Palmer, R.H., McGeary, J.E., Francazio, S., Raphael, B.J., Lander, A.D., Heath, A.C., Knopik, V.S., 2012. The genetics of alcohol dependence: advancing towards systems-based approaches. Drug Alcohol Depend. 125, 179–191.

Ron, D., Messing, R.O., 2013. Signaling pathways mediating alcohol effects. Current Topics Behav. Neurosci. 13, 87–126.

Warren, K.R., Hewitt, B.G., Thomas, J.D., 2011. Fetal alcohol spectrum disorders: research challenges and opportunities. Alcohol Res. Health 34, 4–14.

Xiao J., 1995. China. In: Heath, D.B. (Ed.), International Handbook on Alcohol and Culture. Greenwood Press, Westport, CT, pp. 42–50.

Nicotine

DEFINITIONS

Tobacco is the dried leaves of the cultivated plant *Nicotiana tabacum*, a native of North and South America (*Nicotiana rustica*), and a plant that is a member of the *Solanacae* (nightshade) family. A wide variety of plants, all native to North America, were either combined with tobacco or contain nicotine-like substances, but the only two that were widely cultivated were *Nicotiana tabacum* (common tobacco) and *Nicotiana rustica* (Aztec tobacco; Figure 7.1). The derivation of the word *tobacco* comes from the West Indian (Caribbean) word *tabaco* and Spanish *tobaco* (*tobago* or *tobah*), which actually refer to the pipe or tube with which the Indians smoked the plant. The name was then transferred by the Spaniards to the plant itself. Tobacco is widely used in various products that can be smoked, such as cigars, pipes, and cigarettes, or administered through the oral and nasal cavities, such as via snuff or chewing tobacco.

Cigarette smoke contains more than 4,000 chemicals, many of which could potentially contribute to the addictive properties of tobacco. However, the most well known constituent that causes the acute psychopharmacological properties of tobacco is nicotine, and this has been found to be a major component in tobacco smoke that is responsible for nicotine addiction (Box 7.1).

Nicotine derives its name from the botanical name *Nicotiana*, which in turn was eponymously

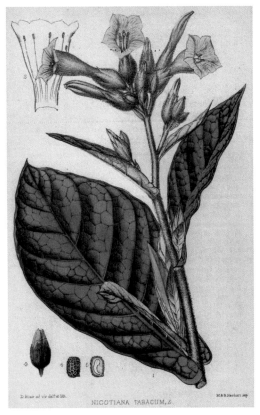

FIGURE 7.1 Parts of the *Nicotiana tabacum* plant: – summit of stem with inflorescence; 2 – corolla split open; 3 – capsule with persistent calyx; 4 – a seed; 5 – section of the same (4 and 5 are greatly enlarged). *[Taken with permission from Bentley R, Trimen H. Medicinal Plants: Being descriptions with original figures of the principal plants employed in medicine and an account of the characters, properties, and uses of their parts and products of medicinal value, vol. 3. J & A Churchill, London, 1880, no. 191.]*

derived from Jean Nicot de Villemain, the French ambassador to Portugal who introduced tobacco to the French court. Mr. Nicot brought tobacco powder via Portugal to Queen Catherine de Medicis after the death of Portugal's King Henri II in 1561. Catherine de Medicis appreciated the pleasurable effects of this *poudre Américaine* ("American powder"). She developed a taste for it, became an enthusiast, and ensured its popularity, first inside and then outside the court.

Nicotine itself was isolated by Posselt and Reimann in 1828. It is a highly toxic alkaloid that is derived from tobacco. It is water-soluble, colorless, and bitter-tasting in the liquid form and is a weak base with pH 8.5. Nicotine is not to be confused with nicotinic acid, which is the fat-soluble vitamin B-3, called niacin, used in the treatment of pellagra, a niacin deficiency syndrome characterized by cutaneous, gastrointestinal, neurologic, and mental symptoms.

Tobacco smoke contains not only nicotine but also carbon monoxide and tar. "Tar" is a generic term for what remains after the moisture and nicotine are removed from tobacco and largely consists of aromatic hydrocarbons, many of which are carcinogens (Table 7.1).

HISTORY OF USE

Tobacco use and cigarette smoking are the most popular and persistent forms of drug taking in the modern age (Figure 7.2). The names ascribed to the plant itself have varied greatly from culture to culture, including *apooke* in Virginia, *yetl* by the Aztecs, *oyngona* by the Huron, *sayri* by the Peruvians, *kohiha* in the Caribbean, and *cogiaba* or *cohiba* by the Spanish. The use of *Nicotiana tabacum* by indigenous people in North and South America can be traced back 8,000 years, both archeologically and ethnopharmacologically, and it has been used for both medicinal and ceremonial purposes (Figure 7.3). Many historians contend that European explorers, such as Columbus in 1492, were the first to record the practice of smoking the dried leaves of the tobacco plant, probably in the form of cigars (Boxes 7.2, 7.3). European travelers to Mexico noted the medical uses of tobacco by the natives:

> "In this country, **tabaco** cures pain caused by cold; taken in smoke it is beneficial against colds, asthma and coughs; Indians and Negroes use it in powder in their mouths in order to fall asleep and feel no pain." (*Stewart GG. A history of the medicinal*

BOX 7.1

SYNOPSIS OF THE NEUROPHARMACOLOGICAL TARGETS FOR NICOTINE

All tobacco products contain nicotine, which is the main psychoactive ingredient in cigarette smoke. Nicotine is considered a psychostimulant, but it can also produce analgesia and anti-anxiety-like (or anxiolytic) effects. Nicotine mimics the actions of the endogenous neurotransmitter acetylcholine and binds as an agonist at nicotinic receptors. These are widely distributed throughout the brain but have high concentrations in reward-related circuits. Nicotinic receptors are ion-gated receptors. The activation of nicotinic receptors opens calcium channels to increase neuronal excitability and promote transmitter release. There are multiple nicotinic receptor subtypes that are composed of different subunits, but most form three broad groups in the brain: α2–6, β2–4, and α7–10 subunits. The α4β2 nicotinic receptor appears to be mostly responsible for the psychostimulant effects of nicotine, in addition to a wide range of behavioral and physiological effects. The psychostimulant and rewarding effects of nicotine are largely mediated by actions on nicotinic receptors in the origin areas (ventral tegmental area) and terminal areas (nucleus accumbens) of the mesocorticolimbic dopamine system and extended amygdala (central nucleus of the amygdala, bed nucleus of the stria terminalis, and a transition zone in the shell of the nucleus accumbens). The addiction potential of nicotine largely derives from powerful within-system neuroadaptations (signal transduction mechanisms) and between-system neuroadaptations (neurocircuitry changes) in the brain motivational and stress systems (see Chapter 2).

use of tobacco, 1492–1860. Medical History, 1967, (11), 228–268.)

Tobacco has been used to prevent fatigue, whiten teeth, treat abscesses, heal wounds, purge nasal passages, relieve thirst, and treat syphilis. English explorers were first made aware of the existence of the plant in Florida in 1565. The plant then proliferated to other countries, including India, Japan, and Turkey. The first American colonial commercial crop was grown for export in Jamestown, Virginia, in 1612 by John Rolfe, husband of Pocahontas (the benevolent Algonquian Native American who helped save the Jamestown colony by supplying it with food during its hard times). Cultivation extended to Maryland in 1631, and Virginia and Maryland were the main producers through the 1700s. By 1630, over 1.5 million pounds of tobacco were being exported from Jamestown every year. Tobacco is now grown in 120 countries worldwide.

As mentioned above, tobacco was introduced to Europe in the 16th century, and its use has survived significant historical attempts at prohibition. Smoking tobacco was considered to be both pleasurable and also a cure for ailments. Tobacco ingestion has fluctuated between smoking, chewing, and snuffing, but one method has often been replaced with another, such as when in the early 18th century the British imported *Nicotiana tabacum* from Virginia in the form of snuff for medical use. By 1726, snuff had nearly eclipsed the other forms of tobacco. In what is probably an apocryphal story, the origin of the cigarette is attributed to serendipity at the siege of Constantinople by the French in the middle of the 19th century:

TABLE 7.1 Major Toxic Agents in Cigarette Smoke (Unaged)

Gas Phase			Particulate Phase		
	Concentration Per Cigarette			**Concentration Per Cigarette**	
Agent	**Range Reported**	**US Cigarettes[1]**	**Agent**	**Range Reported**	**US Cigarettes[1]**
Carcinogen			Carcinogen		
dimethylnitrosamine	1–200 ng	13 ng	N'-nitrosonornicotine	100–250 ng	250 ng
ethylmethylnitrosamine	0.1–10 ng	1.8 ng	polonium-210	0.03–1.3 pCi	nt
diethylnitrosamine	0–10 ng	1.5 ng	nickel compounds	10–600 ng	nt
nitrosopyrrolodine	2–42 ng	11 ng	cadmium compounds	9–70 ng	nt
other nitrosamines	0–20 ng	nt	arsenic	1–25 µg	nt
hydrazine	24–43 ng	32 ng	Cocarcinogen		
vinyl chloride	1–16 ng	12 ng	pyrene	50–200 ng	150 ng
arsine	nt	nt	fluoranthene	50–250 ng	170 ng
nickel carbonyl	nt	nt	benzo(g,h,i)perylene	10–60 ng	30 ng
Cocarcinogen			naphthalenes	1–10 µg	6 µg
formaldehyde	20–90 µg	30 µg	1-methylindoles	0.3–0.9 µg	0.8 µg
Tumor initiator			9-methylcarbazoles	5–200 ng	100 ng
urethane	10–35 ng	30 ng	catechol	40–460 µg	270 µg
Cilia toxic agent			3- & 4-methyl-catechols	30–40 µg	32 µg
formaldehyde	20–90 µg	30 µg	Tumor initiator		
hydrogen cyanide	30–200 µg	110 µg	benzo(a)pyrene	8–50 ng	20 ng
acrolein	25–140 µg	70 µg	5-methylchrysene	0.5–2 ng	0.6 ng
acetaldehyde	18–1400 µg	800 µg	benzo(j)fluoranthene	5–40 ng	10 ng
Toxic agent			benz(a)anthracene	5–80 ng	40 ng
hydrogen cyanide	30–200 µg	110 µg	dibenz(a,j)acridine	3–10 ng	8 ng
nitrogen oxides (NO_x)[2]	10–600 µg	350 µg	dibenz(a,h)acridine	nt	nt
ammonia[3]	10–150 µg	60 µg	dibenzo(c,g)carbazole	0.7 ng	0.7 ng
pyridine[3]	9–93 µg	10 µg	Cilia toxic agent		
carbon monoxide	2–20 mg	17 mg	phenol	10–200 µg	85 µg
Other			cresols	10–150 µg	70 µg
volatile chlorinated olefins & nitro-olefins	nt	nt	Toxic agent		
			nicotine	0.1–2.0 mg	1.5 mg
			minor tobacco alkaloids	10–200 µg	100 µg
			Bladder carcinogen		
			β-naphthylamine	0.25 ng	20 ng

nt: not tested.
[1] 85 mm cigarettes without filter tips bought on the open market 1973–1976.
[2] $NO_x > 95\%$ NO; remainder, NO_2.
[3] Not toxic in smoke of blended US cigarettes because pH < 6.5; therefore, ammonia and pyridines are present only in protonated form.
[Adapted from Wynder EL, Hoffmann D. Tobacco and health: a societal challenge. New England Journal of Medicine, 1979, (300), 894–903.]

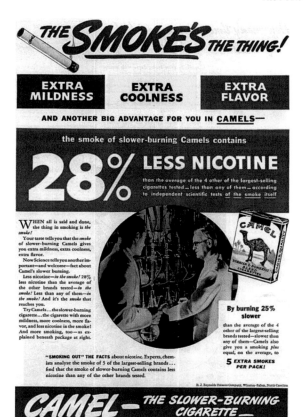

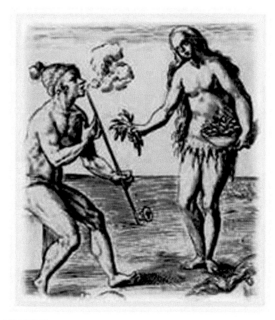

FIGURE 7.3 **Hand-colored engraving of tobacco smoking as a Floridian Native American health remedy.** *(de Bry T, Le Moyne de Morgues J. Brevis narratio eorvm qvae in Florida Americae Provicia Gallis acciderunt [A brief narration of those things which befell the French in the Province of Florida in America]. Francoforti ad Moenvm, Typis I. Wecheli, sumtibus vero T. de Bry, venales reperiutur in fficina S. Feirabedii, 1591.)*

FIGURE 7.2 **Marlboro cigarette advertisement, circa 1958.** Notice the smoke in the photograph – absent now from contemporary advertisements. Notice also the conspicuous lack of the now-ubiquitous Surgeon General's warning, which did not appear on cigarette packages until 1966.

BOX 7.2

CIGARS

Cigars can be defined as any roll of tobacco wrapped in leaf tobacco. Cigars are a tightly rolled bundle of dried and fermented tobacco that is formulated so that its smoke may be drawn into the mouth and absorbed by the mucosal lining there. Cigar smoke is more alkaline than cigarette smoke and therefore is absorbed more readily by the mucous membranes in the mouth, making it easier for the smoker to absorb nicotine without having to inhale. Some individuals inhale cigar smoke, but this is rare. Cigars allegedly date back to the time of the Mayans, and the word is derived from the Mayan "sikar" (to smoke rolled tobacco leaves). Cigars preceded cigarettes in the history of tobacco use (for further reading, see de Assis Viegas, 2008).

BOX 7.3

Elihu Root thinks that a cigar after breakfast is the smoke of the day, and there are many smokers who will agree with him. He is reported as saying: "My breakfast is a very simple meal, and consists of a cup of coffee or chocolate and a roll. When I have finished it, I light my cigar. I find that it assists me in my work. It does not aid me in the creation of ideas so much, nor in reading or actual writing; but when I want to prepare my plans for the day, when I want to arrange and put in shape the work I have before me, I find that smoking is a valuable assistant. I never smoke a large cigar in the morning, and usually do not prolong the smoke beyond the time it takes me to arrange my day's programme. Altogether I should say that I smoke five cigars a day. I have smoked steadily for the past thirty years, and during the first ten years I smoked a pipe. It has been my experience that smoking relieved me at any time when I felt overworked. Consequently, if I find at any time of day that my brain is getting tired, and that my ideas are getting muddled, I stop and light a cigar. I don't think that smoking has a sedative effect upon me, but it composes my thoughts and soothes me to some extent."

From: Bain J Jr., Tobacco Leaves, *H.M. Caldwell Company, Boston, 1903.*

"It is told in Alsace, France, the following story that if apocryphal, has nevertheless the merit to be plausible. At the siege of Constantinople (today's Istanbul) in 1854, an Alsacian Zouave soldier had his pipe pulled out of his teeth by a shell fragment. Not knowing how to smoke his remaining tobacco, he had the idea of rolling it into a tube made of paper. Therefore, it was an accident of war that gave birth to the cigarette, and we all know the comfort it would bring to all soldiers and civilians during the coming wars, whiling away the long hours of anticipation, hunger, and depression." (*Translated from Haug H.* Petite Histoire du Tabac en Alsace, Strasbourg, 1961.)

However, reference is also made to another form of smoking that also resembles the cigarette. An early 16th century expedition to Mexico noted that the natives would pack tobacco and liquid ambar (a herb) into a hollow reed that was allowed to smolder on one end, with the smoke inhaled from the other. According to some, this wrapping evolved from reeds to corn husks to paper used for manufacturing cigars in Spain. The Peninsular War fought by France against the Portuguese, British, and Spanish in the early 19th century disseminated these new, smaller cigars from Spain to France. The French renamed it the "cigarette." The Crimean War of the mid-19th century introduced it in England, where, in 1856, Robert P. Gloag set up a factory in Walworth for mass production. Aromatic tobaccos were used in these new cigarettes because they were the only types of tobacco suitable for smoking in this form. Flue-cured aromatic tobacco and air-cured Burley tobacco were introduced in 1864 for further mildness. These flue- and air-cured tobaccos were substituted for some of the aromatic tobaccos to form the blended cigarette in America in the late 1800s. The first cigarette-making machine was introduced in 1880. From there, tobacco and cigarette production accelerated through the end of the century, attributable to the convenience of the smoking vehicle, ease of production, transportation, distribution, mass media advertising, and demand (Figure 7.4).

Tobacco smoking continues to be a worldwide health problem. The high addictive potential of nicotine is reflected by the vast number of people who habitually smoke and relapse (Box 7.4). The 2011 United States *National Survey on Drug Use and Health* from the Substance Abuse and Mental Health Services Administration estimated that 173.9 million people aged 12 and older (67.5%) had ever engaged in tobacco use, and 81.9 million people aged 12 and older (31.8%) were last-year users of tobacco. Additionally, 161.8 million people aged 12 and older (62.8%) had ever engaged in cigarette use, and 67.1 million people aged 12 and older (26.1%) were last-year users of cigarettes. Notable statistics from the survey included the following. In 2011, of those people aged 12 or older who ever used in the last year, 22.9 million (34.2%) showed cigarette dependence (*Diagnostic and Statistical Manual of Mental Disorders*, 4th edition [DSM-IV], criteria). There is no abuse category for tobacco or cigarettes, so any statistics for substance dependence will be identical to those for tobacco use disorders (see Chapter 1). The World Health Organization has reported that more than 1.3 billion people smoke daily worldwide.

The cost to society is significant in terms of health problems that frequently lead to death, high medical costs, and human suffering. Tobacco smoking is the leading, *avoidable* cause of disease and premature death in the United States. In 2008, the US Centers for Disease Control and Prevention reported that cigarette smoking and exposure to secondhand smoke caused an estimated 443,000 deaths and 5.1 million years of potential life lost during 2000–2004. A 2008 CDC report found that smoking was implicated in 41% of the deaths from cancer, 32.7% of the deaths from cardiovascular disease, and 26.3% of the deaths from respiratory disease. On average, smoking shortens life span by 13 years in males and 15 years in females. Tobacco addiction accounts for 3.7% of DALYs worldwide, and this percentage increases to 10.7% in high-income countries (see Chapter 6 for a description of DALYs).

Maternal smoking during pregnancy is associated with lower birth weight, with heavy smokers reducing the birth weight of their offspring by 226 grams on average. Much more seriously, maternal smoking is now the

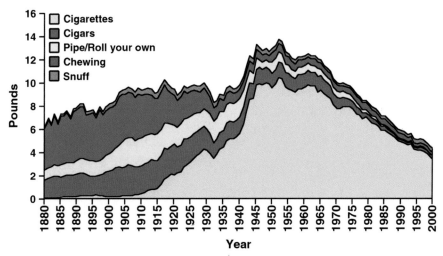

FIGURE 7.4 **Trends in per capita consumption of various tobacco products in the United States (in pounds) from 1880 to 2000 among persons aged 18 years or older.** After the year 2000, the latest data indicate the following per capita consumption for all tobacco products (the latest comparable data end in 2006): 4.3 in 2001, 4.2 in 2002, 4.0 in 2003, 3.9 in 2004, 3.7 in 2005, and 3.7 in 2006. *[Data from the US Department of Agriculture* Tobacco Situation and Outlook Report *series. Figure from Koob GF, Le Moal M.* Neurobiology of Addiction. *London: Academic Press, 2006.]*

BOX 7.4

Edwin Booth was a fierce smoker. His favorite was a pipe, not a cigar. He smoked in his dressing-room, between acts, in his own room, constantly, and I am not sure that he did not smoke in bed. He loved tobacco as another man might love food and drink. His system was full of nicotine, for he overdid it, and he would be alive today if he had been a moderate smoker, as would General Grant...

...The fiercest smoker whom I have ever known was the late Francis Saltus, the marvelous linguist, musician, composer, writer, and traveler. He would smoke (surely) fifty cigarettes a day. You talk about fellows smoking in bed and between courses at a dinner? Well, Frank Saltus would smoke between *mouthfuls*. I have seen him smoke fifty cigarettes in a day, while turning out two or three hundred dialogs ("squibs," he called them) for the papers and magazines. He was a wonder, look at him how you will, and some day the world will know it.

From: Bain J Jr., Tobacco Leaves, H.M. Caldwell Company, Boston, 1903.

BOX 7.5

SUDDEN INFANT DEATH SYNDROME

Definition: Death from the sudden cessation of breathing (apnea) of a seemingly healthy infant, almost always during sleep, sometimes traceable to chronic oxygen deficiency.

---

single most important preventable risk factor for Sudden Infant Death Syndrome. Sudden Infant Death Syndrome results from developmental delays in the neural control of cardiopulmonary function (Box 7.5). The children of smokers are also more likely to have respiratory diseases, such as asthma, and maternal smoking is significantly associated with increased risks of addiction to both tobacco and other drugs of abuse during adolescence, which is likely mediated by alterations in drug reward circuitry (see Chapter 2 and below). Some of these effects may be directly related to nicotine itself. Neurobiological bases exist for the toxic effects of nicotine on the brain, and they follow the transient increases in nicotinic acetylcholine receptor (nAChR) expression within a given brain structure that coincides with the most crucial phases of development. For example, nAChRs critically regulate catecholamine and autonomic development in the prenatal period, hippocampal and cerebellar development during the early postnatal period, and limbic and postnatal catecholamine development during the adolescent period, providing the substrates by which nicotine can alter cardiopulmonary function, immune function, and motivational function, respectively (for further reading, see Dwyer et al., 2009).

An even more surprising finding in the neurotoxicity of tobacco is that a grandmother's tobacco use is associated with an increased risk of early childhood asthma, even if the mother

---

BOX 7.6

EPIGENETICS

Definition: The study of the way in which the *expression* of heritable traits is modified by environmental influences or other mechanisms without a change in the DNA sequence.

---

did not smoke while pregnant. In an animal model of prenatal nicotine exposure, maternal nicotine exposure exerted adverse effects on lung development, not only for the immediate offspring *but also for the next generation.* Such a phenomenon is termed an epigenetic effect (Box 7.6), further emphasizing the important deleterious effects of smoking during pregnancy (for further reading, see Leslie, 2013).

A study sponsored by the World Health Organization and the World Bank estimated that in the United States, smoking-related healthcare expenses accounted for 6% of all annual healthcare costs. Overall, nicotine addiction costs the United States $155 billion annually. A graphic summary of the health toll of tobacco addiction is that:

> "Smokers lose at least one decade of life expectancy, as compared with those who have never smoked. Cessation before the age of 40 years reduces the risk of death associated with continued smoking by about 90%." *(Jha P, Ramasundarahettige C, Landsman V, Rostron B, Thun M, Anderson RN, McAfee T, Peto R. 21st-century hazards of smoking and benefits of cessation in the United States. New England Journal of Medicine, 2013, (368), 341–350.)*

Other forms of nicotine delivery include waterpipe smoking, smokeless tobacco, and electronic cigarettes. A non-cigarette mode of tobacco ingestion, waterpipe smoking, has its roots in ancient India and has been used for over 400 years. Waterpipe smoking has been steadily spreading among young people around the world in the past 10 years. Studies at universities in the United States reported in 2010 that the proportion of people who had ever used water pipes ranged up to 30%, and current waterpipe use ranges up to 20%. A "waterpipe" generally refers to the device or the tobacco use method in which smoke passes through water before it is inhaled. Many different names are associated with waterpipe smoking, including argileh, goza, shisha, and hubble-bubble, but the name *hookah* has gained generic status. A typical waterpipe consists of four main parts (Figure 7.5): the bowl, where the tobacco is burned; the base, filled with water; the stem, which connects the bowl to the base; and the hose and the mouthpiece, through which smoke is inhaled. A different type of tobacco preparation is used in waterpipes, which is both flavored and sweetened, and is referred to as Massel. Various flavors, including apple, blackberry, cappuccino, and mint, provide smokers with distinct cues of a pleasant smoking experience because of the sweet smell and smooth taste of the sweetened tobacco. The attraction of this type of method of tobacco use among young people may be related to its pleasant smooth smoke, social ambience, and the perception of reduced harm. One form of waterpipe involves placing burned charcoal pieces on top of a perforated aluminum foil that separates it from a flavored tobacco mixture. When the smoker draws air through the hose's mouthpiece, charcoal-heated air becomes smoke as it passes the tobacco mixture and cools as it bubbles through the water of the waterpipe before inhalation by the smoker. This alleged "filtering" is the basis for the misconception of "reduced" harm and "reduced" addiction potential. Waterpipes are smoked at "hookah bars,"

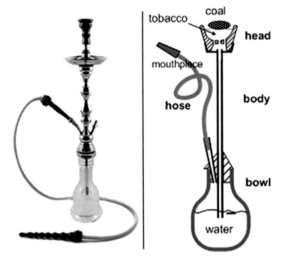

FIGURE 7.5 **A waterpipe and its main parts.** *[Taken with permission from Maziak W. The global epidemic of waterpipe smoking. Addictive Behaviors, 2011, (36), 1–5.]*

establishments that are becoming widespread in large cities across the United States. Recent research suggests that waterpipe smoking can be addictive and produce a substance use disorder-like syndrome. For example, although data are limited, waterpipe smoking is linked to the same cardiovascular and pulmonary diseases as cigarette smoking, with the addition of communicable diseases from sharing waterpipes and mouth pieces (for further reading, see Maziak, 2011; Noonan and Kulbok, 2010; Eissenberg and Shihadeh, 2009).

Smokeless tobacco can be defined as either chewing tobacco or snuff and is also a significant health concern. Adverse health consequences of smokeless tobacco use include oral (gum and buccal mucosa) cancer in smokeless tobacco users who chew quid or tobacco. According to the US National Survey on Drug Use and Health, in 2011, 8.2 million people aged 12 and older (3.2%) used smokeless tobacco, and 1.9 million people aged 18–25 had used a smokeless tobacco product in the past month.

The rapid growth of electronic cigarette use worldwide points to another potential health problem associated with nicotine. Electronic cigarettes deliver nicotine through the battery-powered vaporization of a nicotine/propylene-glycol solution; thus, electronic cigarettes (e-cigarettes) are hypothesized to be less harmful than regular cigarettes because they deliver nicotine without the various toxic constituents of tobacco smoke. Currently, 3.4% of the total population, including 11.4% of current smokers, 2.0% of former smokers, and 0.8% of never-smokers, reported using e-cigarettes (for further reading, see Pearson et al., 2012). Most smokers claim to use e-cigarettes for smoking cessation/reduction, and their use appears to enhance the motivation to quit. To date, studies show that blood nicotine levels generated by e-cigarettes are low to moderate, but e-cigarette use reduced craving and partially alleviated withdrawal symptoms. The compulsive-like use of e-cigarettes remains to be investigated.

MEDICAL USE AND BEHAVIORAL EFFECTS

Evidence indicates that people smoke primarily to experience the psychopharmacological properties of nicotine and that the majority of smokers eventually become dependent on nicotine if they start as adolescents. Numerous preclinical animal studies have demonstrated nicotine's reinforcing properties in many species. In humans, nicotine produces positive reinforcing effects, including mild euphoria, increased energy, heightened arousal, reduced stress, reduced anxiety, and reduced appetite. Cigarette smokers report that smoking produces arousal, particularly with the first cigarette of the day, but also relaxation when under stress (see Behavioral Mechanism of Action).

Nicotine reduces pain in humans and raises pain thresholds. Nicotine nasal spray or transdermal nicotine at low doses has been shown to reduce postoperative pain or reduce postoperative opiate requirements (see also Behavioral Mechanism of Action below).

The positive reinforcing effects of acute nicotine administration through tobacco smoking are considered to be critically important in the initiation and maintenance of tobacco smoking that ultimately leads to dependence. Nevertheless, factors other than nicotine contribute to smoking in human smokers, including sensory and conditioned reinforcing effects. For example, cigarette smoke has monoamine oxidase-inhibiting properties, similar to monoamine oxidase inhibitor antidepressants, which might contribute to its psychotropic effects and addiction potential.

Nicotine also decreases appetite, particularly the desire for sweet-tasting food and carbohydrates in both rats and humans, and this has been linked to the motivation to continue smoking in women and their higher rates of relapse compared with men. This appetite suppression is accompanied by decreases in blood insulin and changes in serotonin function. Nicotine also increases metabolism and fat oxidation.

Nicotine is well known to improve attention, learning, reaction time, and problem solving abilities in abstinent smokers and is particularly effective in enhancing selective attention and vigilance when performing repetitive tasks, a classic stimulant effect. Nicotine has also been shown to enhance cognitive performance in non-smokers.

Nicotine has numerous physiological effects that are mainly attributed to its ability to activate ganglionic receptors in the autonomic nervous system, including the adrenal medulla. However, this activation is only short-lasting, followed by persistent depression of all autonomic ganglia, depending on the dose and history of nicotine intake. In humans, cigarette smoking increases heart rate and blood pressure. It also stimulates the gastrointestinal tract, followed by inhibition, indicating parasympathetic activation. It causes bronchial dilation and stimulates the salivary glands.

Nicotine in a nicotine-naive individual can cause vomiting through activation of an emetic chemoreceptor trigger zone in the area postrema of the medulla and activation of vagal and spinal nerves that form the sensory component of the vomiting reflex. Thus, nicotine has numerous acute activating effects, reinforcing effects, and anxiolytic effects in humans.

PHARMACOKINETICS

When smoked in cigarettes and inhaled, nicotine is quickly absorbed in the lungs, with the freebase largely suspended on tiny tar particles. Inhaled nicotine reaches the brain within eight seconds, almost as quickly as an intravenous injection (Figure 7.6). Tobacco in oral products is more basic (has a high pH) and is better absorbed via the mouth than cigarette smoke, which is more acidic. Cigarettes contain 1–2% nicotine or approximately 10–20 mg of nicotine each. Most of the nicotine in inhaled smoke is absorbed in the lungs; much less is absorbed through the mouth. Dependent cigarette smokers tend to titrate their intake over time within the confines of the rapid rise and fall associated with each cigarette, but they average approximately 1 mg of delivered nicotine per cigarette (Figure 7.7). Dependent smokers will maintain relatively stable blood nicotine levels over the course of their waking hours (Figure 7.8). Plasma nicotine levels range from 4–6 ng/ml for pipe smoking to 20–50 ng/ml for cigarette smoking. Tobacco smokers can accumulate substantial levels of carboxyhemoglobin (7–10%) produced by 12 h of tobacco exposure (Figure 7.8). These carboxyhemoglobin levels produced by exposure to carbon monoxide are sufficient to meet and exceed the Environmental Protection Agency occupational threshold limit of 50 ppm of carbon monoxide

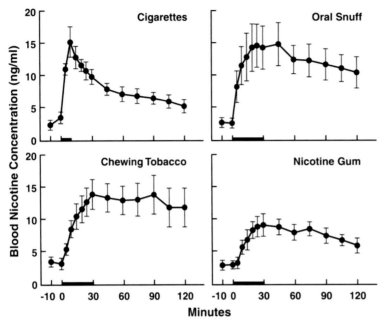

FIGURE 7.6 **Blood concentrations of nicotine in subjects who smoked cigarettes for 9 min (1.33 cigarettes), used oral snuff (2.5 g), used chewing tobacco (mean 7.0 g), or chewed nicotine gum (two 2 mg pieces). Shaded bars indicate the period of exposure to tobacco or nicotine gum.** *These data show that smoking cigarettes produces the most rapid rise in blood nicotine levels. Notice also, however, that oral snuff, chewing tobacco, and nicotine gum also have relatively rapid absorption, more than one sees with the oral administration of other drugs. This is attributable to the more basic pH in these preparations (see Chapter 2 for details on pH and absorption). [Taken with permission from Benowitz NL. Drug therapy: pharmacologic aspects of cigarette smoking and nicotine addiction. New England Journal of Medicine, 1988, (319), 1318–1330.]*

(which produces 5% carboxyhemoglobin). For example, in both males and females with an average cigarette consumption of 36 and 32 cigarettes per day, respectively, who had smoked 21 and 18 cigarettes, respectively, by the time of sampling, venous blood nicotine levels were approximately 32 ng/ml, and average carboxyhemoglobin levels were 8% (Table 7.2). Nicotine can also be passively absorbed, and non-smokers who live with a 40-cigarette-per-day smoker will achieve levels of urinary cotinine (a nicotine metabolite) that are equivalent to smoking approximately three cigarettes. The minimal acute fatal dose of oral nicotine appears to be about 65 mg, but some individuals have ingested much larger quantities and recovered.

About 80–90% of nicotine is metabolized in the liver, and nicotine and its metabolites, mainly cotinine and nicotine-1'-N-oxide, are excreted in the urine. Approximately 4% of nicotine is converted to nicotine N-oxide, which is largely excreted in urine without further metabolism.

Approximately 70% of nicotine is metabolized to cotinine, which is then further metabolized (Figure 7.9). The half-life of nicotine is about 2 h after inhalation or parenteral administration, and the half-life of cotinine is 19 h. The metabolite cotinine has been shown to have psychoactive effects. Intravenously administered cotinine (30 mg) produced blood cotinine levels similar to those of smoking (378 mg/ml) and significantly decreased tobacco withdrawal symptoms in abstinent cigarette smokers.

USE, ABUSE, AND ADDICTION

Tobacco smoking typically begins in adolescence, which significantly increases the likelihood of smoking in adulthood. Adolescents report being able to obtain tobacco easily. Most adolescents (95%) are aware of the health risks associated with smoking, but they report that this is of little concern. The prevalence of adolescent smoking increases with age: 12 (2%), 13 (5%), 14

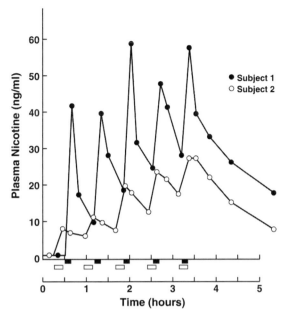

FIGURE 7.7 **Effects of five consecutive cigarettes on plasma nicotine concentration in two human subjects.** Thirty minutes elapsed between the end of one cigarette and the start of the next. The periods of smoking each cigarette are shown as solid bars (Subject 1) and open bars (Subject 2) beneath the X-axis. The curves coincide at the end of smoking the fifth cigarette. Blood samples were taken before smoking, 0.5, 10, and 30 min after the last puff of each cigarette, and 60 and 120 min after the fifth cigarette. *These data show that individuals vary in their absorption of the absolute amount of nicotine but show similar peak and trough patterns after each cigarette, increasing blood nicotine levels overall during the course of smoking five cigarettes each. [Taken with permission from Isaac PF, Rand MJ. Cigarette smoking and plasma levels of nicotine. Nature, 1972, (236), 308–310.].*

(9%), 15 (14%), 16 (22%), 17 (28%). Of adolescent smokers, 75% attempt to quit, but only 30% are able to abstain for more than one month.

Parental smoking, older sibling and peer smoking habits, the self-medication of emotional states, and the self-medication of withdrawal have all been linked to the rapid escalation in nicotine addiction in adolescents.

Prospective studies have found that up to 50% of adolescents and young adults who had initiated smoking showed an escalation in daily smoking within 4–5 years. Various

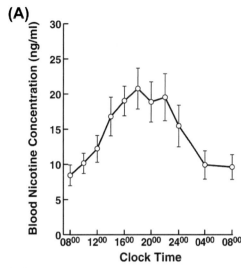

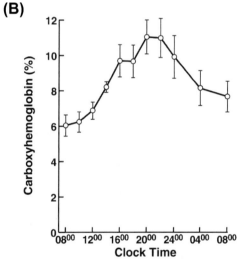

FIGURE 7.8 Venous blood nicotine (A) and carboxyhemoglobin (B) concentrations in human subjects throughout the day while smoking their usual brand. The subjects smoked at least one pack per day (mean, 28 cigarettes; range, 20–40 cigarettes). *These data show that individuals maintain a steady level of nicotine intake over the course of the waking day. Notice the high levels of carboxyhemoglobin that accompany such smoking. [Taken with permission from Benowitz NL, Jacob P 3rd. Nicotine and carbon monoxide intake from high- and low-yield cigarettes. Clinical Pharmacology and Therapeutics, 1984, (36), 265–270.]*

TABLE 7.2   Cigarette Consumption, Type of Cigarette Smoked (Average), and Blood Nicotine and Carboxyhemoglobin Concentrations (Averages) in Men and Women

	Men (*n* = 124)	Women (*n* = 206)
% smoking filtered cigarettes	61.3%	70.9%
% smoking unfiltered cigarettes	13.7%	1.9%
% smoking low-nicotine cigarettes (<1.0 mg)	25.0%	27.2%
Cigarette consumption per day	36.2 cigarettes	32.6 cigarettes
Cigarette consumption on day of test	20.7 cigarettes	18.2 cigarettes
Tar yield per cigarette	17.3 mg	15.8 mg
Nicotine yield per cigarette	1.3 mg	1.2 mg
Nicotine level in blood	33 ng/ml	32 ng/ml
Carboxyhemoglobin level in blood	7.8%	8.6%

Taken with permission from Russell MA, Jarvis M, Iyer R, Feyerabend C. Relation of nicotine yield of cigarettes to blood nicotine concentrations in smokers.
British Medical Journal, 1980, (280), 972–976.

psychosocial factors, such as peer smoking and parenting style, have been suggested to contribute to the escalated smoking behavior. Studies also suggest that the symptoms of nicotine dependence, most commonly craving for tobacco and withdrawal symptoms, can develop at very early stages of initial smoking, and this early appearance of symptoms of nicotine dependence was found to predict future escalation to daily chronic smoking. In contrast, individuals who engage in non-daily smoking without escalation ("chippers") had very few or no symptoms of dependence, and their smoking experience is primarily associated with positive rather than negative reinforcement. Thus, early tobacco use associated with withdrawal symptoms can promote the escalation of smoking behavior, which in turn accelerates the appearance of additional symptoms of dependence. The importance of negative emotional states associated with the withdrawal from tobacco use in the escalation of smoking is also suggested by the calming effects of nicotine when given after even a short period of abstinence, a primary reason given

by both adults and adolescents for smoking (see Behavioral Mechanism of Action). Thus, escalation may be more common among individuals with difficulties regulating negative affect, who are prone to develop withdrawal symptoms, and who have high expectancy of the calming effects of smoking, supporting a key role for negative reinforcement in tobacco addiction (see Chapter 1; for further reading, see Tucker et al., 2003; Heinz et al., 2010).

As smoking progresses, tolerance develops to the autonomic side effects of smoking. Several trajectories of cigarette use and dependence then follow (Figure 7.10). Once regular smoking is established, dependence rapidly follows, and regular smokers find quitting particularly difficult.

As with some other drugs, the trajectories of cigarette use have revealed a category of non-dependent smokers called *chippers*. Chippers are defined as those who smoke fewer than five cigarettes per day. Some people remain chippers, and some become *converted chippers* (those who were heavy smokers previously but currently smoke fewer than five cigarettes

(A)

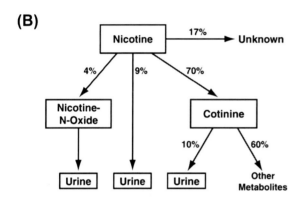

(B)

FIGURE 7.9 **Nicotine metabolism in humans.** (A) Oxidative metabolism of nicotine. (B) Quantitative disposition of nicotine in smokers.
[Taken with permission from Jacob P 3rd, Benowitz NL, Shulgin AT. Recent studies of nicotine metabolism in humans. Pharmacology Biochemistry and Behavior, *1988, (30), 249–253.]*

per day; for further reading, see Shiffman et al., 1994). One study of the smoking behavior of chippers compared their smoking history and dependence with regular smokers. Chippers did not meet the criteria for Substance Dependence (addiction) on nicotine (Table 7.3). When they first started smoking, regular smokers went through a phase of approximately 2 years when they engaged in light smoking (<5 cigarettes per day). Once they reached 15 cigarettes per day for at least 2 years (a frequency more or less defining Substance Dependence or Addiction), regular smokers never returned to chipping. In contrast, chippers smoked ≤5 cigarettes per day for 16 years. However, some converted chippers (29%) had previously smoked daily at a rate of ≥15 cigarettes per day for at least two consecutive years. The converted chippers who were previously regular smokers began their habit like regular smokers but remained chippers for 6 years. They showed a lack of dependence and decreased craving profiles, similar to non-converted chippers.

A nicotine abstinence syndrome after chronic nicotine exposure has been characterized in humans and rats, with both somatic and affective components. In humans, acute nicotine withdrawal is characterized by somatic symptoms, such as bradycardia, gastrointestinal discomfort, and increased appetite that leads to weight gain. Withdrawal is also associated with affective symptoms, including depressed mood, dysphoria, irritability, anxiety, frustration, increased reactivity to environmental stimuli, and difficulty

(A)

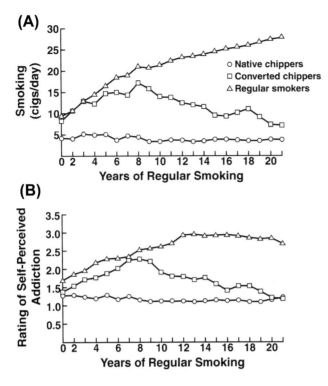

○ Native chippers
□ Converted chippers
△ Regular smokers

(B)

FIGURE 7.10 **Different patterns of smoking that evolve over time as measured by (A) the number of cigarettes smoked and (B) the self-rating of addiction in subjects.** Chippers were arbitrarily defined as individuals who smoked 1–5 cigarettes per day and reported no dependence. Chippers reported casual abstinence without any withdrawal symptoms or any evidence of tolerance. Converted chippers were individuals who met the criteria for chipping but had experienced extended periods of heavy smoking. *These data show multiple patterns of cigarette intake and emphasize the point that not all cigarette smoking meets the criteria for dependence (see discussion of dependence and substance use disorders in* Chapter 1). *[Provided with permission by Dr. Saul Shiffman, Department of Psychology, University of Pittsburgh.]*

concentrating. Anxiety, difficulty concentrating, hunger, irritability, restlessness, weight gain, and decreased heart rate are all validated signs of nicotine withdrawal in self-quitters. These symptoms begin 6–12 h after cessation, peak in 1–3 days, and then return to normal within 7–30 days (for further reading, see Hughes, 1992; Figure 7.11).

Enduring symptoms of nicotine withdrawal (protracted abstinence) in humans include a continued powerful craving that can last up to 6 months. Rates of depression did not increase with spontaneous nicotine withdrawal, but subjects who did experience an increase in depression were more likely to relapse. The somatic symptoms of withdrawal from chronic drug intake are unpleasant and annoying, but avoidance of the *affective* components of drug withdrawal may play a more important role in the maintenance of the tobacco habit. Although many smokers who attempt to quit

are successful early on, relapse rates are high in the long-term, with only 10–20% of individuals remaining abstinent after 1 year.

Nicotine replacement therapy, including nicotine gum, nicotine patches, and sublingual nicotine tablets, reduce the occurrence of withdrawal symptoms in abstinent smokers. The efficacy of nicotine replacement therapy in smoking cessation trials is related to the ability to prevent the onset and reduce the duration of nicotine withdrawal, increasing the percentage of individuals who succeed in quitting smoking permanently. Nonetheless, only 20–30% of smokers who use nicotine replacement therapy remain abstinent after 1 year.

The strong relationship between withdrawal and negative affect, including anxiety, frustration, anger, and depressed mood, has led to another therapeutic approach to smoking cessation: antidepressant treatment. Some estimates indicate that up to 60% of smokers have a history of clinical

TABLE 7.3 Fagerstrom Tolerance Questionnaire Items

Variable[a]	Chippers		Regular Smokers		Effect size[b]
	Mean	SD	Mean	SD	
Latency to first cigarette of the day (min)	347.4	286.2	18.2	27.8	41.1****
Rate-adjusted latency to first cigarette of the day[c]	124.1	276.3	-16.2	24.4	12.0***
Smoking when awakes during night[d] (monthly frequency)	0.2	0.7	1.8	5.0	32.6**
Most hate to give up first cigarette in the morning (%)	4.6	–	9.4	–	5.0*
Smoking or craving more or less in the morning (1–5 scale)	1.7	1.1	3.4	1.1	38.6****
Difficulty refraining when forbidden (1–5 scale)	1.3	0.6	2.6	1.0	39.7****
Smoking when ill in bed (1.5 scale)	1.1	0.4	2.9	1.1	54.2****

Questionnaire from Fagerstrom KO. Measuring degree of physical dependence to tobacco smoking with reference to individualization of treatment. Addictive Behaviors, 1978, (3), 235–241.

[a] *Canonical correlation = 0.81, Wilks' $\lambda = 0.35$, $F_{6,130} = 40.4$, $p < 0.0000001$.*

[b] *Effect size is expressed as percentage of variance accounted.*

[c] *Adjustment made for differences in smoking frequency; lag to first cigarette compared to average inter-cigarette interval. Positive values indicate smoking later than expected; negative values indicate smoking sooner than expected.*

[d] *This item is not part of the original Fagerstrom Tolerance Questionnaire but relates to similar content. Analyzed with nonparametric statistics because of highly skewed distribution.*

* $p < 0.01$,

** $p < 0.001$,

*** $p < 0.00005$,

**** $p < 0.0000001$.

[Taken with permission from Shiffman S, Paty JA, Kassel JD, Gnys M, Zettler-Segal M. Smoking behavior and smoking history of tobacco chippers. Experimental and Clinical Psychopharmacology, 1994, (2), 126–142.]

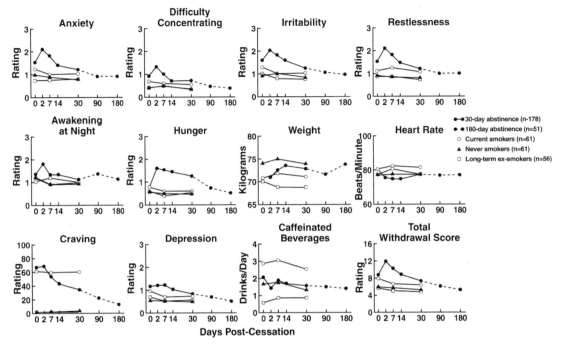

FIGURE 7.11 **Self-reported symptoms before and after the cessation of tobacco use.** The zero value on the X-axis indicates pre-cessation. *These data show a comprehensive assessment of the different symptoms of cigarette smoking during withdrawal in humans. Notice that many of the symptoms are of a motivational nature, such as anxiety, irritability, difficulty concentrating, and depression. [Taken with permission from Hughes JR. Tobacco withdrawal in self-quitters.* Journal of Consulting and Clinical Psychology, *1992, (60), 689–697.]*

depression, and the incidence of clinically diagnosed Major Depressive Disorder among smokers was twice as high as non-smokers. Smokers with a history of clinical depression were also significantly less likely to succeed in quitting than smokers without depressive histories (14% vs. 28%). Unknown is whether individuals who suffer depressive symptoms are more likely to become smokers or whether depressive symptoms are induced or exacerbated by long-term smoking. Tricyclic antidepressants like imipramine have shown some promise in aiding smoking cessation, but selective serotonin reuptake inhibitors like fluoxetine did not affect smoking behavior in heavy smokers. Bupropion (Wellbutrin, Zyban), an atypical antidepressant that facilitates norepinephrine and dopamine neurotransmission but not serotonin neurotransmission, was proven effective in double-blind, placebo-controlled trials. Twice the number of subjects who received 300 mg bupropion per day for 2 months remained abstinent compared with subjects treated with placebo (for more information, see Chapter 9).

BEHAVIORAL MECHANISM OF ACTION

The behavioral mechanism of action of nicotine has been related to "mood titration": the regulation of an individual's mood by adding known amounts of nicotine over circumscribed periods of time until a given mood state occurs. Nicotine produces both attentional and autonomic arousal, and smoking one or two cigarettes increases resting heart rate by about 5 to 40 beats/min, increases blood pressure 5–20 mmHg, and increases epinephrine and cortisol levels. One representative study found that most smokers report that smoking is pleasurable (81%), helps them concentrate (63%), calms them down when stressed or upset (90%), and helps them deal with difficult situations (82%).

Nicotine paradoxically produces decreases in tension and an anxiolytic-like effect. The basis for such tension reduction is still unknown but may be linked to decreases in skeletal muscle tone, a subsequent reduction of muscle tension, and possibly an analgesic effect. Called *Nesbitt's paradox*, smokers allowed to smoke during a stressful experience (for example, in a laboratory setting where they receive painful shocks to the left forearm and upper arm) showed more arousal (an increase in pulse rate) but reported less emotion (more pain endurance and more shocks taken) than smokers who were not allowed to smoke but simulated smoking. These results were interpreted as a paradox, in which smokers exhibit an increase in physiological arousal, but they self-report that they are calmer and more relaxed. A majority of smokers have reported that they smoke to reduce negative mood or to achieve pleasurable relaxation.

Cigarette smokers titrate their level of nicotine intake over the course of a smoking bout, in which the intensity and interval of taking puffs of a single cigarette remain fairly stable and regular while smoking the cigarette. Dependent smokers titrate both their smoking bouts and the number of cigarettes smoked during waking hours. Cigarette smokers will compensate for a reduction of the number of cigarettes smoked by altering the topography of their smoking behavior, with longer and more frequent drags from the cigarette. Low-nicotine cigarettes also lead to similar compensation through increased inhalation and an increase in the number of cigarettes smoked.

Another example of such regulation of nicotine intake is "vent blocking." To lower the smoke and nicotine content of cigarettes, the filter on the end of a low-yield cigarette is ventilated with holes so that each puff is diluted with ambient air. Smokers unconsciously negate the benefit of this ventilation by blocking the air holes with their lips or fingers. Similar titration can be seen when cigarette smokers are allowed to self-administer nicotine intravenously. When subjects were allowed access to 1.5 mg nicotine per intravenous injection, they all self-administered 18–27 μg/kg, despite wide variations in the number of injections (range, 6–25). The number of injections per session was inversely related to the μg/kg administered. The subjects adjusted their intake to compensate for body mass and presumably the volume of distribution of nicotine in the blood.

The *boundary model* (for further reading, see Herman and Kozlowski, 1979) explains the mood titration mentioned above. This model proposes three zones of behavioral effects associated with smoking behavior which are delimited by an aversive state of withdrawal when plasma nicotine levels fall below a certain point (the lower boundary) and the noxious aversive state associated with toxic high doses of nicotine (the upper boundary). The zone between the two is called the *zone of indifference* to nicotine's pharmacological effects, which can be very large for a nondependent smoker and very small for a heavily dependent smoker (Figure 7.12). A narrow zone of indifference explains the regulation of mood that is hypothesized to be the basis of behavioral mood titration.

NEUROBIOLOGICAL EFFECTS

Binge/Intoxication Stage

Nicotine as a Nicotinic Acetylcholine Receptor Agonist

The initial molecular site of action for the physiological effects of nicotine is the nicotinic acetylcholine receptor (nAChR). nAChRs are cationic ligand-gated ion channels that are expressed

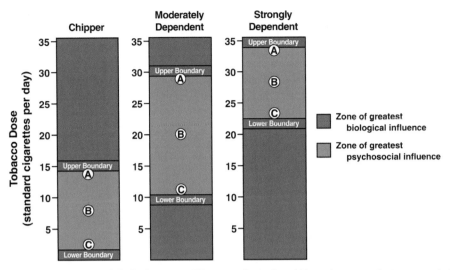

FIGURE 7.12   **The boundary model of tobacco use.** The upper boundary (A) marks a zone that represents the weighted sum of all of the aversive biological consequences of smoking cigarettes. The intermediate zone (B) represents the relative range of indifference to the pharmacological properties of the drug. The lower boundary (C) marks a zone that represents the weighted sum of all of the biologically based pressures to smoke. The zones represent different rates of smoking sustained by an individual, varying from high psychosocial pressure to smoke (light blue) to very low psychosocial pressure (purple). *[Modified with permission from Kozlowski LT, Herman CP. The interaction of psychosocial and biological determinants of tobacco use: more on the boundary model.* Journal of Applied Social Psychology, *1984, (14), 244–256.]*

throughout the central nervous system. Neuronal nAChRs can be presynaptic or postsynaptic and activate other neurons by increasing the influx of calcium, so producing neurotransmitter release. The influx of calcium on postsynaptic neurons can also trigger many cellular signal transduction processes, including the activation of protein kinase and calmodulin-dependent kinase. nAChRs are pentameric structures with at least two ligand-binding sites at the interface between subunits (Figure 7.13). A wide variety of nAChR subtypes with different pharmacological and electrophysiological properties exists. The genes that encode nAChR subunits have been identified and cloned in mammals (α1-α10 and β1-β9), and several subunits have been found in the central nervous system (α2-α7 and β2-β4). These subunits co-assemble to form functional pentameric receptors. Three distinct families of nAChRs are represented in the body and brain. The α1, β1, γ, δ, and ϵ subunits represent the muscle acetylcholine

receptor family. The α2–6 and β2–4 subunits represent one central nervous system family. A third family can form homopentameric acetylcholine receptors composed of α7–10 subunits. All high-affinity binding sites for nicotine include the β2 subunit, a critical subunit for the reinforcing effects of nicotine.

Acute Reinforcing and Stimulant-Like Effects of Nicotine

In animals, nicotine lowers brain reward thresholds, similarly to other drugs of abuse (Figure 7.14). Nicotine sustains intravenous self-administration in both animals and humans. In rats, the dose range at which the animal will self-administer nicotine is relatively narrow (Figure 7.15). Animals and humans titrate their intake of nicotine to maintain stable blood nicotine levels.

Probably not surprisingly, nicotine has less efficacy than cocaine as a reinforcer in nondependent animals, reflected by much higher

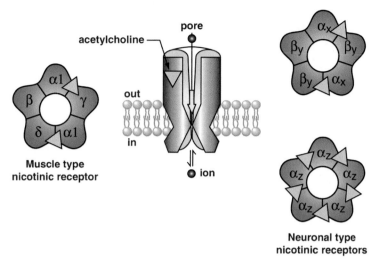

FIGURE 7.13   **Schematic diagram of the structural organization of the nicotinic acetylcholine receptor (nAChR).** The structure of the muscular receptor (left) of the nAChR is well characterized, and much of what we know about the structure of the neuronal receptor (right) is based on studies of the muscular receptor. nAChRs cross the membrane, and the binding of acetylcholine (or nicotine) causes the receptor to change shape and open a channel that allows ions to flow into and out of the cell. The nAChR in adult muscle is made up of the α_1, β_1, γ, and δ subunits, and there are two different families of nAChRs expressed in neurons. One family is made up of a combination of the α and β subunits (in this subtype, $\alpha_x = \alpha_{2-6}$ and $\beta_y = \beta_{2-4}$), whereas the other family can form active receptors made up of only one type of subunit (in this homomeric subtype, $\alpha_z = \alpha_{7-9}$). The five binding sites on the α_7 subtype are hypothesized based on a symmetry argument. Because all five subunits of the complex are identical, the structural elements involved in binding ligands (gray triangles) should be identical on each subunit that provides five binding sites. *[Taken with permission from Picciotto MR, Zoli M, Changeux JP. Use of knockout mice to determine the molecular basis for the actions of nicotine.* Nicotine and Tobacco Research, *1999, 1 (suppl 2): s121–s125.]*

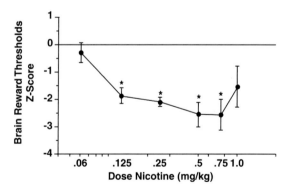

FIGURE 7.14   **Mean z-score (standard score) ± SEM changes in intracranial self-stimulation reward thresholds from pre- to post-drug after administration of various doses of nicotine in rats.** Saline post-drug minus pre-drug threshold is indicated by a z-score of 0. *$p < 0.025$, doses of nicotine that significantly lowered threshold. *These data show that nicotine, like other drugs of abuse, can facilitate brain stimulation reward (for details of intracranial self-stimulation, see* Chapter 3*). A z-score is a statistical measure (also called a "standard score"), representing a standard distribution around a mean of zero. A +1.96 or −1.96 z-score represents close to two standard deviations away from the mean and is considered a statistically significant difference. [Taken with permission from Huston-Lyons D, Kornetsky C. Effects of nicotine on the threshold for rewarding brain stimulation in rats.* Pharmacology Biochemistry and Behavior, *1992, (41), 755–759.]*

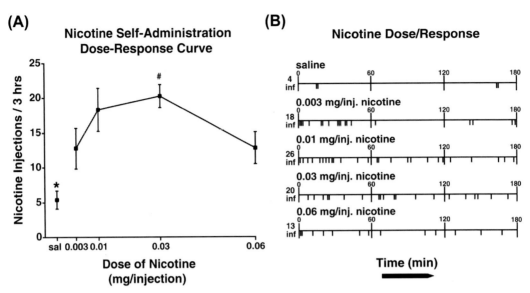

FIGURE 7.15   (A) Mean number of nicotine infusions earned during 3 hour sessions of intravenous nicotine self-administration in rats (*n* = 5–7). The data are expressed as the mean of the second and third days of 3 days of self-administration at each nicotine dose (0, 0.003, 0.01, 0.03, and 0.06 mg/kg/infusion, i.v.). The saline (sal) dose represents the mean of the second and third days after substitution of saline for nicotine. All of the rats were initially trained on 0.03 mg/kg/infusion nicotine. *p < 0.05, responding for saline was significantly different from responding for all nicotine doses; #*p* < 0.05, responding for the 0.03 mg/kg dose was significantly higher than responding for the 0.003 and 0.06 mg/kg doses. (B) Event record of responding for nicotine for each dose tested. *These data show that nicotine is reinforcing in rats. Animals without any deprivation will learn to intravenously self-administer nicotine. The function that relates the unit dose per injection with self-administration shows an inverted U-shaped function, similar to other intravenously self-administered drugs in the psychostimulant class, but the function for nicotine has more of an ascending limb and less of a descending limb for such a fixed-ratio 1 schedule of reinforcement compared with cocaine. Notice in the event recordings that the animals "load up" at the beginning of the session, similarly to human cigarette smokers (see Figure 7.7), but then settle down with regular intervals between infusions.* [Taken with permission from Watkins SS, Epping-Jordan MP, Koob GF, Markou A. Blockade of nicotine self-administration with nicotinic antagonists in rats. Pharmacology Biochemistry and Behavior, 1999, (62), 743–751.]

breakpoints for cocaine than nicotine on a progressive-ratio schedule of reinforcement (Figure 7.16). Similarly to its actions in humans, nicotine produces locomotor activation, analgesia, appetite suppression, and improvements in learning and memory in rats.

In rats, nicotine produces a stimulant effect that can show either tolerance or sensitization, depending on the nature of exposure to the drug. In nicotine-naive rats, acute nicotine administration decreased exploratory locomotor activity, whereas repeated nicotine administration produced rapid tolerance to this locomotor-depressant effect, followed by an increase in locomotor activity. With repeated intermittent nicotine administration, sensitization to the locomotor-activating effects of nicotine develops (Figure 7.17).

Acute nicotine administration can produce an anxiolytic-like effect in the social interaction test, in which two rats are placed in the same cage and allowed to engage in social contact, but high doses can have an opposite effect. Anxiolytic-like effects have also been observed in the potentiated startle paradigm (skeletomuscular response to an abrupt noise or stimulation) and elevated plus maze, both of which are animal models used to test anxiety-like behavior.

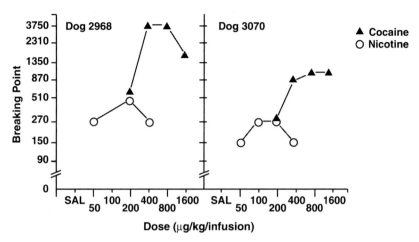

FIGURE 7.16 **The highest fixed-ratio completed by two dogs responding for intravenous infusion of nicotine, cocaine, or saline under a progressive-ratio schedule of reinforcement.** Each point represents a single determination at the selected dose and drug. Dog #2968 was tested twice with saline. Notice the logarithmic scale used for the ordinate. *These data are one of the only direct comparisons of the relative efficacy of given drugs of abuse measured by progressive-ratio responding (see Chapter 3 for details on progressive-ratio schedules of reinforcement). Notice that nicotine under these conditions has much less efficacy as a reinforcer than cocaine.* [*Taken with permission from Risner ME, Goldberg SR. A comparison of nicotine and cocaine self-administration in the dog: fixed-ratio and progressive-ratio schedules of intravenous drug infusion.* Journal of Pharmacology and Experimental Therapeutics, 1983, (224), 319–326.]

Nicotine can reduce pain in humans, and activation of nicotinic receptors elicits an antinociceptive effect in a variety of nonhuman species in a variety of pain tests. Nicotine may act at the spinal cord level of pain processing, in the brain itself. Supraspinally administered nicotine (in the area of the brain above the spinal cord) is more effective than spinally administered nicotine. Nicotine is hypothesized to reduce pain by interacting with several neurotransmitter systems through the release of norepinephrine, the release of endogenous opioids, and through the suppression of inflammatory actions. Nicotine appears to act through both the $\alpha4\beta2$ and $\alpha7$ subunits of the nAChR to produce analgesia (for further reading, see Benowitz, 2008).

Animal studies of the acute reinforcing effects of nicotine using intravenous self-administration have predominantly focused on nAChR activation in the mesocorticolimbic dopamine system that projects from the ventral tegmental area to the nucleus accumbens and prefrontal cortex (Figure 7.18). The presence of nAChRs throughout the mesocorticolimbic dopamine

system suggests that any of the regions that comprise this system could mediate the effects of nicotine, but the ventral tegmental area seems to play a more important role than the nucleus accumbens. Microinjection of nicotine directly into the nucleus accumbens or ventral tegmental area increases extracellular levels of dopamine in the nucleus accumbens (Figure 7.19).

Nicotine-induced dopamine release and the nicotine-induced activation of dopamine neurons depend on the $\beta2$ subunit. Knockout mice that lack the $\beta2$ subunit will not self-administer nicotine (Figure 7.20), indicating that the $\beta2$ subunit is critically involved in nicotine reinforcement.

$\beta2$-selective nAChR antagonists also block nicotine self-administration in rats, indicating that nAChR activation is involved in the reinforcing actions of nicotine. The ventral tegmental area has been shown to have nAChRs on cell bodies and dendrites of dopamine neurons. Infusions of the nAChR antagonist dihydro-β-erythroidine directly into the ventral tegmental area but not nucleus accumbens significantly decreased

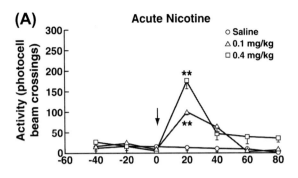

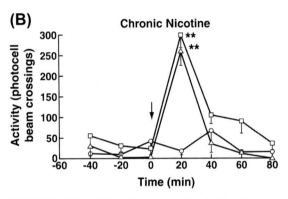

FIGURE 7.17 **Effect of acute and subchronic injections of nicotine on spontaneous locomotor activity in rats.** Rats were habituated to the testing environment for 80 min prior to the injection. (A) For acute treatment, subcutaneous injections of saline ($n = 6$), 0.1 mg/kg nicotine ($n = 6$), or 0.4 mg/kg nicotine ($n = 8$) were given at the point indicated by the arrow (time 0). **$p < 0.01$. (B) For chronic treatment, rats were pretreated with daily subcutaneous injections of saline ($n = 6$), 0.1 mg/kg nicotine ($n = 6$), or 0.4 mg/kg nicotine ($n = 10$) for 5 days before the test day. On the test day, the animals were given injections of saline or nicotine (0.1 or 0.4 mg/kg), respectively, at the time indicated by the arrow (time 0). **$p < 0.01$. *These data show that nicotine, similar to other drugs of abuse, can show locomotor sensitization with repeated administration. Some have argued that this locomotor sensitization has motivational significance for the acquisition and reinstatement of drug-seeking behavior (see Chapter 1). [Taken with permission from Benwell ME, Balfour DJ. The effects of acute and repeated nicotine treatment on nucleus accumbens dopamine and locomotor activity. British Journal of Pharmacology, 1992, (105), 849–856.]*

nicotine self-administration in rats. Dihydro-β-erythroidine is relatively selective for the α4 and β2 subunits of the nAChR. Chemical lesions

with 6-hydroxydopamine (see Chapter 4) of the nucleus accumbens and systemic administration of selective dopamine D_1 and D_2 receptor antagonists also decreased nicotine self-administration (Figure 7.21). Direct administration of the nAChR antagonist methyllycaconitine into the ventral tegmental area also attenuated the nicotine-induced lowering of brain reward thresholds. Such data indicate that one of the primary sites of action for the acute positive reinforcing properties of nicotine is the mesocorticolimbic dopamine system, and these pharmacological data suggest that α4 and β2 subunits of the nAChR play important roles in nicotine reinforcement (for further reading, see Fowler et al., 2008).

Cholinergic neurons from the pedunculopontine tegmental and laterodorsal tegmental nuclei project to dopamine neurons in the substantia nigra and ventral tegmental area and may link important components of the nicotine reward circuit. Myelinated axons in the medial forebrain bundle (an area that supports high rates of electrical self-stimulation behavior; see Chapter 2) that project to the pedunculopontine nucleus activate cholinergic neurons that in turn activate dopamine neurons in the ventral tegmental area by stimulating both nicotinic and muscarinic receptors. The nicotine-induced stimulation of cholinergic neurons in the pedunculopontine tegmental nucleus increases the release of endogenous acetylcholine, which excites dopamine neurons in the substantia nigra and ventral tegmental area. This nicotine-induced activation can by blocked by the nAChR antagonist mecamylamine. Chemical lesions of the pedunculopontine tegmental nucleus or direct administration of the nAChR antagonist dihydro-β-erythroidine into this region blocked nicotine self-administration. Similarly, lesions of the pedunculopontine tegmental nucleus blocked the rewarding effects of nicotine in a conditioned place preference paradigm.

Nicotine also interacts with opioid peptides. High densities of μ opioid receptors are found in the nucleus accumbens. Systemic nicotine

Neurochemical Neurocircuits in Drug Reward
Nicotine

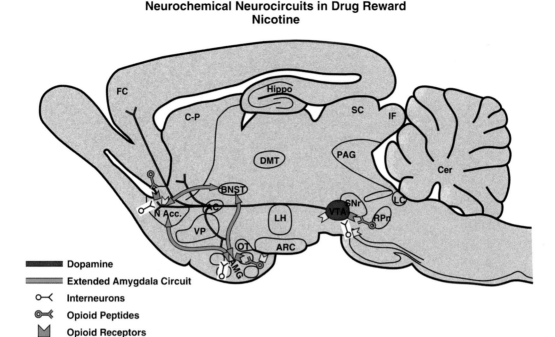

	Dopamine
	Extended Amygdala Circuit
○⊰	Interneurons
⊙⊰	Opioid Peptides
M	Opioid Receptors
M	Nicotine Receptors

FIGURE 7.18   **Sagittal section through a representative rodent brain illustrating the pathways and receptor systems implicated in the acute reinforcing actions of nicotine.** Nicotine activates nicotinic acetylcholine receptors in the ventral tegmental area, nucleus accumbens, and amygdala either directly or indirectly via actions on interneurons. Nicotine may also activate opioid peptide release in the nucleus accumbens or amygdala independent of the dopamine system. The blue arrows represent the interactions within the extended amygdala system hypothesized to play a key role in nicotine reinforcement and dependence. AC, anterior commissure; AMG, amygdala; ARC, arcuate nucleus; BNST, bed nucleus of the stria terminalis; Cer, cerebellum; C-P, caudate-putamen; DMT, dorsomedial thalamus; FC, frontal cortex; Hippo, hippocampus; IF, inferior colliculus; LC, locus coeruleus; LH, lateral hypothalamus; N Acc., nucleus accumbens; OT, olfactory tract; PAG, periaqueductal gray; RPn, reticular pontine nucleus; SC, superior colliculus; SNr, substantia nigra pars reticulata; VP, ventral pallidum; VTA, ventral tegmental area. *[Taken with permission from Koob GF, Le Moal M.* Neurobiology of Addiction. *Academic Press, London, 2006.]*

administration increases opioid peptide levels in the nucleus accumbens. Some clinical studies found that the opioid receptor antagonist naltrexone blocked or lessened the reinforcing effects of nicotine, and μ opioid receptor knockout mice did not exhibit reinforcing effects of nicotine in the conditioned place preference paradigm. μ Opioid receptor knockout mice also exhibited a reduction of the analgesic effects of nicotine and a reduction of nicotine withdrawal in dependent mice. These results suggest that

endogenous opioids may be involved in the reinforcing effects of nicotine.

Other neurochemical systems also modulate certain components of nicotine reinforcement, including glutamatergic and γ-aminobutyric acid (GABA) systems, at the cellular level (see below). Regardless of the extent to which each of these systems modulates nicotine reinforcement, they all appear to interact with the midbrain dopamine system, although dopamine-independent reinforcing actions have also been demonstrated

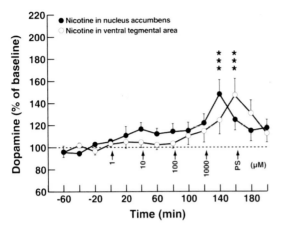

FIGURE 7.19 Temporal changes in extracellular concentrations of dopamine in rats after nicotine infusion (1, 10, 100, and 1000 µM, 40 min each concentration) in the nucleus accumbens ($n = 5$) and ventral tegmental area ($n = 7$). The arrows indicate the start of the infusion of each drug concentration or perfusion solution (PS). ***$p < 0.001$. *These data show that nicotine infused directly into either the ventral tegmental area or nucleus accumbens can activate the mesocorticolimbic dopamine system. Notice that the dose-effect function (see Chapter 2) is shifted to the right for the nucleus accumbens (that is, more nicotine is required at that site to elicit the same response produced by nicotine in the ventral tegmental area). [Taken with permission from Nisell M, Nomikos GG, Svensson TH. Systemic nicotine-induced dopamine release in the rat nucleus accumbens is regulated by nicotinic receptors in the ventral tegmental area. Synapse, 1994, (16), 36–44.]*

using conditioned place preference (for further reading, see Laviolette and van der Kooy, 2004).

Cellular Mechanism of Action

At the cellular level, one hypothesis for the mechanism by which nicotine activates the mesocorticolimbic dopamine system may also involve *N*-methyl-D-aspartate (NMDA) receptors (in the ventral tegmental area). Acute nicotine administration activates nAChRs located presynaptically on glutamatergic terminals, leading to increased glutamate release. In turn, glutamate increases the firing rate of dopamine neurons and increases subsequent dopamine release in the nucleus accumbens. The blockade of NMDA receptors with an NMDA receptor antagonist injected systemically or directly into the ventral

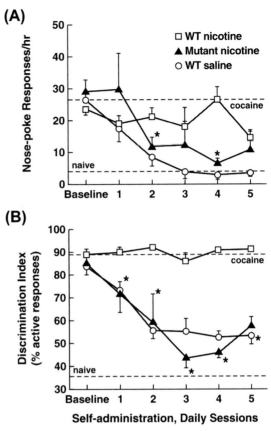

FIGURE 7.20 Intravenous self-administration of cocaine and nicotine in $\beta_2^{-/-}$ knockout mice (mutant nicotine) and their wildtype (WT) siblings with a history of cocaine self-administration. (A) Number of active nosepoke responses per session. Dashed lines represent the average of the last three sessions of cocaine self-administration in all of the groups of mice (cocaine) or spontaneous nosepoke behavior in naive, sham-operated mice (naive). (B) Percentage of the number of active responses compared with the sum of active and inactive responses per session. Values of 50% indicate a lack of discrimination between active and inactive detectors. $\beta_2^{-/-}$ mice differed significantly from wildtype mice that self-administered nicotine in either the active nosepoke ($p < 0.05$) or discrimination ($p < 0.01$) index but did not differ from wildtype mice during saline-induced extinction. The increase in the variability of nosepoke responses in $\beta_2^{-/-}$ mice on the first day of nicotine treatment was attributable to the increased responding of some mice, usually interpreted as a transient overresponse to reinforcer devaluation. *$p < 0.05$, significant difference between $\beta_2^{-/-}$ group and wildtype nicotine group. *These data show that mice with knockout of the β_2 nicotinic receptor will not self-administer nicotine, establishing this receptor subtype as a key initial site for the actions of nicotine. [Taken with permission from Picciotto MR, Zoli M, Rimondini R, Lena C, Marubio LM, Pich EM, Fuxe K, Changeux JP. Acetylcholine receptors containing the $\beta2$ subunit are involved in the reinforcing properties of nicotine. Nature, 1998, (391), 173–177.]*

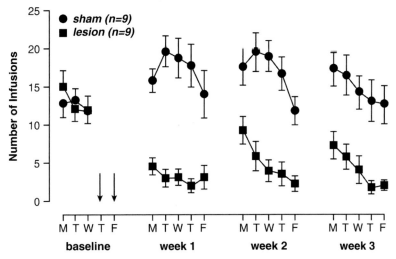

FIGURE 7.21 **Effects of bilateral 6-hydroxydopamine lesions or ascorbate vehicle infusions into the dopamine terminal field in the nucleus accumbens on nicotine self-administration in rats.** Each rat was lesioned on one of two days, as indicated by the arrows. Notice that although the number of nicotine infusions increased at the beginning of the second and third weeks of testing, this increase was not sustained. Over the 3 week test period, a marked difference was observed between the control and lesion groups. *These data show that the removal of dopaminergic terminals in the mesocorticolimbic dopamine system in the nucleus accumbens with a neurotoxin that selectively destroys monoamine axons and terminals causes rats to stop taking nicotine. The rats extinguished their drug-seeking behavior although nicotine was readily available (see Chapter 3 for a definition of extinction). [Taken with permission from Corrigall WA, Franklin KBJ, Coen KM, Clarke PBS. The mesolimbic dopaminergic system is implicated in the reinforcing effects of nicotine.* Psychopharmacology, 1992, (107), 285–289.]

tegmental area dose-dependently attenuated nicotine-induced dopamine release in the nucleus accumbens. The blockade of NMDA receptors also decreased intravenous nicotine self-administration and the nicotine-induced lowering of brain reward thresholds. Such data indicate that the activation of nAChRs on glutamatergic terminals may be a key component of the nicotine/mesocorticolimbic dopamine interaction in the ventral tegmental area that is important for the acute reinforcing properties of nicotine.

Inhibitory GABA neurotransmission may also play a role in nicotine/dopamine interactions. GABAergic afferents to dopaminergic neurons in the ventral tegmental area and medium spiny GABAergic neurons in the nucleus accumbens inhibit mesocorticolimbic dopamine release. Pharmacological enhancement of GABAergic neurotransmission blocked the reinforcing effects of nicotine in conditioned place preference and self-administration studies and blocked nicotine-induced increases in dopamine in the nucleus accumbens (Figure 7.22).

As noted above, nicotine increases the firing rate of dopaminergic neurons in the ventral tegmental area, and substantia nigra, and this excitatory effect appears to occur through the $\alpha4\beta2$ subtype. In an *in vitro* study in which nicotine was directly applied onto a midbrain dopamine neuron in a slice preparation of the ventral tegmental area at a concentration that was equivalent to the nicotine concentration that a smoker would achieve, nicotine activated and then desensitized nicotinic receptors. Also in slice preparations, nicotine enhanced the firing of both dopamine and non-dopamine (presumably GABAergic) neurons, but the non-dopamine neurons desensitized more rapidly. This may contribute to prolonged activation of dopamine neurons through a disinhibitory effect.

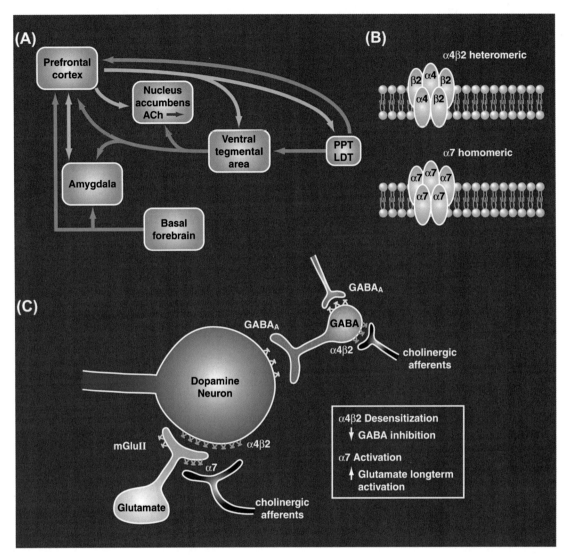

FIGURE 7.22 **Interconnecting brain pathways, receptors, and synapses mediate neuroadaptive changes that accompany nicotine addiction.** (A) Neural systems implicated in addiction and behavioral sensitization. Dopamine neurons (*pink*) located in the midbrain ventral tegmental area project to the limbic forebrain and cortical regions, such as the prefrontal cortex, amygdala, and nucleus accumbens. These structures are connected by glutamatergic pathways (*green*). The cholinergic pathways (*blue*) include cell bodies in the pedunculopontine nucleus (PPT) and lateral dorsal tegmentum (LDT) that project to the ventral tegmental area and cortical regions. A second major cholinergic pathway arises from the basal forebrain and reaches widespread cortical and limbic regions. A third source of forebrain acetylcholine constitutes the intrinsic neurons of the nucleus accumbens, a brain reward region. (B) Two different types of neuronal nicotinic receptors commonly found in the cholinergic pathways described above and proposed to be involved in the brain's response to drugs of abuse. (C) Potential interactions between acetylcholine, glutamate, and dopamine cells in the midbrain. Acetylcholine release in this area could activate both presynaptic nicotinic α_7 receptors located on glutamatergic terminals (GLU) and postsynaptic $\alpha_4\beta_2$ nicotinic receptors located on dopamine cell bodies. Complex interactions between the acetylcholine, dopamine, and glutamate systems are likely to set the addiction process in motion. *[Panels A and B taken with permission from Kelley AE. Nicotinic receptors: addiction's smoking gun?* Nature Medicine, *2002, (8), 447–449.] [Based on Mansvelder HD, McGehee DS. Cellular and synaptic mechanisms of nicotine addiction.* Journal of Neurobiology, *2002, (53), 606–617.]*

Another cellular hypothesis that may explain the overall actions of nicotine in the ventral tegmental area is that nicotine binds to α7 nAChRs on presynaptic glutamate terminals in the ventral tegmental area and induces long-term potentiation of excitatory glutamate transmission in midbrain dopamine neurons. Thus, nicotine's combined effects on glutamate and GABA neurons can produce powerful and prolonged activation of dopamine neurotransmission in the mesocorticolimbic dopamine system (Figure 7.22).

Another motivation-related brain area that is activated by nicotine is the dorsal raphe. Nicotine has shown some stimulatory effects on dorsal raphe serotonin neurons, which may involve both direct effects on serotonin neurons and indirect effects on glutamate/GABA interactions as above. Such effects of nicotine on serotonin neurotransmission may be part of the reason why nicotine apparently has antidepressant-like effects in animal models and humans.

Molecular Mechanism of Action

The most widely expressed subtypes of nAChRs in the brain contain the α4, α7, and β2 subunits. Various nAChR α and β subunit combinations, notably the α4β2 subtype, are present throughout the mesocorticolimbic dopamine pathway, including the ventral tegmental area, prefrontal cortex, amygdala, septal area, and nucleus accumbens. The α4 subunit is critical for the relatively slow electrical currents associated with the slow desensitization component of nAChRs and the release of dopamine produced by systemic nicotine. Knockout of the α4 and β2 subtypes blocks the reinforcing effects of nicotine, as does knockout of the α7 subtype.

In summary, intravenous nicotine self-administration is blocked by dopamine receptor antagonists and lesions of the midbrain dopamine system. Nicotine increases dopamine release in the nucleus accumbens and acutely activates the mesocorticolimbic dopamine system through three possible actions:

1) Direct action on dopamine neurons,
2) Acting through presynaptic activation of glutamate release, and
3) Acting through the activation of GABA interneurons that desensitize more rapidly.

The combined activation of glutamate and deactivation of GABA presumably prolongs the dopaminergic response in the ventral tegmental area. Glutamate (NMDA) receptor antagonists block nicotine self-administration and nicotine-induced dopamine release. GABA receptor agonists have similar effects. Thus, glutamate and GABA appear to modulate nicotine reward. Opioid peptides may also be involved in the reinforcing effects of nicotine, independent of dopamine activation.

Withdrawal/Negative Affect Stage

As described above, animals will regularly self-administer nicotine intravenously, supporting the hypothesis that nicotine is the active ingredient for producing the rewarding effects of tobacco. Adult rats will self-administer nicotine in continuous access situations (24 h/day) to the point of dependence and will show an escalation in drug intake with intermittent access (Figure 7.23). This suggests that intermittent daily use with concomitant daily withdrawal from nicotine contributes to the excessive nicotine intake associated with compulsive use and addiction.

Nicotine Withdrawal

As with other drugs of abuse, such as opiates and alcohol, the nicotine withdrawal syndrome in nonhuman animals has both somatic and affective signs. The somatic syndrome associated with nicotine withdrawal has been modeled in rats (Table 7.4). The somatic signs of nicotine withdrawal after exposure to 3.16 mg/kg nicotine base via a minipump implanted under the skin for 6 days resemble those seen in opiate withdrawal in rats, including abdominal constrictions, facial fasciculation, and ptosis. These signs are called *somatic* because they are expressed as responses of the body (e.g., gasps and writhes). This syndrome has been observed after spontaneous nicotine withdrawal (in which access to nicotine is simply removed) and when withdrawal is induced by a nicotinic acetylcholine receptor antagonist.

Affective and motivational measures of nicotine withdrawal have been modeled in animals using intracranial self-stimulation. Nicotine produces a pronounced elevation in brain reward

thresholds, similar to the elevations seen during withdrawal from all drugs of addiction, including cocaine, amphetamine, morphine, ethanol, and Δ^9-tetrahydrocannabinol (Figure 7.24). One remarkable aspect of nicotine withdrawal is the pronounced and prolonged elevation in brain reward thresholds that is in marked contrast to its efficacy as a reinforcer and the lack of intensity of somatic withdrawal signs. The magnitude of the elevation in reward thresholds produced by nicotine withdrawal depends on the nicotine dose, with higher doses producing greater elevations, and continuous drug administration producing longer-lasting reward elevations during withdrawal than intermittent administration, even when the total dose administered is the same. This parallels the human condition, in

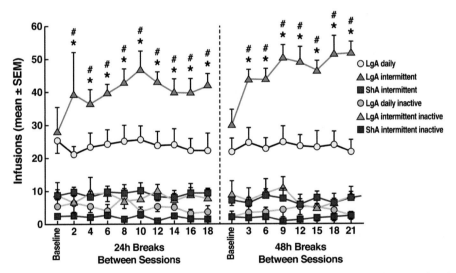

FIGURE 7.23 **Mean nicotine intake in rats that self-administered nicotine under a fixed-ratio 1 (FR1) schedule in either 21 h (long access [LgA]) or 1 h (short access [ShA]) sessions.** LgA rats increased their nicotine intake on an intermittent schedule with 24–48 h breaks between sessions. (left) Total number of nicotine infusions per session when the intermittent schedule included 24 h breaks between sessions. (right) Total number of nicotine infusions per session when the intermittent schedule included 48 h breaks between sessions. *These data show that rats that were allowed to self-administer nicotine intravenously showed a compulsive-like pattern of escalation in nicotine intake, similar to other drugs of abuse when nicotine access was intermittent. Given that this is a pattern of nicotine use in human adolescents who initiate smoking behavior, this animal model has face validity with the human condition (see* Chapter 3 *for descriptions of the different types of validity). [Taken with permission from Cohen A, Koob GF, George O. Robust escalation of nicotine intake with extended access to nicotine self-administration and intermittent periods of abstinence.* Neuropsychopharmacology, 2012, (37), 2153–2160.]

which the predominant symptoms of nicotine withdrawal are high irritability, malaise, and high craving. One hypothesized neurochemical basis of the dramatic elevations in brain reward thresholds during nicotine withdrawal includes effects in systems known to mediate acute nicotine reward, including alterations in nicotinic receptor function, decreased dopamine activity, alterations in dopamine-glutamate and dopamine-GABA interactions, changes in serotonergic function, and changes in opioid peptide function.

Decreases in the extracellular levels of dopamine in the nucleus accumbens and amygdala have been observed during precipitated nicotine withdrawal in rats chronically exposed to nicotine (Figure 7.25). Decreased neuronal firing in

TABLE 7.4   Frequencies of Individual Categories of Abstinence Signs (mean ± SEM) Observed in Rats Over 15 min, 16 hours after the End of Nicotine Infusion

Category	Prior Infusion Rate of Nicotine Tartrate		
	0 mg/kg/day	*3 mg/kg/day*	*9 mg/kg/day*
Teeth-chattering/chews	2.6 ± 1.5	7.0 ± 2.5	15.9 ± 4.9*
Gasps/writhes	3.2 ± 1.4	7.2 ± 1.4	17.1 ± 4.6*
Ptosis	0.6 ± 0.4	1.4 ± 0.5	6.5 ± 1.2*
Shakes/tremors	2.0 ± 0.6	7.0 ± 1.8 †	4.1 ± 1.7
Yawns, dyspnea, seminal ejaculation	0.1 ± 0.1	0.8 ± 0.3	1.3 ± 0.7‡

* p < 0.01 vs. saline-infused controls (Dunnett's t test).
† p < 0.05 vs. saline-infused controls (Dunnett's t test).
‡ 0.05 < p < 0.10 vs. saline-infused controls (Dunnett's t test).
[Taken with permission from Malin DH, Lake JR, Newlin-Maultsby P, Roberts LK, Lanier JG, Carter VA, Cunningham JS, Wilson OB. Rodent model of nicotine abstinence syndrome. Pharmacology Biochemistry and Behavior, 1992, (43), 779–784.]

the ventral tegmental area has also been reported during chronic continuous nicotine infusion.

Another part of the neuronal circuit that drives nicotine reward during withdrawal may occur at the level of pedunculopontine tegmental nucleus cholinergic neurons that terminate on dopamine neurons. One hypothesis is that after nAChR desensitization and upregulation in the absence of sufficient agonist to stimulate the receptors, reduced cholinergic activation of dopamine neurons occurs. A reduction of the cholinergic input to dopamine neurons in the mesocorticolimbic dopamine system may result in decreased brain reward function.

These proposed neuroadaptations that involve dopamine, however, may only partially contribute to nicotine withdrawal symptomatology. Alterations in GABAergic, opioidergic, serotonergic, and corticotropin-releasing factor (CRF) systems may also contribute to the negative affective aspects of nicotine withdrawal. Pharmacological studies have implicated the opioid peptide systems in nicotine dependence. The somatic signs of nicotine withdrawal can be precipitated by the opioid receptor antagonist naloxone. Interestingly, acute injections of the opioid agonist morphine reversed the somatic signs of nicotine withdrawal. Naloxone administration in nicotine-dependent humans dose-dependently increases self-reported affective and somatic signs of nicotine withdrawal, providing evidence that long-term exposure to nicotine is associated with alterations in endogenous opioid peptide systems. Chronic nicotine exposure may release opioid peptides, thus leading to the downregulation of opioid receptor transduction mechanisms. During nicotine abstinence, the downregulation of μ opioid receptors or opioid receptor transduction mechanisms may contribute to some, but not all, aspects of nicotine withdrawal.

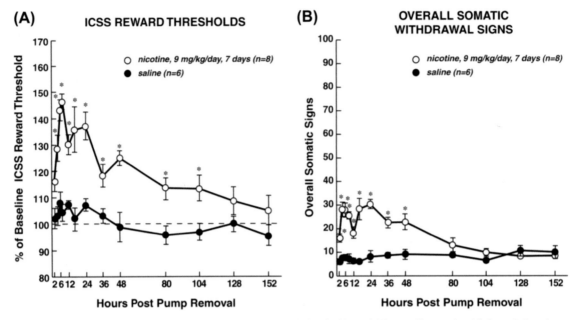

FIGURE 7.24   (A) Intracranial self-stimulation (ICSS) reward thresholds and (B) overall somatic withdrawal signs in rats during spontaneous withdrawal from chronic nicotine administration (9.0 mg/kg/day for 7 days; $n = 8$) or saline ($n = 6$). *$p < 0.05$, significant difference between nicotine and saline groups after removal of the minipumps. *These data show that rats made dependent on nicotine show elevations in reward thresholds measured by intracranial self-stimulation during withdrawal from nicotine (see Chapter 3 for details on the intracranial self-stimulation procedure). These increases can be interpreted as "dysphoric-like" effects, last more than 4 days, and outlast any significant increases in the somatic signs of nicotine withdrawal. [Adapted with permission from Epping-Jordan MP, Watkins SS, Koob GF, Markou A. Dramatic decreases in brain reward function during nicotine withdrawal.* Nature, 1998, (393), 76–79.]

Alterations in serotonin neurotransmission may also be observed in nicotine withdrawal. Chronic nicotine treatment decreases serotonin concentrations in the hippocampus and increases the number of hippocampal serotonin 5-HT_{1A} receptors in chronic smokers. This receptor upregulation may reflect a reduction of the activity of serotonergic neurons in the median raphe nucleus, which innervates the hippocampus, amygdala, and several other forebrain structures. Deficits in serotonin neurotransmission have been implicated in human depression and anxiety. One hypothesis is that decreases in serotonin function during chronic nicotine exposure and nicotine withdrawal play a role in negative affective withdrawal symptoms, including depressed mood, impulsivity, and irritability. nAChRs are located in the somatodendritic region in the median raphe nucleus and terminal fields in the forebrain and may facilitate serotonin release. Chronic nicotine treatment desensitizes nicotinic receptors, decreases serotonin release, and increases postsynaptic serotonin 5-HT_{1A} receptors to maintain functional activity in the terminal regions. At the neuronal level, nicotine withdrawal increases the inhibitory influence of somatodendritic 5-HT_{1A} autoreceptors in raphe nuclei, contributing to decreases in serotonin release in forebrain sites. Serotonergic antidepressant treatment can reverse the elevation in brain stimulation reward thresholds but not somatic signs in rats during nicotine withdrawal.

During nicotine abstinence, decreases in serotonin, combined with upregulated postsynaptic 5-HT$_{1A}$ receptors, may contribute to the depressed mood often reported during nicotine withdrawal.

Alterations in brain stress systems also contribute to the negative affective symptoms associated with nicotine withdrawal (see Figure 7.25). Acute withdrawal from nicotine increases circulating corticosterone, and CRF is increased in the central nucleus of the amygdala. CRF receptor antagonist administration directly into the central nucleus of the amygdala or systemically blocks the increase in nicotine self-administration observed during nicotine abstinence. CRF antagonists also block the escalation in nicotine intake in rats with extended access to nicotine. A common thread between various drugs of abuse, including nicotine, is that CRF levels are increased during withdrawal. Thus, overactivity of brain CRF may underlie the anxiety, increased stress, and irritability often reported by abstinent smokers.

Molecular Changes during Withdrawal from Chronic Nicotine

At the molecular level, the effects of nicotine on central nAChRs have been described as being paradoxical. Chronic nicotine exposure leads to receptor desensitization and inactivation, followed by an upregulation of nicotinic receptors during withdrawal. As mentioned above, acute nicotine administration stimulates nAChRs, leading to the brief opening of the ion channel (receptor activation). The receptor then becomes unresponsive to further agonist exposure (receptor inactivation and desensitization). Consequently, the desensitization process leads to an increase in the number of nAChRs (receptor upregulation). Nicotinic receptor activation, desensitization, and upregulation can be presumed to be a neuronal response that attempts to maintain the baseline level of synaptic activity within cholinergic and other neurotransmitter systems during chronic nicotine exposure. nAChRs may exist in many different functional states within the brain. Differential activation could be a driving force for the neuroadaptive changes associated with dependence. The α2, α4, and α7 subunits become inactive and desensitized with chronic nicotine exposure, but the α3 and α6 subunits do not show inactivation, suggesting that some nAChR subunits are more sensitive to nicotine than others. The differential effects of chronic nicotine exposure on the release of various neurotransmitter systems may be explained by a balance between receptor density, desensitization, and functionality.

During nicotine abstinence, changes in nAChR function may mediate some of the negative affective states and somatic symptoms associated with nicotine withdrawal. For example, nicotine abstinence leads to decreased plasma nicotine levels. The previously desensitized or inactive nAChRs may then begin to recover to their normal functional states at different rates, depending on the brain region and receptor subtype. During chronic nicotine exposure, nAChR upregulation may also occur along non-reward-related cholinergic pathways. nAChR dysregulation in both reward (desensitized) and non-reward (upregulated) circuits may contribute to the negative affective or somatic symptoms of withdrawal. The development and perpetuation of nicotine addiction may involve self-medication to effectively control the number of functional nAChRs along the various pathways affected by nicotine.

Smokers report that the first cigarette of the day is the most pleasurable, possibly because of nicotine-induced activation of recovered nAChRs in the ventral tegmental area, leading to greater dopamine release compared with later time-points during the day. Throughout the day, smokers maintain steady blood nicotine levels and are exposed to nicotine concentrations

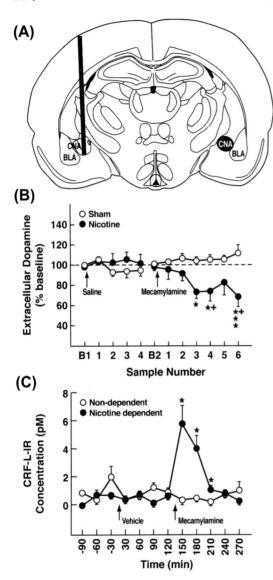

FIGURE 7.25 **Decreased dopamine release and increased CRF release in the central nucleus of the amygdala in nicotine-dependent rats.** (A) The placement of a microdialysis probe in the rat central nucleus of the amygdala (CNA, left side) and a region where Fos-immunoreactive nuclei were counted (CNA, shaded area, right side). BLA, basolateral amygdala. (B) Temporal changes in extracellular dopamine concentrations in the central nucleus of the amygdala after systemic injections (indicated by the arrows) of saline and mecamylamine (1 mg/kg, s.c.) in animals infused for 14 days with nicotine (●, n = 5–6) and control animals (○, Sham, n = 5–8). B1 indicates baseline 1, which is the sample that immediately preceded the saline injection (100% in the figure is the average of the two samples that preceded the saline injection). B2 indicates baseline 2, which is the sample that immediately preceded mecamylamine injection (100% is defined as the average of the two samples that preceded the mecamylamine injection [Taken with permission from Panagis G, Hildebrand BE, Svensson TH, Nomikos GG. Selective c-fos induction and decreased dopamine release in the central nucleus of amygdala in rats displaying a mecamylamine-precipitated nicotine withdrawal syndrome. Synapse, 2000, (35), 15–25.] (C) Effect of mecamylamine (1.5 mg/kg, i.p.)-precipitated withdrawal on extracellular levels of corticotropin-releasing factor in the central nucleus of the amygdala measured by in vivo microdialysis in chronic nicotine-treated rats (nicotine-dependent, n = 7) and chronic saline-treated rats (nondependent, n = 6). *p < 0.05, compared with nondependent rats. [Taken with permission from George O, Ghozland S, Azar MR, Cottone P, Zorrilla EP, Parsons LH, O'Dell LE, Richardson HN, Koob GF. CRF-CRF1 system activation mediates withdrawal-induced increases in nicotine self-administration in nicotine-dependent rats. Proceedings of the National Academy of Sciences USA, 2007, (104), 17198–17203.]

These data show that animals made dependent on nicotine show a decrease in dopamine release in the central nucleus of the amygdala and a concomitant increase in corticotropin-releasing factor release from the central nucleus of the amygdala during precipitated withdrawal measured by in vivo microdialysis.

that cause nAChR desensitization in the ventral tegmental area. If different nAChRs in the ventral tegmental area are differentially sensitive to nicotine as suggested above, then periodic re-administration of nicotine engages nAChRs that are only activated by high nicotine doses once a steady-state of nicotine is reached.

In summary, the same neurotransmitter systems hypothesized to mediate the acute reinforcing effects of nicotine are compromised during the development of dependence, reflected by aberrant or decreased function during withdrawal. Dopamine and serotonin activity decreases during withdrawal. CRF activity increases during withdrawal. These changes appear to contribute to the negative affective state that drives negative reinforcement in nicotine dependence.

Preoccupation/Anticipation Stage

Nicotine-, Cue-, and Stress-Induced Reinstatement

Nicotine, cues, and contexts will cause reinstatement of nicotine seeking behavior in mice and rats that have been trained to intravenously self-administer nicotine and then subjected to extinction. In rats, the visual cues paired with intravenous nicotine self-administration appear to be as important as nicotine in sustaining a high rate of responding once self-administration has been established. Similarly to other drugs of abuse, stress and intermittent footshock caused the reinstatement of nicotine seeking behavior in rats trained to intravenously self-administer nicotine and subsequently extinguished (see Chapter 3 for details of drug, cue-, and stress-induced reinstatement).

The cue-induced reinstatement of nicotine seeking in mice and rats that have been trained to intravenously self-administer nicotine self-administration and then subjected to extinction is blocked by drugs that block nicotinic receptors, most notably varenicline (an $\alpha 4\beta 2$ nAChR antagonist that is on the market for the treatment of nicotine addiction; see Chapter 9). The cue-induced reinstatement of nicotine seeking in mice and rats that have been trained to intravenously self-administer nicotine self-administration and then subjected to extinction is also blocked by drugs that block dopamine receptors, cannabinoid receptors, metabotropic and ionotropic glutamate receptors, opioid receptors, and serotonin receptors.

Nicotine withdrawal in animals treated with chronic nicotine results in lower corticosterone levels during restraint stress, suggesting subsensitivity of the hypothalamic–pituitary–adrenal axis to stress, similar to other drugs of abuse and to parallel studies that have reported the sensitization of extrahypothalamic CRF systems, suggesting a key role for activation of the brain stress systems during the *preoccupation/anticipation* stage of the addiction cycle. Stress-induced reinstatement of nicotine seeking in rodents that have been trained to intravenously self-administer nicotine and then subjected to extinction has been shown to be blocked by CRF receptor antagonists, an $\alpha 2$ adrenergic receptor agonist, and a κ opioid receptor antagonist.

Neuroanatomical Substrates of Nicotine "Craving"

A human neurological study of individuals with stroke-induced destruction of the insula cortex revealed that in the group who smoked prior to stroke stopped smoking abruptly following damage to the insula. Preclinical studies have subsequently shown that destruction of the insula blocks the cue-induced reinstatement of nicotine seeking in mice and rats that have been trained to intravenously self-administer nicotine and then subjected to extinction. Deep-brain stimulation of the insula has similar effects.

Another likely driving force for craving is the nucleus accumbens. In a rat study, 2 weeks after nicotine self-administration, activated α-amino-3-hydroxy-5-methyl-4-isoxazole propionic acid and NMDA receptors and a reduction of glutamate transporters were observed in the nucleus accumbens. Cues paired with nicotine elicited glutamate release. The blockade of NMDA receptors blocked cue-induced reinstatement (Table 7.5). Notably, this pattern of low basal glutamate tone (decreased glutamate transporters) in the nucleus accumbens but the phasic release of glutamate in the presence of nicotine cues is identical to observations of protracted cocaine abstinence.

TABLE 7.5 Neuropharmacological Agents that Block Nicotine-, Cue, and Stress-Induced Reinstatement in Rodents that Have Been Trained to Intravenously Self-Administer Nicotine and then Subjected to Extinction

Nicotine-induced reinstatement	Dopamine D_4 receptor antagonist α-type peroxisome proliferator-activated receptor agonist
Cue-induced reinstatement	noncompetitive nicotinic receptor antagonist (mecamylamine) $\alpha 4\beta 2$ nicotinic receptor partial agonist (varenicline) GABA agonist (GABA transaminase inhibitor) $GABA_B$ receptor agonist dopamine D_1, D_2, D_3, and D_4 receptor agonists dopamine D_2 receptor partial agonist cannabinoid CB_1 receptor antagonist anandamide transporter inhibitor opioid receptor antagonist (naltrexone) metabotropic glutamate 5 receptor antagonist metabotropic glutamate 2/3 receptor antagonist metabotropic glutamate 1 receptor antagonist NMDA subunit antagonist cystine-glutamate antiporter system agonist (N-acetylcysteine) glutamate modulator (acamprosate) $\alpha 1$ adrenergic receptor antagonist β adrenergic receptor antagonist serotonin $5\text{-}HT_{2C}$ receptor antagonist serotonin $5\text{-}HT_6$ receptor antagonist T-type calcium channel antagonist
Stress-induced reinstatement	CRF receptor antagonist $\alpha 2$ adrenergic receptor agonist (clonidine) κ opioid receptor antagonist

Molecular Changes during Protracted Abstinence from Chronic Nicotine

Another mechanism of neuroadaptation that may have long-term consequences includes alterations in gene transcription through changes in the activity of transcription factors. Nicotine exposure, nicotine self-administration, and nicotine withdrawal activate immediate early genes in the ventral tegmental area and projection areas of the mesocorticolimbic dopamine system. Nicotine self-administration and nicotine cues increase Fos-like immunoreactivity in the prefrontal cortex (a marker of neuronal activation). Decreased phosphorylated cyclic adenosine monophosphate (cAMP) response element binding protein (CREB) levels in the cingulate gyrus, cerebral cortex, medial and basolateral amygdala, and nucleus accumbens have been observed during withdrawal. In rodent studies, decreased CREB in the amygdala during nicotine withdrawal was shown to be correlated with increased anxiety-like responses in the elevated plus maze (Figure 7.26).

Genetic Vulnerability to Tobacco Addiction?

A single-nucleotide polymorphism within the $\alpha 5$ gene of the nicotinic receptor reduces $\alpha 5$ nAChR function and in humans is associated with a greater risk of nicotine dependence, heavier smoking, and increased rewarding effects from cigarettes. Subunit expression is high in the medial habenula, interpeduncular nucleus, and ventral tegmental area. The habenula projects to the interpeduncular nucleus, which is adjacent to dopaminergic cells in the ventral tegmental area (see Chapter 2). The blockade of $\alpha 5$ receptors blunts nicotine withdrawal, and $\alpha 5$ subunit knockout mice self-administer nicotine at high doses that otherwise limit intake in wildtype mice with normal $\alpha 5$ subunit expression. Thus, one hypothesis is that the $\alpha 5$ habenula-interpeduncular pathway mediates some of the aversive effects of nicotine and is involved in nicotine withdrawal symptoms.

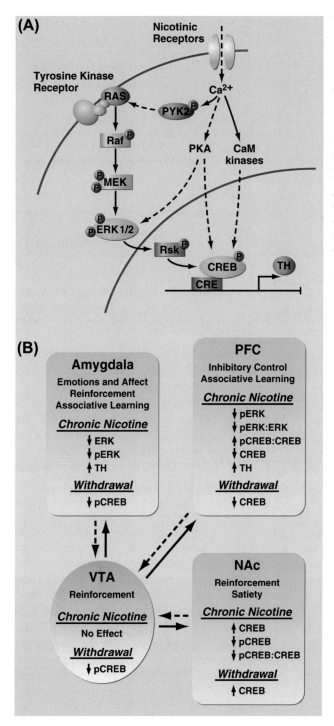

FIGURE 7.26 **Signaling pathways related to extracellular signal-regulated kinase (ERK) activation that may be involved in nicotine dependence and withdrawal.** (A) Nicotine could affect ERK/CREB (cyclic adenosine monophosphate response element binding protein) signaling by direct activation of nicotinic receptors or indirectly via changes in tyrosine kinase receptor activation. Dashed lines indicate multi-step processes. (B) Summary of changes in response to chronic nicotine exposure and withdrawal in the amygdala, prefrontal cortex (PFC), nucleus accumbens (NAc), and ventral tegmental area (VTA). Each of these brain areas is connected by reciprocal connections to the ventral tegmental area. Changes in signaling within these pathways are likely to alter communication between brain areas involved in drug dependence. [*Taken with permission from Brunzell DH, Russell DS, Picciotto MR. In vivo nicotine treatment regulates mesocorticolimbic CREB and ERK signaling in C57Bl/6J mice. Journal of Neurochemistry, 2003, (84), 1431–1441.*]

SUMMARY

Although declining in the United States, tobacco addiction remains the most prevalent addiction of all drugs of abuse. Nicotine is an alkaloid derived from the *Nicotiana tabacum* (common tobacco) plant, which has been cultivated for centuries for ceremonial and medicinal uses. The dried leaves of the plant are generally smoked, although oral administration in the form of snuff or chewing tobacco is also widespread. Cigarettes began to be manufactured in the mid-19th century. Since 1940, they have been the most prevalent form of administration.

Nicotine produces euphoria characterized by arousal and a stimulant effect, including cognitive activation, autonomic activation, and increases in heart rate and blood pressure. Paradoxically, it also reduces perceived tension and stress. Nicotine also produces analgesia and decreases appetite. Animal studies have shown that nicotine lowers brain reward thresholds, increases locomotor activity, and is intravenously self-administered. Nicotine can produce anxiolytic-like effects in various animal models of anxiety. It is rapidly absorbed by smoking and oral administration and has a short half-life of 2 hours. Tobacco smoke produces high carboxyhemoglobin levels and has significant amounts of carcinogens that have been linked to the toxic effects of smoking.

The behavioral mechanism of action of nicotine is linked to its mood titration effects via Nesbitt's paradox, in which smokers maintain a certain blood nicotine level over the course of a smoking bout that is extended to waking hours in dependent smokers. The boundary model explains such titration, in which the upper boundary delimits the aversive effects of high nicotine doses, and the lower boundary delimits the aversive effects of nicotine withdrawal.

Much information has been gleaned from animal work about the neurobiology of the acute reinforcing and stimulant effects of nicotine. Nicotine binds to nAChRs and activates the mesocorticolimbic dopamine system, including the ventral tegmental area and nucleus accumbens. The molecular site of action for the acute reinforcing effects of nicotine involves interactions with the $\alpha 4\beta 2$ and $\alpha 6\beta 2$ subunits. Mutant mice that lack the b2 subunit do not self-administer nicotine. In the ventral tegmental area, nAChRs are localized to dopaminergic cell bodies and GABAergic and glutamatergic afferents. The combination of effects of nicotine on nAChRs at these locations facilitates the actions of dopamine neurons. There is evidence of opioid peptide interactions with nicotine reinforcement. μ Opioid receptor knockout mice show no nicotine-induced conditioned place preference. The neurobiological bases for the dependence-inducing properties of nicotine involves within-system decreases in reward-related neurotransmitter function, including dopamine, opioid peptides, and serotonin, and the recruitment of the between-system brain CRF stress system, similar to other drugs of abuse.

At the molecular level, differential receptor desensitization may underlie negative reinforcement, in which self-medication is used to control the functional recovery of nAChRs. At the neurocircuitry level, decreases in dopaminergic neurotransmission in the ventral tegmental area and nucleus accumbens are associated with the malaise associated with acute nicotine withdrawal. Losses of the functional activity of glutamate, serotonin, and likely opioid peptides and the recruitment of the brain stress systems (CRF) are also associated with nicotine withdrawal and by extrapolation also drive negative reinforcement. Chronic nAChR activation alters CREB activity. Decreased CREB activity has been observed in the amygdala, nucleus accumbens, and prefrontal cortex during withdrawal. These changes may alter gene expression and trigger long-term neuroadaptive responses that are similar to other drugs of abuse.

Suggested Reading

Benowitz, N.L., 2008. Nicotine and postoperative management of pain. Anesth. Analg. 107, 739–741.

de Assis Viegas, C.A., 2008. Non-cigarette forms of tobacco use. Jornal Brasileiro de Pneumologia 34, 1069–1073.

Dwyer, J.B., McQuown, S.C., Leslie, F.M., 2009. The dynamic effects of nicotine on the developing brain. Pharmacol. Ther. 122, 125–139.

Eissenberg, T., Shihadeh, A., 2009. Waterpipe tobacco and cigarette smoking: direct comparison of toxicant exposure. Am. J. Prev. Med. 37, 518–523.

Fowler, C.D., Arends, M.A., Kenny, P.J., 2008. Subtypes of nicotinic acetylcholine receptors in nicotine reward, dependence, and withdrawal: evidence from genetically modified mice. Behav. Pharmacol. 19, 461–484.

Heinz, A.J., Kassel, J.D., Berbaum, M., Mermelstein, R., 2010. Adolescents' expectancies for smoking to regulate affect predict smoking behavior and nicotine dependence over time. Drug. Alcohol. Depend. 111, 128–135.

Herman, C.P., Kozlowski, L.T., 1979. Indulgence, excess, and restraint: perspectives on consummatory behavior in everyday life. J. Drug. Issues. 9, 185–196.

Hughes, J.R., 1992. Tobacco withdrawal in self-quitters. J. Consult. Clin. Psychol. 60, 689–697.

Laviolette, S.R., van der Kooy, D., 2004. The neurobiology of nicotine addiction: bridging the gap from molecules to behavior. Nat. Rev. Neurosci. 5, 55–65.

Leslie, F.M., 2013. Multigenerational epigenetic effects of nicotine on lung function. BMC Medicine 27 (11).

Maziak, W., 2011. The global epidemic of waterpipe smoking. Addict. Behav. 36, 1–5.

Noonan, D., Kulbok, P.A., 2010. New tobacco trends: waterpipe (hookah) smoking and implications for healthcare providers. J. Am. Acad. Nurse. Pract. 21, 258–260.

Pearson, J.L., Richardson, A., Niaura, R.S., Vallone, D.M., Abrams, D.B., 2012. e-Cigarette awareness, use, and harm perceptions in US adults. Am. J. Public. Health. 102, 1758–1766.

Shiffman, S., Paty, J.A., Kassel, J.D., Gnys, M., Zettler-Segal, M., 1994. Smoking behavior and smoking history of tobacco chippers. Exp. Clin. Psychopharmacol. 2, 126–142.

Tucker, J.S., Ellickson, P.L., Klein, D.J., 2003. Predictors of the transition to regular smoking during adolescence and young adulthood. J. Adolesc. Health. 32, 314–324.

DEFINITIONS

Source of the Drug

Cannabis is a highly adaptive annual plant that grows throughout temperate and tropical zones worldwide. Cannabis in the form of hemp likely originated in central Asia or near the Alai and Tian Shan mountain ranges that extend from Kyrgyzstan through Tajikistan to the China-Mongolia border. It has been a familiar agricultural crop since the beginning of civilization. Archaeologists have found evidence of hemp plant use in the late Neolithic era, dating back at least 6,000 years to the New Stone Age. *Ma* is the Chinese word for *hemp*, defined by the Merriam-Webster dictionary as a tall, widely cultivated Asian herb (*Cannabis sativa*) of the mulberry family with tough phloem fiber used especially for cords and ropes. It is composed of two Chinese written characters (Figure 8.1). Reference to hemp (*ta ma*) as a medicinal herb dates back to 2,838 B.C. in Emperor Shen Nung's compilation of the *Pen Ts'ao* (or *The Herbal*), a kind of herbal standard. Emperor Nung experimented with various herbs and listed *ta ma* as medicinal:

> "...ma-fen (fruits of hemp)...if taken in excess will produce hallucinations (literally 'seeing devils'). If taken over a long term, it makes one communicate with spirits and lightens one's body" (*Li, 1974a, b*).

Hua T'o, a Chinese physician from the 2nd century A.D., used an oral preparation of cannabis called *ma-fei-san* (hemp-boiling compound, combined with wine) to anesthetize patients who were undergoing abdominal surgery. The Swedish botanist Carl Linnaeus named the plant *Cannabis sativa* in 1753. Although accounts of the etymology of the word *cannabis* differ, it may have derived from the Greek and Latin *kannabis*, the Assyrian *kunnapu* (a way to produce smoke), or perhaps the Sanskrit *cana* (hemp or cane). The word *kan* referred to hemp or cane in many ancient languages, and *bis* can be linked to the word *aromatic*. Thus, cannabis is the "fragrant cane." The French naturalist Jean Baptiste Lamarck argued that the hemp plant grown in Europe was sufficiently different from that grown in India to be a different species. The plant grown for fiber use was called *Cannabis sativa*, and the plant grown for psychoactive properties was called *Cannabis indica*. The Russian botanist Janischevski recognized a third wild species in Asia called *Cannabis ruderalis*.

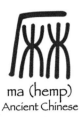 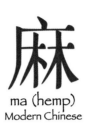

ma (hemp)   ma (hemp)
Ancient Chinese   Modern Chinese

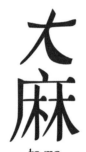

ta ma
(*Cannabis sativa*)

FIGURE 8.1 **Evolvement of the Chinese character for hemp, or ma, from the archaic chuan script (dating from 1766–1122 B.C. during the Shang Dynasty), to the contemporary cursive hsing script (emerging in the 3rd century A.D.).** The ideogram is composed of the *madare* radical (top and left) which represents a tilted roof and is used in the characters for words such as *house, shop, to live*, etc. Under the "roof" are two small characters for *tree* which by themselves mean "small forest." Literally, the character for *hemp* expresses the idea of a "small forest in or at one's house," or a "domestic forest." The part beneath and to the right of the straight lines represents hemp fibers dangling from a rack. The horizontal and vertical lines represent the home in which they are drying (*Abel EL. Marijuana: The First Twelve Thousand Years. Plenum Press, New York, 1980*). The pictograph at the bottom combines *big* (*ta*) with *ma* to form the Chinese ideogram (*ta ma*) for psychoactive marijuana from cannabis. [*Taken with permission from Koob GF, Le Moal M. Neurobiology of Addiction. Academic Press, London, 2006.*]

The relationships between an individual plant and its environment are complex and determine the representative phenotypes of the species; therefore, the genetic plasticity of *Cannabis sativa* enables wide phenotypic variability for adapting to diverse conditions.

Marijuana is the dry, shredded, green or brown mixture of flowers, stems, seeds, and leaves of the hemp plant *Cannabis sativa*. The word *marijuana* may have been derived from the Spanish *Mariguana*, one of the islands that form the Bahamas, but others have suggested it derived from the Spanish prenomes *Maria*

(Mary) and *Juana* (Jane). This claim, however, has not been substantiated.

The dried mixture can be smoked like a cigarette (termed a *joint*) or in a pipe (*bong*) or in a cigar from which the tobacco has been removed (*blunt*). Other preparations include hash or hashish (the dried sticky resin of the flowers of the female plant) or hash oil (a sticky black liquid).

The marijuana plant contains numerous chemical species, but the active constituent mainly responsible for its pharmacological effect is $(-)\Delta^9$-6a,10a-trans-tetrahydrocannabinol, simply referred to as Δ^9-THC (Box 8.1). The term *cannabinoid* originally referred to Δ^9-THC and related phytocannabinoids of the marijuana plant *Cannabis sativa* with a typical 21-carbon chemical structure and any products derived from these structures. A broader definition based on pharmacology and chemistry "encompasses kindred structures, or any other compound that affects cannabinoid receptors" (Pate DW. Taxonomy of cannabinoids. In: Grotenhermen F, Russo E (eds.) *Cannabis and Cannabinoids: Pharmacology, Toxicology, and Therapeutic Potential*. Haworth Integrative Healing Press, New York, 2002, pp. 15–26) or "all ligands of the cannabinoid receptor and related compounds including endogenous ligands of the receptors and a large number of synthetic cannabinoid analogs" (Grotenhermen

---

BOX 8.1

SYNOPSIS OF THE NEUROPHARMACOLOGICAL TARGETS FOR CANNABINOIDS

Cannabinoids are found in all *cannabis* preparations, and the principal psychoactive ingredient is Δ^9-tetrahydrocannabinol (Δ^9-THC). All cannabinoid drugs, both natural and synthetic, have pharmacological actions that are similar to Δ^9-THC. All cannabinoids bind as direct agonists to cannabinoid receptors in the brain to produce their behavioral effects. Endogenous cannabinoids bind as agonists to cannabinoid receptors and include anandamide and 2-arachidonylglycerol (2-AG), which are widely distributed throughout the brain and have high concentrations in reward- and pain-related neurocircuits. Cannabinoids act as retrograde neuromodulators that are synthesized in postsynaptic elements of neurons as required. This occurs in response to depolarization by receptor-stimulated synthesis from membrane lipid precursors, and they are released from cells immediately after their production. The behavioral effects of cannabinoids are transduced by two transmembrane G-protein-coupled opioid receptors – cannabinoid-1 (CB_1) and cannabinoid-2 (CB_2) – and subsequent second-messenger gene transcription changes. The CB_1 receptor is hypothesized to be largely responsible for the intoxicating effects of cannabinoids, in addition to a wide range of behavioral and physiological effects. The intoxicating effects of cannabinoids are hypothesized to be mediated by actions on cannabinoid receptors in the origin areas (ventral tegmental area) and terminal areas (nucleus accumbens) of the mesocorticolimbic dopamine system and extended amygdala (central nucleus of the amygdala, bed nucleus of the stria terminalis, and a transition zone in the shell of the nucleus accumbens). The addiction potential of cannabinoids is hypothesized to derive from powerful within-system neuroadaptations (signal transduction mechanisms) and between-system neuroadaptations (neurocircuitry changes) in the brain motivational and stress systems.

F. Pharmacokinetics and pharmacodynamics of cannabinoids. *Clinical Pharmacokinetics*, 2003, (42), 327–360).

> "The dried Hemp plant which has flowered, and *from which the resin has not been removed*, is called *Gunjah*. It sells from 12 annas to one rupee seer in the Calcutta bazars, and yields to alcohol twenty per 100 of resinous extract, composed of the resin (*churrus*) and green coloring matter (*Chloro-phille*). Distilled with a large quantity of water, traces of essential oil pass over, and the distilled liquor has the powerful narcotic odor of the plant. The *gunjah* is sold for smoking chiefly. The bundles of *gunjah* are about two feet long, and three inches in diameter, and contain 24 to 36 plants. The color is dusky green – the odor agreeably narcotic – the whole plant resinous and adhesive to the touch. The larger leaves and capsules without the stalks are called *'Bangh Subjee or Sidhee.'* They are used for making an intoxicating drink, for smoking, and in the conserve or confection termed *Majoon. Bang* is cheaper than *gunjah*, and though less powerful, is sold at such a low price, that for one pice enough can be purchased to intoxicate an experienced person" (*O'Shaughnessy WB. On the preparations of the Indian hemp, or gunjah.* Transactions of the Medical and Physical Society of Bengal, *1838–1840, pp. 421–461*).

Concentrations of Δ^9-THC

In the cannabis plant, Δ^9-THC content is highest in the oil from the flowering tops and lowest in the seeds, declining in concentration in the following order: flowering tops > bracts > leaves > stems > roots > seeds (Table 8.1). Cannabis is able to survive in very hot, arid climates because of the resin film that protects it from losing moisture caused by evaporation. This sticky coating is called hashish:

> "The means by which cannabis accomplishes this amazing feat is by producing a thick, sticky resin that coats its leaves and flowers. This protective canopy prevents life-sustaining moisture from disappearing into the dry air. But this thick sticky resin is not an ordinary goo. It is the stuff that dreams are made of, the stuff that holds time suspended in limbo, the stuff that makes men forgetful, makes them both sad and deliriously happy, makes them ravenously

hungry or completely disinterested in food. It is a god to some and a devil to others. It is all of these things and more. This resin, this shield against the sun, this sticky goo... hashish" (*Abel EL*. Marihuana: The First Twelve Thousand Years. *Plenum Press, New York, 1980*).

The term *hashish* has an even more interesting derivation and has been related to a particular sect of one of the main branches of Islam (Shiite branch) known as Nizari Ismaili. Led by a famous Islamic dissident, Hasan ibn-Sabah (1050–1124), the movement extended into the period of the Crusades and was marked by terrorist-like secret assassinations of prominent leaders within both Islam and Christianity. Known as the Hashshahin or Heyssessini, two accounts exist which indicate that the followers of this sect may have used cannabis, one by Marco Polo (although he only referred to the drug as an unidentified potion) and another by 12th century friar Arnold von Lubeck (who did refer to it as *hemp*). Though the state of cannabis intoxication does not lend itself to acts of violence (quite the contrary; see below) the legend begot the name and was embellished by the writings of Marco Polo. Eventually the word *assassin* came to define a perfidious murderer, and hashish came to be considered a drug that turned normal individuals into assassins. This myth continues to be perpetuated even in modern times. The word *hashish* itself may have derived from the Arabic *asas* or "foundation" (which applied to Islam's religious leaders) and *hassas*, meaning either "to kill," or the followers of Hasan ibn-Sabah.

The taxonomic classification of cannabis continues to be in flux, with discussions often referring to either two or three species. The two-species formulation includes *Cannabis sativa* (not very psychoactive and used mainly for fiber) and *Cannabis indica* (psychoactive). Another formulation supports a three-species formulation (*Cannabis sativa, Cannabis indica*, and *Cannabis ruderalis*). A recent two-species formulation of

TABLE 8.1 Levels of Cannabinoids in Various Plant Parts

	Fetterman et al., 1971a	ElSohly and Holley, 1983	Fetterman et al., 1971b	Fairbairn et al., 1971
Δ^9-THC CONTENT				
Bracts*	0.37%	–	3.7%	–
Buds[†]	–	3.6–4.6%	–	–
Flowers	–	–	1.6%	1.56%
Leaves	0.32%	–	1.0–1.4%	0.83–1.56%
Stems	0.02%	–	0.89%	0.07–0.11%
Roots	0.002%	–	–	–
Seeds	0.00057%	–	0.01%	–
Sinsemilla	–	3.6–4.6%	–	–
Hashish	–	2.4–3.4%	2.1%	–
Hash oil	–	11.5–21.6%	10%	–
CANNABIDIOL CONTENT				
Bracts	5.55%	–	0.15%	–
Leaves	1.6%	–	0.079–0.085%	–
Stems	0.19%	–	0.055%	–
Roots	0.015%	–	–	–
Seeds	0.00887%	–	trace	–
Hashish	–	–	9.8%	3.5%
Hash oil	–	–	0.88%	–
CANNABINOL CONTENT				
Bracts	0.038%	–	0.18%	–
Leaves	0.088%	–	0.047–0.051%	–
Stems	trace	–	0.076%	–
Roots	0.002%	–	nt	–
Seeds	trace	–	0.01%	–
Hashish	–	–	3.5%	–
Hash oil	–	–	3.5%	–

Note that variability exists due to methods of analysis, species of plant, and plant origin (see Fetterman PS, Doorenbos NJ, Keith ES, Quimby MW. A simple gas liquid chromatography procedure for determination of cannabinoidic acids in *Cannabis sativa* L. *Experientia*, 1971, (27), 988–990.)

* A bract is a leaflike plant part, usually small, located just below a flower, a flower stalk, or an inflorescence.

[†] Buds include flowering tops, smaller leaves and seeds.

Fetterman PS, Keith ES, Waller CW, Guerrero O, Doorenbos NJ, Quimby MW. *Mississippi-grown Cannabis sativa L: preliminary observation on chemical definition of phenotype and variations in tetrahydrocannabinol content versus age, sex, and plant part. Journal of Pharmaceutical Science, 1971, (60), 1246–1249.*

ElSohly MA, Holley JH. Potency Monitoring Project *(series title:* University of Mississippi Quarterly Report, *vol 5). University of Mississippi, Jackson MS, 1983.*

Fairbairn JW, Liebmann JA, Simic S. *The tetrahydrocannabinol content of cannabis leaf. Journal of Pharmacy and Pharmacology, 1971, (23), 558–559.*

Fetterman PS, Doorenbos NJ, Keith ES, Quimby MW. *A simple gas liquid chromatography procedure for determination of cannabinoidic acids in* Cannabis sativa L. Experientia, *1971a, (27), 988–990.*

Traditional *Cannabis* Gene Pools

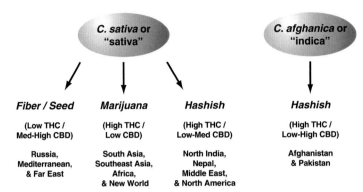

FIGURE 8.2   **The four major *Cannabis* gene pools.**   Most modern medical cannabis varieties are a blend of traditional *sativa* marijuana varieties with *indica* hashish varieties. The traditional *Cannabis* gene pools originate either from *Cannabis sativa*, which comprises the vast majority of naturally occurring hemp and drug land races, or from *Cannabis afghanica* from Afghanistan and Pakistan, which is commonly called "indica" and has become a component in many modern drug *Cannabis* cultivars. Also, all taxonomists recognize the species *Cannabis sativa*. Schultes et al. (1974) divided *Cannabis* into three species: *Cannabis sativa*, *Cannabis indica*, and *Cannabis ruderalis*. Clarke and Watson (2002) consider *Cannabis sativa* to describe all wild hemp and drug *Cannabis* races with the possible exception of the races used for hashish production in Afghanistan and Pakistan which they term *Cannabis afghanica* and others refer to as *indica*. THC, Δ^9-tetrahydrocannabinol; CBD, cannabidiol. [*Adapted from Clarke RC, Watson DP. Botany of natural* Cannabis *medicines. In: Grotenhermen F, Russo E (eds)* Cannabis and Cannabinoids: Pharmacology, Toxicology and Therapeutic Potential. *Haworth Integrative Healing Press, New York, 2002, pp. 3–13.*]

Cannabis sativa includes all wild, hemp, and drug cannabis races, and *Cannabis indica* includes cannabis races used for hashish production (also termed *Cannabis afghanica*; Figure 8.2). For growing hemp for fiber or seeds (sativa or indica), both male and female plants are left undisturbed until harvest. However, in the 1970s, marijuana cultivators in North America and Europe began to grow *sinsemilla* (Spanish for "without seed"). Sinsemilla preparations can effectively be implemented by eliminating staminate (male) plants from the fields and keeping only the unfertilized pistillate (female) plants to mature for later harvest. The female plants continue to produce flowers, are high in resin glands, and have an increased Δ^9-THC content. More recently, indoor plant growing has become popular for growing cannabis for medical purposes. Plants are reproduced vegetatively by rooting cuttings of only female plants, producing uniform crops of seedless females. Marijuana prepared from the dried flowering tops and leaves have Δ^9-THC

concentrations that average 4.5%. The Δ^9-THC of hashish can range from 12.7% to 15.6%. Hash oil is made by soaking cannabis leaves and flowering tops in a solvent such as isopropanol. The plant material is then removed, and the isopropanol that contains the cannabinoids is heated to allow the isopropanol to evaporate, leaving the pure hash oil. It has the highest Δ^9-THC concentration of marijuana preparations, reaching 14.1–19.5%. Selective breeding has resulted in special varieties of marijuana, such as sinsemilla and "Netherweed" (Dutch hemp), that may have concentrations as high as 11% (Table 8.2).

Types of Cannabinoids

Two numbering systems have been developed for cannabinoids. In the formal numbering system for pyran compounds (the dibenzopyran nomenclature), the main active ingredient is referred to as Δ^9-THC. However, not all cannabinoids are pyran compounds; therefore, a second nomenclature was developed based on biogenetics (monoterpenoid nomenclature). In this older numbering system, Δ^9-THC is actually referred to as Δ^1-THC (which readers will find to be the case when looking at older literature).

Cannabis contains a total of 66 phytocannabinoids spanning several different subclasses of compounds, of which three are known to be psychoactive: Δ^9-THC, Δ^8-THC (67% of the potency of Δ^9-THC as an isomer), and Δ^9-tetrahydrocannabidivarin (25% of the potency of Δ^9-THC as a propyl homolog). However, the latter two probably do not contribute greatly to the psychological or physiological effects of cannabis, representing considerably less than 10% of samples. The chemical structure of Δ^9-THC was determined to be Δ^1-3,4-*trans*-tetrahydrocannabinol (again, Δ^1 is equivalent to Δ^9). Over 483 natural components have been isolated (Table 8.3). Cannabis also frequently contains cannabinoid acids in various amounts relative to Δ^9-THC, but many of these constituents are devoid of psychotropic effects. Cannabichromene has slight Δ^9-THC-like effects. Cannabidiol appears to be largely inactive psychotropically. Cannabidiol does not bind to cannabinoid CB_1 or CB_2 receptors (for more on the receptor subtypes, see below), but it has been shown to have

anti-arthritic properties in a mouse model of arthritis. It may also have anxiolytic-like and antipsychotic like effects in animal models and may attenuate the effects of Δ^9-THC (Table 8.4). Other cannabinoids, such as cannabinol, cannabigerol, cannabichromene, and cannabidiolic acid, appear to exert no major active or potentiating effects. The fiber type of

TABLE 8.2   Average Cannabinoid Concentrations in Cannabis Preparations

	Concentration	
	Δ^9-THC	Cannabidiol
Marijuana	4.5%	0.4%
Sinsemilla	11.0%	0.2%
Hashish	12.7–15.6%	2.5%
Hashish oil	14.1–19.5%	0.5%

Data from Mehmedic Z, Chandra S, Slade D, Denham H, Foster S, Patel AS, Ross SA, Khan IA, ElSohly MA. Potency trends of Δ^9-THC and other cannabinoids in confiscated cannabis preparations from 1993 to 2008. Journal of Forensic Science, 2010, (55), 1209–1217.

TABLE 8.3   Cannabis Constituents

Chemical Class	Known Constituents in Cannabis
Cannabinoids	66
Nitrogenous compounds	27
Amino acids	18
Proteins, glycoproteins, and enzymes	11
Sugars and related compounds	34
Hydrocarbons	50
Simple alcohols	7
Simple aldehydes	12
Simple ketones	13
Simple acids	21
Fatty acids	22
Simple esters and lactones	13
Steroids	11
Terpenes	120
Noncannabinoid phenols	25
Flavonoids	21
Vitamins	1
Pigments	2
Elements	9
Total	483

Taken with permission from ElSohly MA. Chemical constituents of Cannabis. *In: Grotenhermen F, Russo E (eds) Cannabis and Cannabinoids: Pharmacology, Toxicology and Therapeutic Potential. Haworth Integrative Healing Press, New York, 2002, pp. 27–36.*

TABLE 8.4   Approved Medical Uses of Cannabinoids

Dronabinol (Marinol) is the pure isomer of Δ^9-THC. It is available as a prescription drug in the United States and is approved by the Food and Drug Administration for nausea and vomiting in patients who undergo chemotherapy and anorexia in AIDS wasting syndrome. The pharmacokinetics of oral THC are far less conducive to psychotropic effects than those of smoked cannabis. The absorption of smoked THC is very rapid, with peak levels of intoxication reported after ~30 min compared with 90 min or longer for oral administration.

Nabilone (Cesamet) is a synthetic analog of THC and was approved for use in the United States for nausea and vomiting in patients who undergo chemotherapy and anorexia in AIDS wasting syndrome. It is administered orally, so the same pharmacokinetic issues as dronabinol are relevant.

Nabiximols (Sativex) is a patented oromucosal mouth spray that is a cannabinoid-based medicine for multiple sclerosis. It is composed of the two main active ingredients of *Cannabis sativa*: a 1:1 mixture of Δ^9-THC + cannabidiol. The psychotropic effects of Sativex are alleged to be less than smoked cannabinoids. Again, it is administered orally, so the same pharmacokinetic issues as dronabinol are relevant. The levels of THC in the blood are much less after oromucosal use of Sativex at equivalent doses (163 ng/ml smoked; 8.8 ng/ml Sativex spray; for further reading, see Stott et al., 2008). Sativex is being marketed in the United Kingdom, Canada, and a number of European countries for the treatment of spasticity associated with multiple sclerosis.

the cannabis plant contains very little Δ^9-THC. Dronabinol (Marinol) is the (−)*trans*-isomer of Δ^9-THC, which is dissolved in sesame oil to create 2.5, 5.0, and 10 mg capsule formulations (Table 8.4).

"Spice" and Herbal Marijuana Alternatives

Synthetic cannabinoid receptor agonists historically have been synthesized in biomedical research to understand the neuropharmacology of cannabinoid action and to develop new therapeutic agents. However, approximately 10 years ago (around 2004), street chemists began synthesizing alleged herbal products called "Spice" in Europe and "K2" in the United States. Manufacturing such "herbal" products was neither illegal nor controlled. Although little is known about the exact composition of these herbal products, numerous compounds with CB_1 receptor agonistic activity have been used as additives in smokable herbal products to attain psychophysical effects that are similar to those of smoked THC. These compounds are known by the JWH designation (synthesized by John W. Huffman at Clemson University) or CP designation (Pfizer), such as JWH-018, JWH-073,

and CP 47497-C8. Later, numerous chemically similar compounds were identified in such herbal mixtures (for further reading, see Seely et al., 2012; Musshoff et al., 2013). In 2011, the United States Drug Enforcement Administration gave Schedule I status to the synthetic cannabinoids listed above, although preparations of these compounds are still available on the Internet and in local shops that sell drug paraphernalia in the United States.

HISTORY OF CANNABINOID USE

Cannabis is the most commonly used illicit drug in the United States. The 2011 United States *National Survey on Drug Use and Health* from the Substance Abuse and Mental Health Services Administration estimated that 107.8 million people aged 12 and older (42%) had ever engaged in marijuana use, and 29.7 million people aged 12 and older were last-year users of marijuana (11.5%). Notable statistics from this survey included the following. In 2011, of those people aged 12 or older who ever used in the last year, 4.2 million (13.9%) showed cannabis abuse or dependence (Substance Use Disorder based on the *Diagnostic*

BOX 8.2

GATEWAY HYPOTHESIS

The Gateway Hypothesis of the trajectory of the evolution of drug use, particularly in adolescents, was originally formulated as four stages in the sequence of involvement with drugs: beer or wine or both, cigarettes or hard liquor, cannabis, and other illicit drugs (for further reading, see Kandel, 1975). Relevant to the present chapter, the Gateway Hypothesis has been invoked most often in the link between the use of cannabis and the subsequent use of other illicit drugs, with much support generated for such a link but not necessarily causality. Some work now shows a significant association between the *frequency* of cannabis use and *frequency* of the use of other illicit drugs, even when genetic, environmental, and individual variables are controlled, leading some to argue for a causal link between the use of cannabis and the use of other illicit drugs (for further reading, see Fergusson et al., 2006).

and Statistical Manual of Mental Disorders, 5th edition [DSM-5] criteria), and 2.6 million (8.8%) of those who ever used in the last year showed cannabis dependence (DSM-IV criteria; see Chapter 1).

Marijuana has long been argued to be a "Gateway Drug" (Box 8.2). In a report of adolescents referred for conduct and substance abuse problems, cannabis, tobacco, and alcohol had the highest overall prevalence, with a rapid progression from first use to regular use (Figure 8.3). Long-term trends have shown increases in marijuana use in the 1960s and 1970s, declines in the 1980s, and increases again in the 1990s. In the mid-1960s, only 5% of young adults aged 18–25 had ever used marijuana, but this increased to 54% in 1982 (Figure 8.4) and has remained relatively steady since then.

MEDICAL USES

Medical uses for marijuana have been ubiquitous for centuries in Asia, Southeast Asia, and India. Hemp was used to expel flatulence, excite the appetite, and induce eloquence. Both stimulant and sedative effects have been described as being dose-related, with higher doses producing more sedative-like effects. The early explorations of the medical uses of cannabis focused on its ability to cause profound "narcoticism," demonstrating effectiveness in the treatment of a case of infantile convulsions. It also resulted in a "singular form of delirium which the incautious use of the hemp preparations often occasions, especially among young men first commencing the practice" (O'Shaughnessy WB. On the preparations of the Indian hemp, or gunjah. *Transactions of the Medical and Physical Society of Bengal*, 1838–1840, pp. 421–461). Describing a state of intoxication, the user is said to have "a strange balancing gait, perpetual giggling, expressions of cunning and merriment, increased libido and a voracious appetite" (O'Shaughnessy WB. On the preparations of the Indian hemp, or gunjah. *Transactions of the Medical and Physical Society of Bengal*, 1838–1840, pp. 421–461).

Possible indications for the medical use of cannabis preparations are numerous (Table 8.5). Cannabinoids have two currently accepted medical uses in the United States. Dronabinol (Marinol; the pure isomer of Δ^9-THC) and nabilone (Cesamet; a synthetic analog of THC) are approved for use in refractory nausea and vomiting associated with cancer chemotherapy and appetite loss in

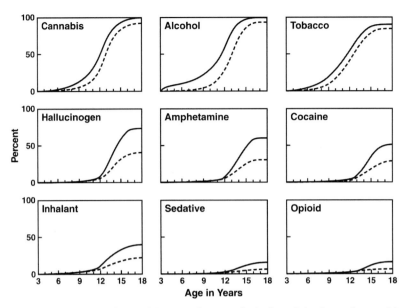

FIGURE 8.3 **Cumulative percentage of 218 subjects aged 13–19 who had used the drugs shown either once (solid line) or at least monthly (dashed line) by various ages.** Subjects for this study were patients admitted to a substance abuse treatment program between 1991 and 1994. All patients had: (1) significant antisocial problems, diagnosed substance problems, and diagnosed conduct disorder, (2) been judged by clinical staff not to be currently psychotic, mentally retarded, homicidal, suicidal, or a current arson risk, (3) no physical illness which would prevent participation in active, group-oriented treatment, (4) written, informed consent from a parent or guardian, (5) assent from the youth. *These data suggest that cannabis, like alcohol and tobacco, is used at significantly earlier ages than other drugs of abuse. Such data can be considered to support a Gateway-like hypothesis or simply that availability is a major factor. Alcohol, tobacco, and cannabis are the most used drugs overall in the population of the United States (see* Chapter 1). *[Data from Crowley TJ, Macdonald MJ, Whitmore EA, Mikulich SK. Cannabis dependence, withdrawal, and reinforcing effects among adolescents with conduct symptoms and substance use disorders.* Drug and Alcohol Dependence, *1998, (50), 27–37. Modified from Koob GF, Le Moal M. Neurobiology of Addiction. London: Academic Press, 2006.]*

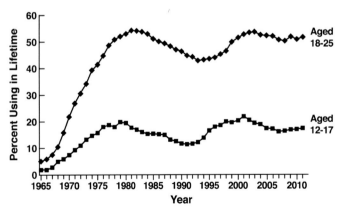

FIGURE 8.4 **Percentage of persons aged 12–17 and 18–25 who had ever used marijuana through the year 2011.** *These data show that the initial rise in marijuana use in the United States occurred in the 1960s, followed by a peak in the 1980s, a decrease in the 1990s, and a resurgence of use that has stabilized from 2000 on. The increases in the use of marijuana over the years correspond to and parallel the inverse of perceived risk over the same period. In other words, during the 1990s when the use of marijuana was low, the perceived risk was high. Conversely, in the years when use was high, the perceived risk was low. [Data from Substance Abuse and Mental Health Services Administration, National Survey on Drug Use and Health.]*

HIV/AIDS patients with anorexia (see Table 8.4). Potential medical effects that have been relatively less well confirmed include the amelioration of spasticity caused by spinal cord injury and multiple sclerosis. Cannabinoids are effective analgesics and have shown some effectiveness in chronic pain conditions. They have also been shown to be effective in asthma and in lowering

TABLE 8.5 Potential Medical Uses of Cannabinoids

WELL CONFIRMED CLINICAL EFFECTS

refractory nausea / vomiting*

anorexia appetite loss*

HIV/AIDS/cancer cachexia*

LESS WELL CONFIRMED CLINICAL EFFECTS

spasticity due to spinal cord injury*

multiple sclerosis*

neurogenic pain, neuropathy, allodynia

movement disorders (Tourette's syndrome; dystonia; dyskinesia)

bronchodilation effects

glaucoma

LARGELY UNEXPLORED BUT POSSIBLE CLINICAL EFFECTS

epilepsy

hiccups

bipolar disorder

Alzheimer's disease

alcohol dependence

BASIC RESEARCH

amyloid formation

opiate withdrawal

ischemia

hypertension

neoplasms

diarrhea

bronchospasms

sleep apnea

colonic inflammation

irritable bowel syndrome

cough

Huntington's disease

optic nerve damage

* *See Table 8.4.*

intraocular pressure in patients with glaucoma. Cannabinoids have been hypothesized for use in the treatment of movement disorders, including dystonias, dyskinesias, and tardive dyskinesia. Other proposed actions of cannabinoids that are largely unconfirmed but are being studied range from the treatment of allergies and inflammation to epilepsy and psychiatric disorders.

BEHAVIORAL EFFECTS

Cannabis produces intoxication in humans that is often labeled as pleasurable and, by definition, rewarding. The subjective effects include euphoria and mood swings characterized by initial feelings of "happiness," sudden talkativeness, a dreaming or lolling state, and general activation and hyporeactivity. Users report feeling fuzzy, dizzy, sleepy, and in a dream-like state. They also feel more friendly toward others and find more pleasure in the company of others. In a group setting, smoking cannabis produces talkativeness among people, with contagious laughing and joking and a particularly high-pitched giggly laughter. In studies of the self-reported effects of cannabis in regular human cannabis users, both in naturalistic studies and laboratory settings, the most frequently reported effect of cannabis was relaxation. Enhanced mood (happiness or laughing more), sensory alterations, enhanced appetite, and greater insight/thinking also ranked high (Table 8.6). Large individual differences have been observed in the response to cannabis, and the effects are heavily influenced by a person's expectations. Decreased talkativeness and decreased sociability are often reported, and these effects may be dose-related and more likely to occur at higher doses. A characteristic effect of marijuana intoxication compared with alcohol intoxication is being "less noisy and boisterous at parties than when drunk or tipsy on alcohol" (Tart CT. *On Being Stoned: A Psychological Study of Marijuana Intoxication*. Science and Behavior Books, Palo Alto CA, 1971).

TABLE 8.6   Ten Most Frequently Reported Effects of Marijuana Intoxication (Based on Open-Ended Questions)

Berke (1974) (n = 522)	%	Goode (1970) (n = 191)	%	Atha (1998) (n = 2794)	%
Enhanced relaxation	25.7	More relaxed	46.1	Relaxation	25.9
Happiness	16.1	Senses more perceptive	36.1	Insight/personal growth	8.7
Appreciation of music	15.5	Think deeper	31.4	Pain relief	6.1
Visual illusions / hallucinations	13.4	Laugh much more	28.8	Antidepressant/happy	4.9
Enhanced insight into others	11.9	Time slowed down	23.0	Respiratory benefit	2.4
Hunger/appetite enhanced	11.9	Become more withdrawn	22.0	Creativity	2.3
Heightened sense perception	11.7	Feels nice, pleasant	20.9	Socializing	2.0
Elation	11.5	Mind wanders	20.9	Sensory perception	1.6
Colors brighter	11.1	Feel dizzy, giddy	20.4	Improved sleep	1.6

Taken with permission from Green B, Kavanagh D, Young R. Being stoned: a review of self-reported cannabis effects. Drug and Alcohol Review, 2003, (22), 453–460.

Sociability can go either way, with self-reports of "I become more sociable" (more likely at lower levels of intoxication) and "I become less sociable" (at higher levels of intoxication; Figure 8.5). In a human laboratory study, in which subjects smoked at least four times per week (average 6.6 times per week) while they participated in a 16 day residential study, smoking marijuana cigarettes varied as a function of Δ^9-THC content. Marijuana cigarettes with Δ^9-THC concentrations of 2.2% and 3.9% were smoked more than placebo cigarettes. Subjects reported significant increases in ratings of *high, stimulated,* and *good drug effect,* but measures of *forgetful* and *can't concentrate* also increased, and performance decreased on a digit-symbol substitution task, divided attention task, rapid information task, and mathematics task. Some of these effects were greater in the subjects who smoked marijuana cigarettes with 3.9% vs. 2.2% Δ^9-THC content.

Human subjects may have a form of disinhibition, with an inclination to increase motor activity and behave impulsively. However, paradoxically, even the simplest tasks appear to require enormous effort. Users generally seek situations where no physical effort is required. Thus, an individual may be disinhibited, but incoordination and clumsiness prevent the individual from attempting many activities. Following is an early clinical description of acute intoxication:

"Walking becomes effortless. The paresthesias and changes in bodily sensations help to give an astounding feeling of lightness to the limbs and body. Elation continues: he laughs uncontrollably and explosively for brief periods of time without at times the slightest provocation: if there is a reason it quickly fades, the point of the joke is lost immediately. Speech is rapid, flighty, the subject has the impression that his conversation is witty, brilliant; ideas flow quickly." *(Bromberg W. Marihuana intoxication: a clinical study of Cannabis sativa intoxication.* American Journal of Psychiatry, 1934, (91), 303–330.)

Psychedelic-like effects are also associated with marijuana intoxication. Subjects report an increased sensitivity to sound and a keener appreciation of rhythm and timing.

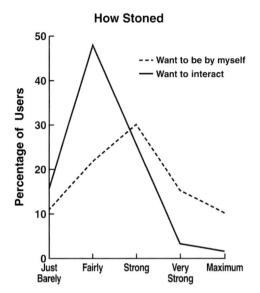

How Stoned

- - - Want to be by myself
—— Want to interact

Percentage of Users

Just Barely | Fairly | Strong | Very Strong | Maximum

FIGURE 8.5 **Effect of level of marijuana intoxication on sociability.** "I become more sociable" is a common effect, but its converse, "I become less sociable; I want to be by myself," is just as common. The latter occurs at higher levels of intoxication than the former. At a party, for instance, people sitting by themselves may often be more intoxicated than the people who are conversing. The intoxication level data will not always add up to 100% because of variable numbers of respondents who skip various questions or because of rounding errors. In interpreting the graph, notice that the percentage of users plotted at each level is the percentage of people who indicated that level as their minimal level of intoxication for experiencing that particular effect. A drop in the curve with an increasing minimal level of intoxication does not mean that fewer users experience that effect at higher levels, but rather that fewer give a higher level as their minimal level for experiencing that effect. *These data suggest that greater intoxication is associated with a greater likelihood that one will not socially interact. Conversely, less intoxication is associated with a greater likelihood that the person will socially interact. [Taken with permission from Tart CT.* On Being Stoned: A Psychological Study of Marijuana Intoxication. *Science and Behavior Books, Palo Alto CA, 1971.]*

TABLE 8.7 Behavioral Effects of Marijuana Intoxication

- Euphoria
- Perceptual changes
  feelings of "unreality"
  lightness or heaviness of the body
  time slowed down
  distorted spatial vision
  more vivid colors
  more intense sounds
  synesthesia (at high doses)
- Sedation
- Motor impairment
- Decreased mental performance
- Increased appetite
- Analgesia

[Taken with permission from Koob GF, Le Moal M. Neurobiology of Addiction. *Academic Press, London, 2006.]*

be seen, or amorphous forms of vivid color may evolve into geometric figures, shapes, or faces. The depth of color is striking, with an apparent increase in auditory faculties (Table 8.7). Users may also have subjective feelings of unreality that border on depersonalization, with various sensations of lightness or heaviness in the body and a sensation of floating in air or walking on waves. One adolescent user reported:

"Man, when I'm up on the weed, I'm really livin'. I float up and up and up until I'm miles above the Earth. Then, Baby, I begin to come apart. My fingers leave my hands, my hands leave my wrists, my arms and legs leave my body and I just flooooooat all over the universe." *(Bloomquist ER.* Marijuana: social benefit or social detriment? *California Medicine. 1967, (106), 346–353.)*

PHARMACOKINETICS

Cannabis is used primarily by the smoking route, although oral marijuana also produces both subjective effects and increases in heart rate. After inhalation, Δ^9-THC is detectable in plasma within seconds, with peak concentrations 3–10 min after smoking and bioavailability that ranges from 10% to 35%, depending

The perception of time often slows, with an exaggeration of the sense of time. The perception of space may broaden, and objects that are near may appear distant. Visual hallucinations, similar to psychedelics such as lysergic acid diethylamide, can include illusionary transformations of the outer world. Flashes of light may

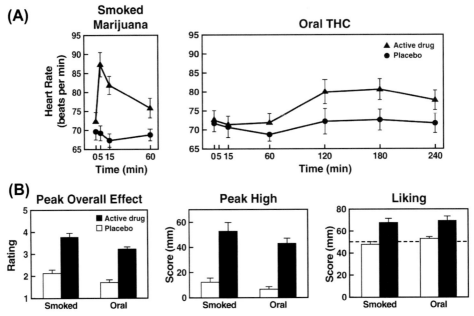

FIGURE 8.6 **Physiological and subjective effects of smoked *vs.* oral administration of Δ⁹-tetrahydrocannabinol.** Smoked marijuana cigarettes contained 2.3–3.6% Δ⁹-THC. Oral administration was via Marinol capsules (2.5, 5, and 10 mg). (A) Heart rate before and after active drug or placebo administration. (B) End-of-session questionnaire scores after active drug or placebo administration. *These data show that similar to other drugs of abuse, smoked marijuana has much faster absorption and is more effective. Notice that it took 1–2 h for significant increases in heart rate to be seen after oral administration, whereas significant increases in heart rate were observed at 5 min with smoked marijuana. [Modified with permission from Chait LD, Zacny JP. Reinforcing and subjective effects of oral Δ⁹-THC and smoked marijuana in humans.* Psychopharmacology, *1992, (107), 255–262.]*

on the experience of the smoker (Figure 8.6). Oral administration results in low bioavailability (6–7%) because of numerous factors, but mainly extensive first-pass liver metabolism. The effects of oral Δ⁹-THC are significantly delayed; by up to 60–120 min compared with the smoking route. These routes of administration correlate well with their relative effectiveness in producing the subjective "high" associated with intoxication (Figure 8.7). Other potential effective, seldom used routes of administration include rectal (13.5% bioavailability), sublingual, transdermal, and opthalmic (6–40% bioavailability). The inhalation of Δ⁹-THC produces dose-dependent blood levels; significantly lower peak blood levels are reached after oral administration (Table 8.8).

Δ⁹-THC has a peculiar distribution because of its high lipophilicity compared with other drugs of abuse. As a result, it rapidly enters highly vascularized tissues. After intravenous administration, only 1% is estimated to enter the brain at the time of peak behavioral effects. The significant accumulation of cannabinoids occurs later in less vascularized tissues and body fat, which is the major long-term storage site.

Δ⁹-THC is broken down in the liver by enzymes of the cytochrome P450 system. In humans, hydroxylation produces 11-OH-THC, and oxidation leads to THC-COOH (Figure 8.8). The elimination half-life for Δ⁹-THC ranges widely, from 20 to 60 h. The half-like in chronic users is shorter (28 h) than in non-users (57 h). The elimination half-life for Δ⁹-THC metabolites

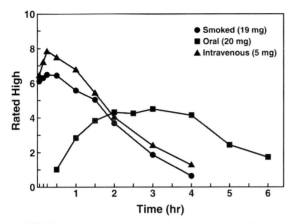

FIGURE 8.7 **Time course of subjective high after smoked (19 mg), oral (20 mg), and intravenous (5 mg) Δ^9-THC administration.** *These data show that the route of administration determines the profile of intoxication produced by marijuana over time. Notice that the onset of the peak levels of intoxication in the blood is delayed with oral administration compared with intravenous and smoked marijuana and that the peak levels of intoxication are higher for intravenous and smoked marijuana compared with oral administration. [Adapted from Hollister LE, Gillespie HK, Ohlsson A, Lindgren JE, Wahlen A, Agurell S. Do plasma concentrations of Δ^9-tetrahydrocannabinol reflect the degree of intoxication?* Journal of Clinical Pharmacology, *1981, 21(8–9 suppl): 171s–177s.]*

TABLE 8.8   Peak Plasma Levels of Δ^9-THC After Smoked vs. Oral Administration

Route	Δ^9-THC Dose	Mean Peak Plasma Level (Range)
Smoked	16 mg	84.3 (50.0–129.0) ng/m (Huestis et al.)
	34 mg	162.2 (76.0–267.0) ng/m (Huestis et al.)
Oral	2.5 mg	2.01 (0.6–12.5) ng/m (Timpone et al.)
	15 mg	3.9 (2.7–6.3) ng/m (Frytak et al.)
	20 mg	6.0 (4.4–11.0) ng/m (Ohlsson et al.)
	30 mg	15.5 ng/m* (Haney et al.)

* *Peak at 1 h.*
Expanded references for column 3 have been added to Suggested Reading.

is longer than for the parent compound, ranging from five to six days.

Δ^9-THC is excreted from the body as acid metabolites, and these metabolites can be detected in the urine for an average of 27 days in chronic users, and positive urine results have been detected up to 46 days after the last administration.

USE, ABUSE, AND ADDICTION

For some time, a common belief was that marijuana abuse and dependence rarely occurred as a primary problem. Many people believed that cannabis did not produce a true dependence syndrome. Beginning in the 1980s, however, an increasing number of individuals who could not stop smoking cannabis on their own have sought treatment primarily for

cannabis dependence. When subjects present for treatment, various rationales for discontinuing marijuana use are given, including fear of the physical consequences of smoking cannabis, difficulty expressing emotions, difficulty experiencing feelings of intimacy or closeness with a partner, and dissatisfaction with a failure in achieving life goals (Box 8.3). Chronic users are described as having mild boredom, a lack of zest, or a low level of depression that resolves during marijuana abstinence. Subjects readily respond to advertisements for the treatment of cannabis dependence, and the majority are not abusing other substances.

Cannabis Use Disorder has a characteristic clinical course that can be identified, is predictable, and has elements common to Substance Use Disorders for other drugs of abuse. A user will typically begin with social use, often enjoying the pleasurable effects of cannabis in a social setting while learning to use the drug to enhance such effects (for example, learning to inhale). Marijuana use can then increase to the point where the drug is no longer used socially,

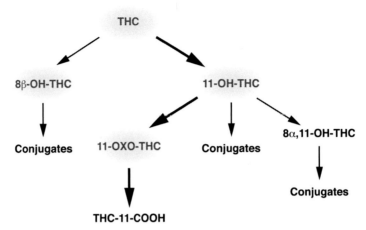

FIGURE 8.8 **Metabolic pathways of Δ⁹-THC.** *The highlighted compounds signify psychoactive metabolites. The bold arrows indicate the predominate metabolic pathway. The 11-OH → COOH pathway is where most of the Δ⁹-THC ends up going. This is why it is often the primary choice for detection in drug testing.*

BOX 8.3

VOLUNTEER WITH UNSUCCESSFUL TREATMENT

JS was an 18-year-old male who voluntarily presented because he "wanted to stop." Consumption of drugs consisted of about 3.5 grams of marijuana and hashish per day for one year prior to seeking treatment. He self-administered every one to four hours while awake and complained of chronic cough, anorexia, depression, and weight loss. When he had tried abruptly to cease marijuana by himself, he had hallucinations, depression, and anergy. Urinalysis testing revealed the presence of marijuana, but no other drugs. The patient entered a counseling program, but received no medications. Only one return appointment was kept, and he was lost to followup.

From: Tennant FS Jr, The clinical syndrome of marijuana dependence, Psychiatric Annals, 1986, (16), 225–234.

---

and users begin smoking whenever possible (for example, on the way to school or even between classes or during work). Tolerance develops, and more and more marijuana is smoked, possibly because of the effect of tolerance. Performance in social settings and occupational/academic functioning decline, and denial and resistance to considering cannabis use as a problem develop. An important criterion for clinically diagnosing Substance Dependence on cannabis, as defined by the DSM-IV and DSM-5, is that marijuana use affects a person's ability to function. Abnormal or compulsive marijuana use is often argued to be the result of a given problem rather than the cause of it, but the converse may also be true (see below). Difficulty sleeping, depression, and stress fall into this category. Both social users and dependent users may use marijuana for the same reasons:

"The reason addicts use marijuana *abnormally* is because marijuana apparently provides an unusual

TABLE 8.9   Two Clinical Forms of Marijuana Dependence

	Frequency of Self-Administration	Likely Dependence Metabolites	Usual Treatment Referral	Self-Perceived Dependence	Severity of Withdrawal Symptoms	Relapse Rate
Type One	multiple times each day	Δ^9-tetrahydro-cannabinol 11-hydroxy-Δ^9-tetra-hydrocannabinol	voluntary; self-referred	significant	moderate	high
Type Two	every 24–48 hr	11-nor-Δ^9-tetrahydro-cannabinol-carboxylic acid	involuntary; detected by mandatory screening	minor-moderate	mild	high

Taken with permission from Tennant FS. The clinical syndrome of marijuana dependence. Psychiatric Annals, 1986, (16), 225–234.

BOX 8.4

MANDATORY WORK-SITE DETECTION AND REFERRAL

HS was a 37-year-old male salesperson. He was reported to the management of his company to be a marijuana user who also sold it to other employees while on company premises. A mandatory urine test revealed the presence of marijuana metabolites, and in order to retain employment he was required to undergo withdrawal and enter a periodic urine-testing program. Upon interview, he stated that he had used marijuana every evening for approximately 22 years. He believed this habit had not been injurious to himself until approximately three months prior to treatment when he began to notice some defects in his short-term memory.

Physical examination was normal. Plasma analysis showed there to be 148 ng/ml of 11-OH THC and 80 ng/ml of THC-C. He was administered desipramine, 25 mg, three times per day and tyrosine. During the first three weeks following cessation of marijuana, he reported mild insomnia, depression, anergy, and craving. Urine analysis showed no marijuana metabolite after about 30 days. After six weeks of abstinence, he reported improvement of short term memory and improved job performance.

From: Tennant FS Jr, The clinical syndrome of marijuana dependence, Psychiatric Annals, 1986, (16), 225–234.

---

reinforcement to those with a vulnerability to marijuana not possessed by others." *(Miller NS, Gold MS. The diagnosis of marijuana (cannabis) dependence.* Journal of Substance Abuse Treatment, *1989, (6), 183–192.)*

Two clinical forms of dependence have been described: Type 1 and Type 2 (Table 8.9). Such a prior distinction seemed to foretell the diagnostic changes adopted by the DSM-5 by considering cannabis use disorder on a continuum of severity. Type 1 involves an individual who smokes or uses marijuana several times per day at approximately 2–4h intervals, except during sleep, and who escalates intake. Such subjects exhibit significant impairment in social and occupational functioning and often ultimately seek treatment. Type 2 presents at mandatory screening and involves individuals who usually use marijuana every 24–36h (Box 8.4). Although they present with impairment in social and occupational functioning, these individuals have less withdrawal symptoms and less perceived dependence.

Most of the DSM-III-R criteria for Substance Dependence were met by individuals diagnosed with Substance Dependence on cannabis. Preoccupation with obtaining and using marijuana is represented by the persistent presence of marijuana in the individual's daily living and choices of activities. Compulsivity is represented by continued use despite marijuana-related consequences. Relapse or the propensity to relapse is reflected by a return to marijuana use after a period of abstinence and may provide confirmation of the suspected diagnosis. In a study of adolescents who were referred for substance abuse and conduct problems, the most frequently observed criteria were a substantial time spent obtaining marijuana, using marijuana, or recovering from its effects, continued use despite problems in social and occupational functioning, and tolerance or withdrawal (Figure 8.9).

The treatment of cannabis dependence has relied almost exclusively on behavioral therapies. No pharmacological treatments for cannabis dependence have been approved by the US Food and Drug Administration (see Chapter 9). Few pharmacological treatments have shown any success. There is some evidence that dronabinol

(Marinol) can be used as a substitution therapy, similar to methadone treatment for heroin dependence, and a successful clinical trial has been conducted with gabapentin. Cognitive behavioral therapy, motivational enhancement therapy, relapse prevention support groups, social support groups, and motivational interviewing have all significantly reduced marijuana use compared with baseline, but no single therapy has stood out as being significantly more effective than any other. A large-scale, multi-site clinical trial found that approximately 23% of the people in an experimental group that received extended cognitive behavioral therapy combined with motivational enhancement therapy remained abstinent at 4 months compared with 9% of people in a brief intervention group and 4% of people in a delayed treatment group, suggesting some semblance of a treatment "dose" response.

Cannabinoid Tolerance

Tolerance readily develops to most of the effects of cannabinoids in humans and is largely attributed to pharmacodynamic (brain neuroadaptation) rather than pharmacokinetic (metabolic or distribution) changes. Chronic cannabinoid administration leads to profound downregulation of cannabinoid receptors in humans,

FIGURE 8.9 **Percentage of patients with various DSM-III-R dependence symptoms, among those dependent on cannabis (**n** = 180), alcohol (**n** = 186), or cocaine (**n** = 51).** *[Taken with permission from Crowley TJ, Macdonald MJ, Whitmore EA, Mikulich SK. Cannabis dependence, withdrawal, and reinforcing effects among adolescents with conduct symptoms and substance use disorders.* Drug and Alcohol Dependence, *1998, (50), 27–37.]*

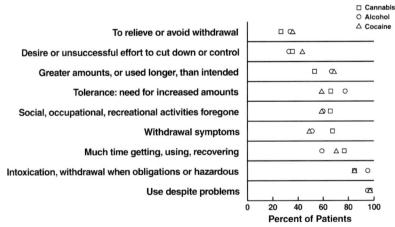

suggesting one of several mechanisms for tolerance (see below for other mechanisms). Tolerance is reflected by changes in the increases in heart rate or subjective high. In an inpatient study of 30 subjects who smoked marijuana, the mean heart rate and subjective "high" decreased over a 94 day smoking period (Figure 8.10). Tolerance to subjective effects but not the effects on food intake have been observed in some studies. Tolerance has also been observed to the effects of Δ^9-THC on intraocular pressure, cardiovascular measures other than heart rate, sedative effects, and autonomic and sleep changes.

Cannabinoid Withdrawal

Cannabis withdrawal in humans has long been described anecdotally and has now been codified by the medical community as a Cannabis Withdrawal Syndrome in the DSM-V. Both inpatient and outpatient studies contributed to the criteria for cannabis withdrawal in humans (Table 8.10). The most common symptoms associated with cannabis withdrawal are decreased appetite/weight loss, irritability, nervousness, anxiety, anger, aggression, restlessness, sleep disturbances, and depressed mood. A substantial percentage of heavy marijuana users (16%)

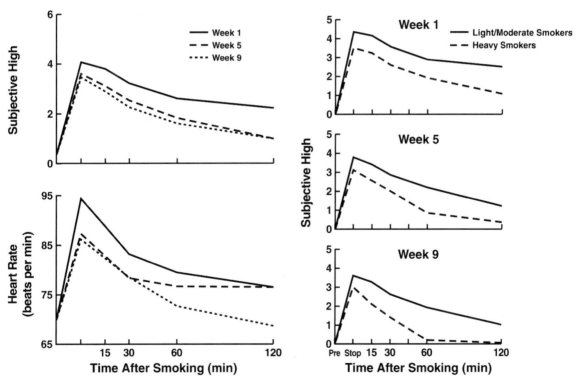

FIGURE 8.10 **Tolerance to the subjective and physiological effects of marijuana intoxication.** (Left) Mean heart rate and subjective high after smoking one marijuana cigarette after 1, 5, and 9 weeks of smoking at least one 900 mg marijuana cigarette per day. (Right) Comparison of light-to-moderate smokers to heavy smokers in ratings of subjective high. *These data show that repeated smoking of marijuana produces tolerance to the increases in heart rate and the subjective high produced by marijuana. Notice that tolerance is reflected by less of a peak response and a faster return to baseline for both heart rate and subjective high. [Taken with permission from Nowlan R, Cohen S. Tolerance to marijuana: heart rate and subjective "high." Clinical Pharmacology and Therapeutics, 1977, (22), 550–556.]*

TABLE 8.10   Cannabis Withdrawal Syndrome in the Diagnostic and Statistical Manual of Mental
Disorders, 5th Edition

Cannabis Withdrawal

A. Cessation of cannabis use that has been heavy and prolonged (i.e., usually daily or almost daily use over a period of at least a few months)

B. Three (or more) of the following signs and symptoms develop within approximately one week after Criterion A:

  1. Irritability, anger, or aggression

  2. Nervousness or anxiety

  3. Sleep difficulty (e.g., insomnia, disturbing dreams)

  4. Decreased appetite or weight loss

  5. Restlessness

  6. Depressed mood

  7. At least one or the following physical symptoms causing significant discomfort: abdominal pain, shakiness/tremors, sweating, fever, chills, or headache

C. The signs or symptoms in Criterion B cause clinically significant distress or impairment in social, occupational, or other important areas of functioning

D. The signs or symptoms are not attributable to another medical condition and are not better explained by another mental disorder, including intoxication or withdrawal from another substance

From American Psychiatric Association. Diagnostic and Statistical Manual of Mental Disorders, *5th edition. American Psychiatric Publishing, Washington DC, 2013.*

exhibit withdrawal symptoms. Outpatient studies in adolescents and adults who sought treatment for cannabis dependence have shown that the majority of users reported histories of repeated marijuana withdrawal. The onset of withdrawal typically occurs within 1–3 days. Peak effects are experienced at 2–6 days, and most of the withdrawal symptoms last 4–14 days (Figure 8.11). The long onset of Δ^9-THC withdrawal appears to be directly related to the long half-life and slow decline of blood Δ^9-THC levels (Box 8.5).

Some clinicians have argued for the existence of a protracted abstinence state, in which the body reconstitutes itself to a normal, pre-drug state that can be quite prolonged and may last up to 15–18 months. Mild flu-like symptoms may occur a week or more later. Other subjective effects of prolonged abstinence include cognitive deficits and sleep disturbances. During this recovery period, subjects report the recovery of behaviors as subtle as being able to better sustain concentration when doing visualizations or meditations within a treatment session, engaging in more difficult reading material, and being less accident prone.

Pathology and Psychopathology

Acute administration of cannabis produces a pleasant experience in most users, associated with intoxication and the subjective high (see above). However, some individuals with existing psychopathology, particularly in naive individuals who ingest cannabis unknowingly, can experience anxiety and panic reactions. Sometimes these reactions can include paranoia, dysphoria, depersonalization, and psychosis in vulnerable individuals (Box 8.6).

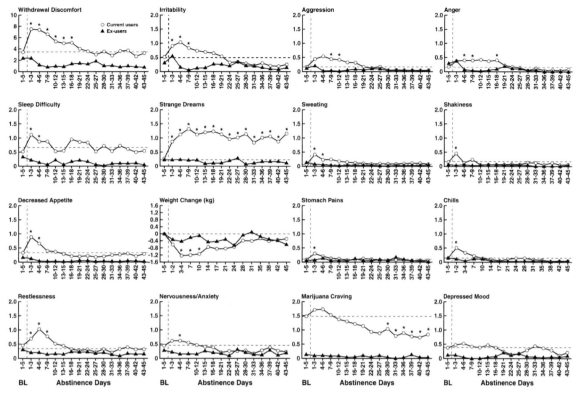

FIGURE 8.11 **Mean withdrawal scores over 45 days of marijuana abstinence in current marijuana users (n = 18) and ex-users (n = 12).** Ranges overall: 0–3. Range for Withdrawal Discomfort: 0–36. The value of the baseline (BL) data point reflects the mean of days 1, 3, and 5. The dotted horizontal line represents the baseline mean score. *$p < 0.05$, significant difference between specific 3 day abstinence periods and baseline mean or between body weight at specific abstinence days and baseline. *These data give a comprehensive assessment of the different symptoms of withdrawal from chronic marijuana use in humans. Notice that many of the symptoms are of a motivational nature, such as discomfort, irritability, anxiety, and strange dreams. Notice also that some symptoms, such as discomfort and strange dreams, persist for weeks. [Taken with permission from Budney AJ, Moore BA, Vandrey RG, Hughes JR. The time course and significance of cannabis withdrawal.* Journal of Abnormal Psychology, 2003, (112), 393–402.]

Cannabis produces numerous physiological effects in the cardiovascular system, including an increase in heart rate. In vulnerable individuals, this increase can contribute to pathology. Δ^9-THC also increases supine blood pressure, produces postural hypotension, and increases cardiac output. Tolerance develops to the increases in heart rate and blood pressure. Although the cardiovascular effects of marijuana are not associated with serious health risks in young healthy users (although

occasional cardiac events have been reported), marijuana smoking by people with cardiovascular disease poses health risks.

The adverse effects of smoking cannabis on the respiratory tract may be similar to the effects of tobacco smoking. Firm conclusions in this regard are limited, however, by a lack of animal models, concomitant tobacco use, and the relatively short period of time that marijuana has been smoked in Western society (30–35 years) compared with tobacco. Common untoward

BOX 8.5

DELAYED WITHDRAWAL SYMPTOMS

A 27-year-old male was admitted to a day-treatment program for marijuana dependence. He had been identified at work for being "under the influence" on more than one occasion and was, therefore, referred for treatment. Drug consumption consisted of intermittent cocaine use and daily use of about one marijuana joint. He perceived that he had been "addicted" to marijuana for about 15 years, and that he had skipped marijuana use on very few days during this time. A physical examination was normal except for mild nasal-septum inflammation and a swollen uvula. Urine analysis showed the presence of marijuana metabolite and marijuana plasma analysis by high performance liquid chromatography (HPLC) showed no 11-OH-THC and THC-C to be 8 ng/ml. A 24-hour urine specimen showed secretion of 2-methoxy-4- hydroxy-phenyglycol (MHPG) to be 143.0 MCG/24 hours (normal is 1164 to 2216). Since his continued employment was dependent upon attending the day-care program until his urine was void of all drugs, compliance with treatment and testing procedures was good. Withdrawal medication consisted of desipramine, 25 mg, administered three times per day, and the amino acid, tyrosine. On the third treatment day, his urine still contained metabolite, and his plasma contained 3 ng/ml of THC-C. On the eighth day of attendance, he complained of a flu-like illness consisting of nausea, vomiting, diaphoresis, chills, myalgia, anorexia, and insomnia. The patient did not relate these symptoms temporally to his marijuana use, since he had ceased use eight days previous. Plasma analysis showed no detectable presence of 11-OH-THC or THC-C, but marijuana metabolite was still present in urine at this time. The apparent withdrawal symptoms resolved within 48 hours. Marijuana metabolite remained in his urine until the 34th day of treatment.

From: Tennant FS Jr., The clinical syndrome of marijuana dependence, Psychiatric Annals, 1986, (16), 225–234.

BOX 8.6

MARIJUANA DEPENDENCE: VOLUNTARY ADMISSION TO TREATMENT

MV was a 25-year-old male who presented with the complaint that he could not "stop marijuana by myself." He was a 12-year user having begun marijuana smoking at 13 years of age. He had used marijuana daily for about five years and was using two to three joints per day at the time of admission to outpatient treatment. The patient was married and held a regular job as a warehouse superintendent. He claimed he was having considerable conflicts with his wife and employer. In addition, he had noticed in the two months just prior to admission that he occasionally heard voices that were not real, did not always have total "control over his mind," and had some thoughts of suicide. He denied use of any other drug or excessive alcohol intake. His treatment admission breath alcohol was negative, and his urine contained marijuana metabolite, but no other abusable drug. The patient was administered desipramine, 25 mg, three times per day and was given weekly psychotherapy for approximately six months. During the first ten days of treatment, he reported insomnia, abdominal cramps, diaphoresis, tachycardia, and anxiety. These symptoms subsided, and he submitted a urine void of marijuana approximately 30 days after admission. Most of the thought disturbances noted above disappeared after about two to six weeks of treatment. He denied any marijuana use during the six months after entering treatment, and he submitted monthly urine tests that showed no marijuana.

From: Tennant FS Jr., The clinical syndrome of marijuana dependence, Psychiatric Annals, 1986, (16), 225–234.

respiratory effects reported by abusers include cough, dyspnea, sore throat, nasal congestion, and bronchitis. The long-term effects on the respiratory tract are likely to be similar to those of tobacco because of the similarities in the composition of smoke between cannabis and tobacco (Table 8.11). Although the number of cannabis cigarettes smoked may be less than the number of tobacco cigarettes smoked in a chronic smoker, several characteristics of marijuana smoking are likely to increase the burden of tar and carbon monoxide. Marijuana cigarettes are not usually filtered, and smokers tend to smoke to the very end of the butt length, which increases the total levels of tar, carbon monoxide, and Δ^9-THC delivered to the lungs. Marijuana smokers also tend to inhale larger puff volumes, draw more deeply, and hold the smoke longer in their lungs. In subjects with both tobacco and marijuana experience, marijuana smoking was associated with a five-fold greater increase in carboxyhemoglobin levels.

Cannabis use at intoxicating doses impairs psychomotor performance in any situation that requires perceptual, cognitive, and psychomotor functioning, including driving an automobile and flying an airplane. Mental and motor performance, including response speed, physical work capacity, fine hand-eye coordination, complex tracking, divided attention tasks, visual information processing, altered sense of time, and impaired short-term memory are dose-related. Impairment can begin with 5–15 mg, which is equivalent to 4–16 puffs on a 3.55% Δ^9-THC cigarette that yields 63–188 ng/ml (Figure 8.12). Automobile driving or flying an airplane in a simulator have shown dose-related deficits, even at doses as low as 5–10 mg, and up to 24 h after smoking (Table 8.12). The actual extent to which cannabis ingestion contributes to road accidents is no longer controversial, and in many countries cannabis is the most common drug detected in individuals involved in reckless driving or traffic accidents with or without alcohol. Significant percentages of impaired drivers or drivers involved in fatal accidents

TABLE 8.11 Comparison of Marijuana and Tobacco Smoke Constituents

Constituent	Marijuana	Tobacco
Whole smoke		
burning rate	11.6 mm/min/g	5.7 mm/min/g
pH (3rd to 10th puffs)	6.56–6.58	6.14–6.02
moisture	10.3%	11.1%
Particulate phase		
total particulate (per puff)	1.6 mg	2.4 mg
phenol	76.8 μg	39.0 μg
o-cresol	17.9 μg	24.0 μg
m-cresol + p-cresol	54.4 μg	65.0 μg
2,4-dimethylphenol + 2,5-dimethylphenol	6.8 μg	14.4 μg
naphthalene	3.0 mg	1.2 mg
benz(a)anthracene	75 μg	43 μg
benz(a)pyrene	31 μg	22 μg
nicotine	–	2.85 mg
Δ^9-tetrahydrocannabinol	820 μg	–
cannabinol	400 μg	–
cannabidiol	190 μg	–
Gas phase		
carbon monoxide (per cigarette)	2600 ppm	4100 ppm
ammonia	228 μg	198 μg
hydrogen cyanide	532 μg	498 μg
isoprene	83 μg	310 μg
acetaldehyde	1.20 mg	0.98 mg
acetone	443 μg	578 μg
acrolein	92 μg	85 μg
acetonitrile	132 μg	123 μg
benzene	76 μg	67 μg
toluene	112 μg	108 μg
dimethylnitrosamine	75 μg	84 μg
methylnitrosamine	27 μg	30 μg

Taken with permission from Huber GL, First MW, Grubner O. Marijuana and tobacco smoke gas phase cytotoxins. Pharmacology Biochemistry and Behavior, *1991, (40), 629–636.]*

FIGURE 8.12 **Number of correct responses on a word recall test as a function of list presentation order and placebo, alcohol (0.25, 0.5, and 1.0 g/kg), and marijuana (3.55% Δ⁹-THC; equivalent to 34 mg).** Each data point represents the mean of five measurements taken at 0, 30, 60, 90, and 120 min post-dosing in five subjects. Filled symbols indicate a significant difference from placebo (p < 0.05). *These data show that marijuana and alcohol in the moderate intoxication range produced equivalent dose-dependent deficits in word recall memory in humans. [Taken with permission from Heishman SJ, Arasteh K, Stitzer ML. Comparative effects of alcohol and marijuana on mood, memory, and performance.* Pharmacology Biochemistry and Behavior, *1997, (58), 93–101.]*

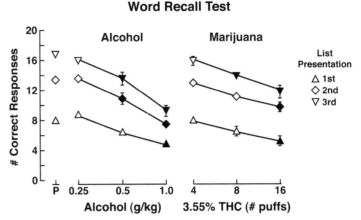

TABLE 8.12   Effects of Cannabis that Impair Driving and Piloting Skills

Slowed complex reaction time

Poor detection of peripheral light stimuli

Poor oculomotor tracking

Space and time distortion

Impaired coordination

Brake and accelerator errors

Poor speed control

Poor judgment

Increased risks in overtaking

Impaired attention, especially for divided attention tasks

Impaired short-term memory

Additive effects with alcohol and other drugs

Taken with permission from Ashton CH. Adverse effects of cannabis and cannabinoids. British Journal of Anaesthesia, *1999, (83), 637–649.*

in the United Kingdom, Canada, Europe, New Zealand, and Australia have been reported, with approximately 47% of 1,842 impaired drivers (driving while intoxicated) having cannabis suspected by drug recognition experts, with most of the opinions confirmed by chemical tests. Another study found that 33% of impaired individuals tested positive for marijuana in a group that was not impaired by alcohol. A meta-analysis

showed that smoking cannabis increases the probability of an automobile accident two-fold (for further reading, see Ashbridge et al., 2012). These studies suggest that cannabis with or without other sedative hypnotics, like alcohol and benzodiazepines, can contribute to automobile accidents.

Daily or chronic cannabis use at intoxicating doses can lead to chronic impairments in social and occupational functioning, including ineffectiveness in school, sports, work, and learning to initiate and sustain healthy relationships. The state of chronic intoxication increases risk-taking behaviors as a result of disinhibition. Such individuals may participate in unprotected sex, driving while intoxicated, or riding with an intoxicated driver.

Even more remarkable is the lack of motivation, lack of direction, lack of ambition, and inability to hold a coherent conversation. As early as the late 1960s, this configuration of effects was termed "amotivational syndrome" (McGlothlin and West, 1968). Most discussions of this topic recognize this syndrome as a state of chronic intoxication rather than a neurotoxic effect of marijuana itself, because the syndrome disappears when the individual ceases to smoke marijuana. Characterized by diminished goal-directed behavior, apathy, and an inability to master new problems, the "amotivational syndrome" has often been used to explain poor school performance in adolescents, personality deterioration, and a general decrease in function. This syndrome is more likely to occur in high-dose compulsive users than in controlled low-dose users and often remits with the cessation of use.

Acute cannabis intoxication can also lead to an acute transient psychotic episode in some individuals. Such psychotic breaks are characterized by delusions, loosening of associations, and marked illusions. Cannabis can also produce a short-term exacerbation or recurrence of pre-existing psychotic symptoms. Accumulating evidence indicates that cannabis can contribute to the causes of a functional psychotic illness or schizophrenia. Although causality has been difficult to prove, several studies have suggested a causal relationship. Cross-sectional national surveys have found that the rates of cannabis use are approximately two times higher among subjects diagnosed with schizophrenia than among the general population. Daily cannabis use has been shown to double the risk of reporting psychotic symptoms. A series of studies in Sweden, The Netherlands, France, and New Zealand examined cannabis use in adolescence with regard to later adult psychotic symptoms. The results of these studies supported the hypothesis that "cannabis use is an independent risk factor for the emergence of psychosis in psychosis-free persons" (van Os J, Bak M, Hanssen M, Bijl RV, de Graaf R, Verdoux H. Cannabis use and psychosis: a longitudinal population-based study. *American Journal of Epidemiology*, 2002, (156), 319–327; Table 8.13). The overall risk (odds ratio) for psychosis in cannabis users was 2.8, meaning that cannabis users are almost three times more likely to develop psychosis than non-cannabis users. Such an association between cannabis use in adolescence and psychosis in adulthood persisted even after controlling for numerous social, gender, age, and ethnic group factors. For example, this association was documented as being dose-related in a meta-analysis and a sibling pair analysis nested within a prospective birth cohort (for further reading, see McGrath

et al., 2010). Overall, cannabis use conveys a three-fold higher risk for later schizophrenia or schizophreniform disorder. Theoretically, without cannabis use, the general population would have an 8% lower incidence of schizophrenia.

Another insidious toxic effect of cannabis use has been revealed by studies that showed possible adverse effects on executive function in young users, particularly users who begin using cannabis during adolescence. During adolescence, prefrontal areas of the brain continue to develop, and these areas are linked to decision making and executive function (Box 8.7). The adolescent period represents a critical phase of development, characterized by specific progressive neurobiological maturational processes in the prefrontal cortex that include myelination and synaptic pruning. This period of maturation also involves the rearrangement of key neurotransmitter systems, such as glutamate, γ-aminobutyric acid, dopamine, and endocannabinoid systems in the frontal cortex. Changes in these systems are believed to support the emergence of adult cognitive processes. Over the course of adolescence and during early adulthood, individuals show normative growth in planning, preference for delayed rather than immediate rewards, resistance to peer pressure, and impulse control. Many of the brain regions that are undergoing these developmental changes may be particularly affected by alcohol and marijuana use.

Cannabis-dependent adolescents typically have cognitive deficits, characterized by short-term memory and verbal fluency impairments, attentional dysfunction, and poor performance in executive functioning. Memory difficulties are one of the most widely reported and most persistent cognitive deficits associated with extensive marijuana use in adolescents. Functional magnetic resonance imaging studies of adult subjects who abuse marijuana have shown altered activation in prefrontal and insular regions while they performed cognitive tasks, such as those that involve attention, working memory inhibitory control, and decision making during acute marijuana use,

TABLE 8.13   Longitudinal Studies in the General Population on the Role of Cannabis as a Risk Factor for Schizophrenia

Study	Authors	Study Design	Number of Subjects	Follow-up Period	Odds Ratio (95% Confidence Interval)
United States	Tien and Anthony, 1990	Population-based	4,494	–	2.4 (1.2–7.1)
Sweden	Andreasson et al., 1987 Zammit et al., 2002	Conscript cohort	50,053	15 years 27 years	2.3 (1.0–5.3) 3.1 (1.7–5.5)
The Netherlands	Van Os et al., 2002	Population-based	4,045	3 years	2.8 (1.2–6.5)
Israel	Weiser et al., 2002	Population-based	9,724	4–15 years	2.0 (1.3–3.1)
New Zealand (Christchurch)	Fergusson et al., 2003	Birth cohort	1,265	3 years	1.8 (1.2–2.6)
New Zealnd (Dunedin)	Arseneault et al., 2002	Birth cohort	1,034	15 years	3.1 (0.7–13.3)
The Netherlands	Ferdinand et al., 2005	Population-based	1,580	14 years	2.8 (1.79–4.43)
Germany	Henquet et al., 2005	Population-based	2,437	4 years	1.7 (1.1–1.50
United Kingdom	Wiles et al., 2006	Population-based	8,580	18 months	1.5 (0.55–3.94)
Greece	Stefanis et al., 2004	Birth cohort	3,500	–	4.3 (1.0–17.9)

Andréasson S, Allebeck P, Engström A, Rydberg U. Cannabis and schizophrenia: a longitudinal study of Swedish conscripts. Lancet, 1987, (2), 1483–1486.
Arseneault L, Cannon M, Poulton R, Murray R, Caspi A, Moffitt TE. Cannabis use in adolescence and risk for adult psychosis: longitudinal prospective study. British Medical Journal, 2002, (325), 1212–1213.
Ferdinand RF, Sondeijker F, van der Ende J, Selten JP, Huizink A, Verhulst FC. Cannabis use predicts future psychotic symptoms, and vice versa. Addiction, 2005, (100), 612–618.
Fergusson DM, Horwood LJ, Swain-Campbell NR. Cannabis dependence and psychotic symptoms in young people. Psychological Medicine, 2003, (33), 15–21.
Henquet C, Krabbendam L, Spauwen J, Kaplan C, Lieb R, Wittchen HU, van Os J. Prospective cohort study of cannabis use, predisposition for psychosis, and psychotic symptoms in young people. British Medical Journal, 2005, (330), 11.
Stefanis NC, Delespaul P, Henquet C, Bakoula C, Stefanis CN, Van Os J. Early adolescent cannabis exposure and positive and negative dimensions of psychosis. Addiction, 2004, (99), 1333–1341.
Tien AY, Anthony JC. Epidemiological analysis of alcohol and drug use as risk factors for psychotic experiences. Journal of Nervous and Mental Disease, 1990, (178), 473–480.
van Os J, Bak M, Hanssen M, Bijl RV, de Graaf R, Verdoux H. Cannabis use and psychosis: a longitudinal population-based study. American Journal of Epidemiology, 2002, (156), 319–327.
Weiser M, Knobler HY, Noy S, Kaplan Z. Clinical characteristics of adolescents later hospitalized for schizophrenia. American Journal of Medical Genetics, 2002, (114), 949–955.
Wiles NJ, Zammit S, Bebbington P, Singleton N, Meltzer H, Lewis G. Self-reported psychotic symptoms in the general population: results from the longitudinal study of the British National Psychiatric Morbidity Survey. British Journal of Psychiatry, 2006, (188), 519–526.
Zammit S, Allebeck P, Andreasson S, Lundberg I, Lewis G. Self-reported cannabis use as a risk factor for schizophrenia in Swedish conscripts of 1(969), historical cohort study. British Medical Journal, 2002, (325), 1199.
[Table from: Casadio P, Fernandes C, Murray RM, Di Forti M. Cannabis use in young people: the risk for schizophrenia. Neuroscience and Biobehavioral Reviews, 2011, (35), 1779–1787.]

BOX 8.7

EXECUTIVE FUNCTION

Definition: Conceptualized as the ability to organize thoughts and activities, prioritize tasks, manage time, and make decisions. Neurobiological substrates include the prefrontal cortex and orbitofrontal cortex.

chronic marijuana use, and abstinence. Growing evidence suggests that marijuana use during adolescence adversely affects normal physiological maturational processes in the frontal cortex, with reduction of cortical thickness in regions of the prefrontal cortex and insula in adolescents measured by magnetic resonance imaging. Such alterations in normal maturational processes possibly contribute to future problems with impulse control, including substance use disorders. As noted above, accumulating evidence from epidemiological studies suggests that cannabis use is a risk factor for the development of psychosis or schizophrenia.

The ingestion of synthetic cannabinoids like THC produces euphoria and relaxation but also unwanted effects, including tachycardia, anxiety, nausea, agitation, an inability to speak, dystonia, and short-term memory deficits. There are also reports of more severe and dangerous adverse reactions, including elevated blood pressure, tremor, convulsions, hallucinations, and paranoid behavior. Numerous driving-under-the-influence-like impairments have been linked to synthetic cannabinoids (e.g., JWH-019, JWH-122, JWH-210, and AM-2201), indicated by positive chemical/toxicological test results (Box 8.8). Some of the adverse clinical-like effects of "Spice" are listed in Table 8.14 (see "Spice" and Herbal Marijuana Alternatives section above). Most of these effects reported to date are acute effects. However, new-onset psychosis has been reported in otherwise healthy individuals who smoked synthetic cannabinoids, and at least one incidence of withdrawal syndromes has been described (Boxes 8.9, 8.10; for further reading, see Seeley et al., 2012).

BEHAVIORAL MECHANISM OF ACTION

Cannabis and its active ingredient Δ^9-THC have behavioral effects that intersect with two drug classes: sedative hypnotics and psychedelics. Sedative-hypnotic drugs disinhibit behavior (i.e., individuals show a release of inhibitions in situations where normally they might be socially constrained). Alcohol is widely used as a social lubricant to promote conversation and social interaction. The disinhibition associated with alcohol is often mistaken for a psychostimulant effect, and alcohol is often labeled as a stimulant at lower doses. The disinhibition produced by cannabis is more cognitive or perceptual, with a pronounced decrease in motivation to exert energy, thus limiting any actual disinhibited behavior that would resemble the stimulant-like effects of alcohol. The increased psychedelic-like perceptual effects,

---

BOX 8.8

CASE HISTORY

A 20-year-old male driver was checked during a general road traffic control. The police noted: "vestibular disorder, disturbance of fine motor skills, enlarged pupils, and blunt mood." A blood sample was taken 80 min later with the following notes being made by the physician: "finger-to-finger test doubtful, obviously enlarged pupils, and delayed reaction of the pupils to light."

Toxicological results [for synthetic cannabinoids with CB_1 receptor agonist activity]:

JWH-019 1.7 ng/ml
JWH-122 7.6 ng/ml
JWH-210 4.4 ng/ml
AM-2201 0.31 ng/ml

From: Musshoff F, Madea B, Kernbach-Wighton G, Bicker W, Kneisel S, Hutter M, Auwärter V. Driving under the influence of synthetic cannabinoids ("Spice"): a case series. International Journal of Legal Medicine, 2013, (128), 59–64.

TABLE 8.14   Spice-Induced Adverse Clinical Effects

Central effects	Psychosis
	Seizures
	Anxiety
	Agitation
	Irritability
	Memory changes
	Sedation
	Confusion
Cardiovascular effects	Tachycardia
	Tachyarrhythmia
	Cardiotoxicity
	Chest pain
Gastrointestinal effects	Nausea
	Vomiting
Other effects	Somnolence
	Dilated pupils
	Brisk reflexes
	Emesis
	Appetite changes
	Tolerance
	Withdrawal
	Drug dependence

From: Seely KA, Lapoint J, Moran JH, Fattore L. Spice drugs are more than harmless herbal blends: a review of the pharmacology and toxicology of synthetic cannabinoids. Progress in Neuropsychopharmacology and Biological Psychiatry, 2012, (39), 234–243.

decreased motivation, and impaired cognitive function associated with high doses of Δ^9-THC lead to a unique behavioral mechanism of action that presumably exaggerates the normal actions mediated by endogenous cannabinoids.

Endogenous cannabinoids (see below) may play a functional role in the brain to temper excessive arousal and excessive cognitive function but increase the response to novelty, thus increasing perceptual function and facilitating hedonic processes. Marijuana may induce variability in information processing by higher brain structures that involve executive function, leading to the retardation of habituation of classical reinforcers and inducing novel experiences. Cannabinoids may also amplify the hedonic aspects of eating. Thus, the behavioral mechanism of action of cannabinoids may involve perceptual disinhibition of both external and internal cues/states without motivational disinhibition. This *perceptual disinhibition* can be pleasant in an appropriate external context with positive valence, ranging from external sensory modalities (visual, auditory, and tactile) to the taste modality (sweet or particularly palatable food), or can be unpleasant in situations with negative emotional valence.

NEUROBIOLOGICAL EFFECTS

Discovery and Neuropharmacology of Endogenous Cannabinoids

The discovery of endogenous cannabinoid substances in the brain has a rich history that began with the synthesis and radiolabeling of synthetic and potent cannabinoids that allowed the identification and characterization of cannabinoid receptors in the rat brain. The pharmacological potency of cannabinoids correlated well with their affinity for the cannabinoid binding site (Figure 8.13). The cannabinoid receptor distribution in rat brain sections showed the densest binding in the basal ganglia and cerebellum, with intermediate levels in the hippocampus, amygdala, and cortex. Low levels were found in brainstem areas. This corresponds well with the low levels of lethality of cannabinoids in terms of respiratory depression (Figure 8.14).

The identification of a brain binding site and early work that showed that cannabinoids inhibited the enzyme adenylate cyclase led to the hypothesis that the cannabinoid receptor

---

BOX 8.9

WITHDRAWAL FROM CHRONIC USE OF SPICE

A single case report describes chronic synthetic cannabinoid use in a 20-year-old man who smoked 3 g of Spice Gold daily for eight months. He found Spice relaxing, sedative, and to have cannabis-like psychoactive effects. However, he developed tolerance and the following signs of withdrawal during his hospital admission:

"inner unrest, drug craving, nocturnal nightmares, profuse sweating, nausea, tremor, headache," hypertension, and tachycardia.

From: Zimmermann US, Winkelmann PR, Pilhatsch M, Nees JA, Spanagel R, Schulz K. Withdrawal phenomena and dependence syndrome after the consumption of spice gold. Deutsches Ärzteblatt International, 2009, (106), 464–467.

BOX 8.10

CANNABIS AS A DOPING DRUG

Should cannabis be considered a "doping" drug in sports and continue to be banned? There are clear arguments that cannabis can have some beneficial effects in reducing anxiety, improving muscle relaxation, and reducing fearful memories. However, cannabis can impair performance and cause memory loss, executive function deficits, and motor impairment, in addition to the possibility of impairing lung function. Thus,

cannabis can both improve performance and pose a health risk, two of the criteria for inclusion in the Prohibited List according to the Code of the World Doping Agency. Presumably, cannabis ingestion also violates the spirit of the sport, the third criterion. Thus, compelling arguments exist for considering cannabis a doping drug (for further reading, see Bergamaschi and Crippa, 2013).

---

was G-protein linked. Serendipitous cloning of the cannabinoid receptor that had homology with other G-protein receptors confirmed this hypothesis. The mRNA distribution of the receptor clone paralleled the distribution of the cannabinoid receptor. This cannabinoid receptor was named CB_1 and belongs to the G-protein-coupled receptor subfamily.

The receptor-mediated action of cannabinoids was based on the synthesis and radiolabeling of potent cannabinoids and the establishment of binding in brain membranes. The initial site of Δ^9-THC binding was hypothesized to be the CB_1 receptor, which is widely distributed throughout the brain but is particularly concentrated

in the extrapyramidal motor system. The CB_1 receptor was the first to be cloned and localized to brain structures. Subsequently, the CB_2 receptor was cloned and initially localized peripherally (outside the brain) and more recently within the brain. CB_1 receptors mediate many of the psychoactive effects of cannabinoids. CB_2 receptors in the periphery are mainly expressed in the immune system. However, CB_2 receptors have recently been identified in the brain and may have functional effects in modulating the mesocorticolimbic dopamine system.

Both CB_1 and CB_2 receptors are coupled to the G-proteins G_i and G_o, and this interaction inhibits adenylate cyclase. This inhibition leads to a

FIGURE 8.13 **ED$_{50}$ values (μmol/kg) plotted against the K$_I$ (nM) value for 29 different cannabinoids.** The potency of these cannabinoid analogs administered intravenously in the mouse was assessed using four pharmacological measures: spontaneous activity, antinociception, hypothermia, and catalepsy. The solid line represents the linear regression of the relationship between the ED$_{50}$ and the K$_I$ for each measure across 29 compounds. The dashed line represents the linear regression that would be obtained if the mean ED$_{50}$ value of the four measures was plotted instead of that shown for each individual behavior, so it is the same in each panel. *These data show the relationships between the ED$_{50}$ for different cannabinoids as a function of their binding to the CB$_1$ receptor. ED$_{50}$ refers to the dose that produces a given effect in 50% of the population. Binding affinity in this study was determined using a radiolabeled ligand (known as a hot ligand). The drug in question in the figure involves binding site competition between a hot ligand and a cold ligand (29 different untagged cannabinoid ligands). K$_i$ (nM) refers to the dose that displaces the binding of a tritiated high-potency synthetic cannabinoid CB$_1$ receptor agonist by 50%. Notice that similar functions are generated for each of the different behaviors, suggesting a common site of action at the CB$_1$ receptor.* [Taken with permission from Compton DR, Rice KC, De Costa BR, Razdan RK, Melvin LS, Johnson MR, Martin BR, Cannabinoid structure-activity relationships: correlation of receptor binding and in vivo activities, Journal of Pharmacology and Experimental Therapeutics, 1993, (265),218–226.]

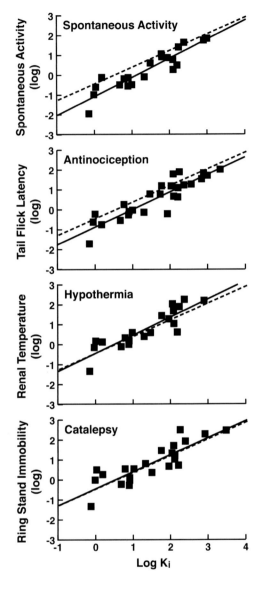

subsequent reduction of cAMP and an increase in mitogen-activated protein kinase. Cannabinoids also enhance the activation of A-type potassium channels, enhance outward potassium current, inhibit voltage-activated N-type calcium channels, and inhibit presynaptic P/Q calcium channels. The activation of CB$_1$ receptors inhibits the presynaptic release of other neurotransmitters via several molecular pathways, including the inhibition of adenylyl cyclase.

The discovery of the cannabinoid receptors immediately raised the possibility that endogenous ligands for this receptor existed, resulting in the discovery of an arachidonic acid derivative called arachidonoylethanolamide (later termed anandamide) that bound to the CB$_1$

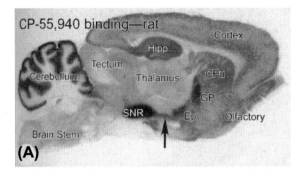

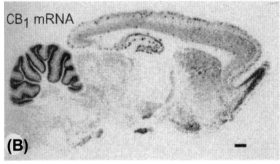

FIGURE 8.14 Autoradiographic film images that show cannabinoid receptor localization (A) in the rat. The sagittal section of the rat brain (B) shows the locations of neurons that express the mRNA at this level. High levels of receptor protein are visible in basal ganglia structures, including the globus pallidus (GP), entopeduncular nucleus (Ep), and substantia nigra pars reticulata (SNR). High binding is also seen in the cerebellum. Moderate binding is found in the hippocampus (Hipp), cortex, and caudate putamen (CPu). Low binding is found in the brain stem and thalamus. Notice that the GP, Ep, and SNR do not contain CB_1 mRNA-expressing cells (B). This is because the receptors in these areas are on axons (large arrows in panel A) and terminals, and the mRNA-expressing cells of origin reside in the caudate and putamen. [Taken with permission from Freund TF, Katona I, Piomelli D. Role of endogenous cannabinoids in synaptic signaling. Physiological Reviews, 2003, (83), 1017–1066.]

receptor (Figure 8.15). Numerous subsequent studies found that anandamide binds competitively to the CB_1 receptor, inhibits adenylate cyclase, inhibits voltage-sensitive calcium channels, and produces various behavioral and pharmacological effects that are similar to the effects of Δ^9-THC, including antinociception, hypomotility, catalepsy, and hypothermia.

However, relative to other cannabinoids, anandamide produces only weak and transient behavioral effects, possibly because of its rapid breakdown.

After the identification of anandamide, a second endogenous cannabinoid (endocannabinoid) was found: 2-arachidonylglycerol (2-AG). 2-AG is an anandamide analog with a glycerol backbone. It has high affinity for the CB_1 receptor and is found in the brain in amounts 1000 times higher than anandamide. Both of these endocannabinoids are lipid-like compounds that are synthesized and released from neurons, bind to cannabinoid receptors, activate transduction mechanisms, and have a reuptake system, although questions remain regarding the alleged anandamide transporter (Figure 8.16). However, endocannabinoids do not fulfill all the requirements of a "classic" neurotransmitter. They are not synthesized in the cytosol of neurons; they are not stored in synaptic vesicles to be secreted by exocytosis following excitation of nerve terminals by action potentials. Instead, endocannabinoids are synthesized in *postsynaptic elements* of neurons when required in response to depolarization by receptor-stimulated synthesis from membrane lipid precursors and released from cells immediately after their production (Figure 8.17). Once released, endocannabinoids act on cannabinoid receptors and may be taken back into cells via an energy-independent transport system. Once inside the cells, both anandamide and 2-AG can be broken down. This non-synaptic release mechanism and the rapid breakdown of both endocannabinoids suggest that these compounds may locally regulate the effects of primary neurotransmitters (Figure 8.18).

Advances in the understanding of the neuropharmacology of endocannabinoids have been aided by the identification of drugs that can block the formation, hypothesized reuptake, and inactivation of both anandamide and 2-AG. Anandamide reuptake is theorized to be blocked

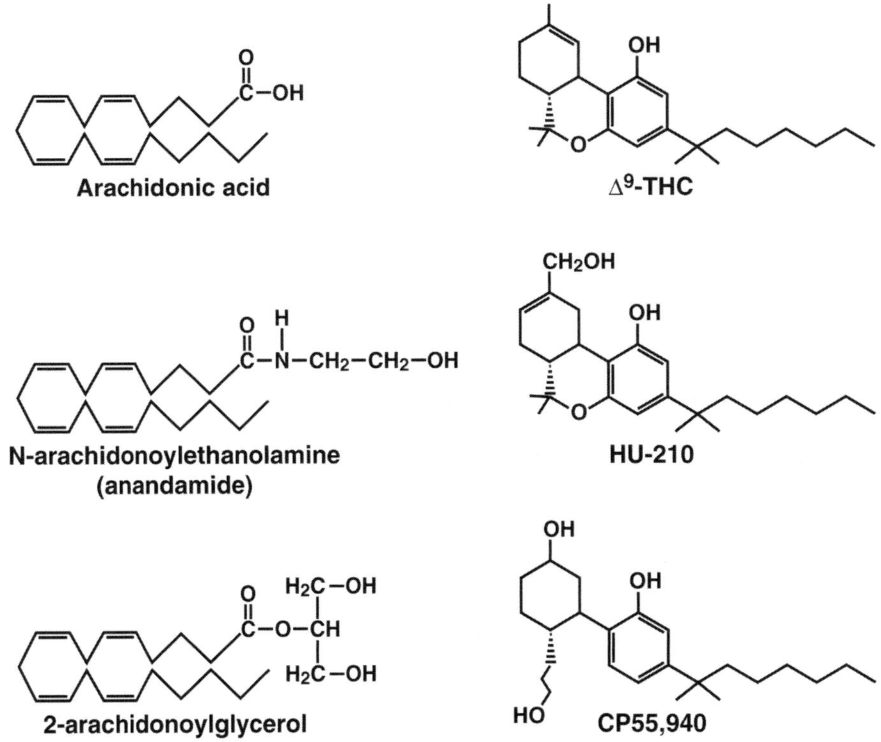

Arachidonic acid

Δ⁹-THC

N-arachidonoylethanolamine (anandamide)

HU-210

2-arachidonoylglycerol

CP55,940

FIGURE 8.15   Chemical structures of 2-arachidonoylglycerol, structural analogs, and synthetic cannabinoids.

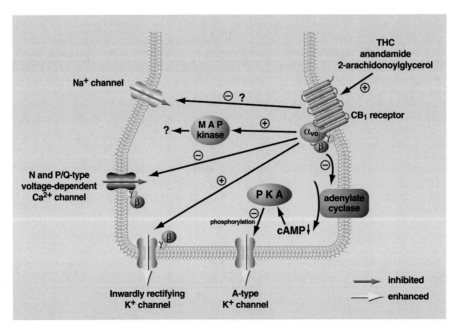

FIGURE 8.16   **Signal transduction mechanisms stimulated by CB₁ receptors in a presynaptic nerve terminal.**   *[Taken with permission from Ameri A. The effects of cannabinoids on the brain.* Progress in Neurobiology, *199, (58), 315–348.]*

by the hypothesized anandamide transport inhibitor N-(4-hydroxyphenyl)-arachidonamide (AM 404). The effects of exogenous anandamide are potentiated by AM 404, which has been shown to elevate the levels of circulating anandamide and produce behavioral effects, but it is not entirely clear that these effects are mediated by reuptake blockade. Inhibitors of anandamide amidohydrolase can also increase the levels of anandamide by blocking its breakdown. Another enzyme implicated in the function of anandamide is fatty acid amide hydrolase (FAAH), a membrane-associated hydrolase that breaks down anandamide. Genetically engineered mice that lack FAAH are unable to degrade anandamide. These mice also show an enhanced response to exogenous anandamide administration, including hypoactivity, analgesia, catalepsy, and hypothermia. In the brain, FAAH is localized in the cell body and dendritic areas of neurons that are postsynaptic to CB_1-expressing axons, suggesting that FAAH may participate in cannabinoid signaling mechanisms by inactivating locally released endocannabinoids (for further reading, see Freund et al., 2003).

Key enzymes that regulate the generation and degradation of the other major endogenous cannabinoid, 2-AG, have been elucidated. The enzyme responsible for the synthesis of 2-AG is diacylglycerol lipase α (see Figure 8.17). The deletion of diacylglycerol lipase α in mice completely eliminated cannabinoid-based neuroplasticity and negative feedback function, suggesting that 2-AG is likely the predominant neurotransmitter for currently identified roles of the endogenous cannabinoid system. The enzyme primarily responsible for the breakdown of 2-AG is monoacylglycerol lipase (MAGL), and the blockade or elimination of this enzyme using a constitutional genetic knockout approach in mice produces an accumulation of excessive 2-AG in the brain and cannabinoid receptor-mediated effects on analgesia, hypothermia, and locomotor activity. Long-term excessive 2-AG accumulation eventually leads to cannabinoid tolerance, receptor downregulation, and even physical withdrawal typically seen with THC. Using a combination of FAAH (the anandamide-metabolizing enzyme) and MAGL inhibition to elevate anandamide and 2-AG simultaneously produces mild THC-like behavioral effects in mice and fully substitutes for THC in the drug discrimination paradigm, suggesting that the two endogenous cannabinoids act on separate but interacting neuronal populations to produce cannabinoid-like effects.

Binge/Intoxication Stage

Acute Reinforcing Effects of Cannabinoids

Δ^9-THC has been shown to have acute reinforcing effects in animal studies, brain stimulation reward, conditioned place preference, and intravenous self-administration. In drug discrimination studies, rats and monkeys will discriminate Δ^9-THC (see Chapter 3). Cannabinoid receptor agonists can substitute for Δ^9-THC, and the effects of these agonists can be blocked by cannabinoid receptor antagonists. No cross substitution has been observed with a wide variety of different neuropharmacological agents, including opioids, anticonvulsants, antipsychotics, serotonergic drugs, psychostimulants, and psychedelics. Only very high doses of anandamide substitute for Δ^9-THC.

Intracranial self-stimulation thresholds are lowered by Δ^9-THC administration in rats with acute administration. This lowering of thresholds is similar to all other major drugs of abuse. Δ^9-THC produces both conditioned place aversion and preference in rodents, depending on the dose and experience of the animals. Place aversion is found with acute administration of moderate to high doses, but place preference is found at low doses and in animals with a history of pre-exposure to Δ^9-THC. The potent synthetic cannabinoid receptor agonist CP 55,940 can produce a marked place preference that is reversed by naloxone.

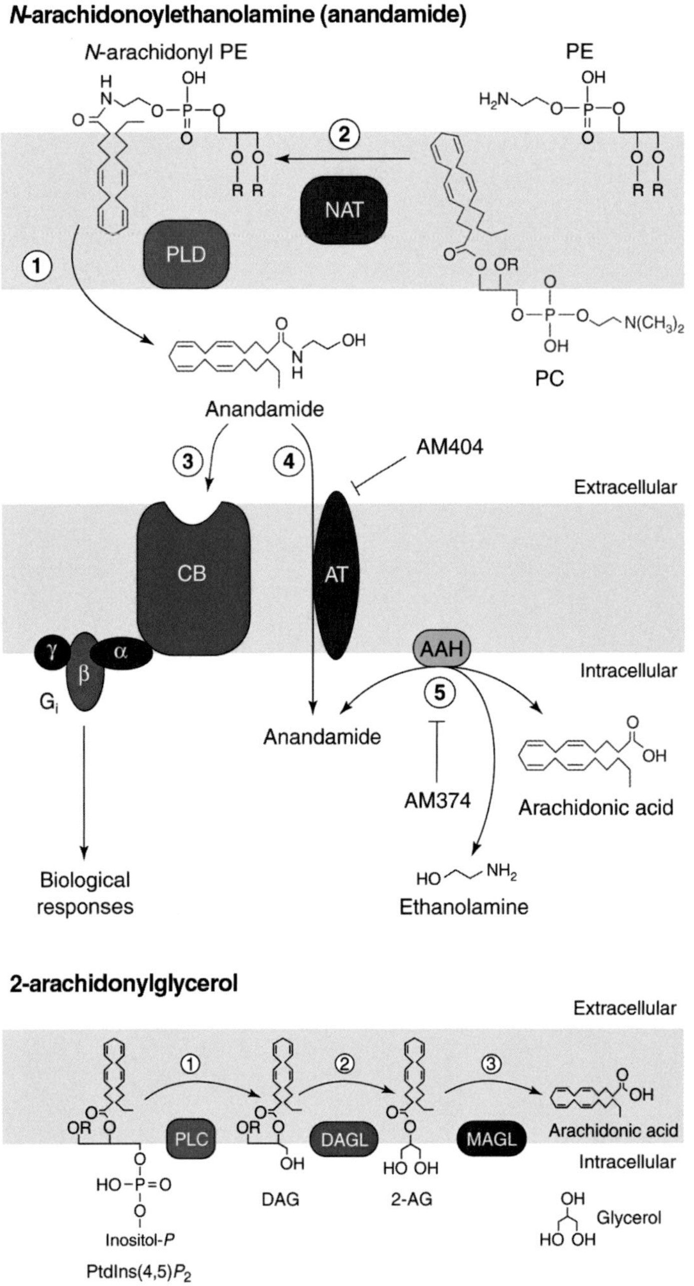

FIGURE 8.17   (Top) **Formation and inactivation of N-arachidonoylethanolamine (anandamide).** Anandamide can be generated by hydrolysis of N-arachidonoyl phosphatidylethanolamine (N-arachidonoyl PE), which is catalyzed by phospholipase D (PLD) ①. The synthesis of N-arachidonoyl PE, depleted during anandamide formation, might be mediated by N-acyl transferase activity (NAT) ②, which detaches an arachidonate moiety (red) from the sn-1 position of phospholipids such as

Early Δ^9-THC self-administration studies in animals were marked by failure. Researchers were unable to achieve reliable self-administration in laboratory animals largely because of its long duration of action and pronounced aversion, even at modest doses. The advent of synthetic cannabinoid agonists, however, allowed researchers to elicit robust intravenous and intracerebroventricular self-administration of synthetic cannabinoid agonists in mice and squirrel monkeys. Additionally, studies have reported intravenous self-administration of low doses of Δ^9-THC in mice and squirrel monkeys (Figures 8.19, 8.20). Squirrel monkeys with unlimited access to food and water were allowed a wide range of doses of Δ^9-THC (1.0–8.0 µg/kg/injection) on a fixed-ratio 10 schedule of reinforcement and showed reliable intravenous self-administration. The self-administration of Δ^9-THC and a synthetic cannabinoid was blocked by the CB_1 receptor antagonist SR141716A.

As with other drugs of abuse, the acute reinforcing effects of Δ^9-THC involve activation of the mesocorticolimbic dopamine system. Δ^9-THC selectively increases the release of dopamine in the shell of the nucleus accumbens, an effect also observed with all major drugs of abuse (Figure 8.21). Similar increases in extracellular dopamine in the nucleus accumbens have been observed with the synthetic cannabinoid receptor agonist WIN 55,212-2.

Another potential neuropharmacological mechanism for the acute reinforcing effects of Δ^9-THC is the release of endogenous opioid peptides. Intravenous Δ^9-THC self-administration and intracerebroventricular CP 55,940 self-administration are blocked by the opioid receptor antagonist naltrexone, suggesting a role for opioid peptides in the reinforcing effects of Δ^9-THC (see Figure 8.20). These studies indicate that cannabinoids increase the synthesis and release of endogenous opioid peptides, possibly by inhibiting the release of an inhibitory neurotransmitter such as γ-aminobutyric acid (GABA; see below). Both cannabinoid and opioid receptors are also colocalized on medium-spiny γ-aminobutyric acid (GABA) neurons in the nucleus accumbens. As with other drugs of abuse, the sites of action of Δ^9-THC may involve actions in the ventral tegmental area, nucleus accumbens, and possibly extended amygdala (Figure 8.22).

◀ phosphatidylcholine (PC) and transfers it to the primary amino group of PE. The membrane localizations of PLD and NAT are speculative. Newly formed anandamide can be released into the extracellular space, where it can activate G-protein-coupled cannabinoid (CB) receptors located on neighboring cells ③ or on the same cells that produce anandamide (not shown). Anandamide release in the external milieu has been demonstrated both *in vitro* and *in vivo*. Anandamide can be removed from its sites of action by carrier-mediated transport (anandamide transport, AT) ④, which can be inhibited by AM404. Transport into cells can be followed by hydrolysis catalyzed by a membrane-bound anandamide amidohydrolase (AAH, also called fatty acid amide hydrolase) ⑤, which can be inhibited by AM374. Arachidonic acid produced during the AAH reaction can be rapidly reincorporated into phospholipid and is unlikely to undergo further metabolism. *In vitro*, AAH also can act in reverse, catalyzing the formation of anandamide from arachidonic acid and ethanolamine. The physiological significance of this reaction in anandamide formation is unclear. Abbreviation R indicates a fatty acid group. (Bottom) **Formation and inactivation of 2-arachidonylglycerol (2-AG).** Hydrolysis of phosphatidylinositol(4,5)-bisphosphate [PtdIns(4,5)P₂] by phospholipase C (PLC) produces the second messengers 1,2-diacyl-glycerol (DAG) and inositol (1,4,5)-trisphosphate [Ins(1,4,5)P₃] ①. DAG serves as a substrate for DAGlipase (DAGL), which catalyzes the production of 2-AG ②. This pathway also gives rise to free arachidonic acid. 2-AG can be released into the external milieu, measured *in vitro*, allowing it to interact with cannabinoid receptors, and its effects can be terminated by uptake into cells (not shown). However, extracellular release of 2-AG has not yet been reported *in vivo*. Intracellular 2-AG can be hydrolyzed to arachidonic acid and glycerol by an uncharacterized esterase such as monoacylglycerol lipase (MAGL) ③. *[Taken with permission from Piomelli D, Giuffrida A, Calignano A, Rodriguez de Fonseca F. The endocannabinoid system as a target for therapeutic drugs. Trends in Pharmacological Sciences, 2000, (21), 218–224.]*

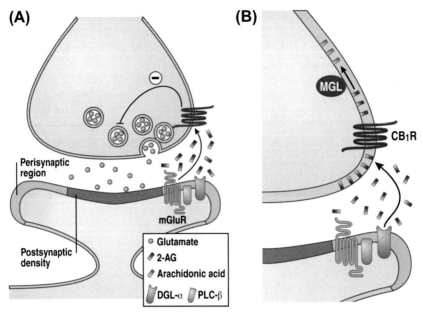

FIGURE 8.18 **Specialized lipid-signaling junctions in the brain.** (A) The endocannabinoid lipid 2arachidonoyl-*sn*-glycerol (2-AG) is thought to mediate retrograde signaling in the hippocampus, cerebellum, and other brain regions. Glutamate (blue circles) released from excitatory axon terminals activates postsynaptic type I metabotropic glutamate receptors (mGluR), stimulating 2AG production through the phospholipase C-β (PLC-β)/diacylglycerol lipase (DGL) pathway. Type 1 mGluR, PLCβ, and DGLα are localized at the perisynapse (light red), a region of the dendritic spine that borders the postsynaptic density (purple). 2AG crosses the synaptic cleft and activates presynaptic CB_1 cannabinoid receptors (CB1R), which suppress glutamate release. (B) Hypothetical model of a specialized lipid-signaling junction at hippocampal glutamate-containing synapses. Endocannabinoid-synthesizing enzymes (PLCβ and DGLα) and CB1R are positioned to optimize the transsynaptic actions of 2AG. These may be further facilitated by the ability of this lipid messenger to reach CB_1 receptors by lateral diffusion through the lipid bilayer. The cleavage of 2AG by monoacylglycerol lipase (MGL), leading to the production of arachidonic acid, might terminate the effects of this messenger. The flipping of 2AG across the bilayer, which may be rather slow, might occur either before or after the interaction of the lipid with CB_1 receptors. *[Taken with permission from Piomelli D, Astarita G, Rapaka R. A neuroscientist's guide to lipidomics.* Nature Reviews Neuroscience, *2007, (8), 743–754.]*

Neurobiological Mechanisms – Cellular and Molecular

Much work has focused on the interactions between cannabinoids and brain circuitry in the basal ganglia because of the high density of cannabinoid receptors in this region and the complex effects of cannabinoids on movement. Low doses have activating effects on movement, and high doses have inhibitory effects. CB_1 receptors are expressed by the axons of striatal GABAergic medium-spiny neurons. Cannabinoids inhibit GABA-mediated inhibitory postsynaptic potentials in the cell bodies of striatal medium-spiny neurons, possibly by decreasing presynaptic GABA release from medium-spiny axon collaterals. This ultimately could result in a disinhibitory effect by increasing the firing rate of striatal medium-spiny neurons. Similar to their actions in the basal ganglia, cannabinoids in the periaqueductal gray may inhibit presynaptic GABA release or glutamate release and may mediate the well-documented analgesic effects of cannabinoids. In the periaqueductal gray, electrical

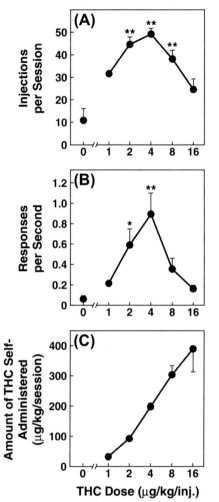

FIGURE 8.19 Δ^9-**THC dose–response curves for intravenous self-administration in squirrel monkeys with no history of exposure to other drugs** ($n = 3$). (A) Numbers of injections per session. (B) Overall rates of responding in the presence of a green light signaling Δ^9-THC availability. (C) Total Δ^9-THC intake per session. Each panel is presented as a function of the injection dose of Δ^9-THC. Each symbol represents the mean of the last three sessions under each Δ^9-THC injection dose condition and under a vehicle condition from three monkeys, with the exception of the values for the 1 µg/kg per injection dose, which represent means from two monkeys. *$p < 0.05$, **$p < 0.01$, significant differences compared with vehicle conditions. *These data show that Δ^9-THC is reinforcing in squirrel monkeys. Animals without any deprivation or history of self-administration of other drugs will learn to intravenously self-administer Δ^9-THC. The function that relates the unit dose per injection with self-administration shows an inverted U-shaped function, similar to the one seen with other intravenously self-administered drugs in the psychostimulant class. Despite the inverted U-shape function as the unit dose per injection of Δ^9-THC increased, the total amount of Δ^9-THC self-administered per session increased.* [Taken with permission from Justinova Z, Tanda G, Redhi GH, Goldberg SR. Self-administration of Δ^9-tetrahydrocannabinol (THC) by drug-naive squirrel monkeys. Psychopharmacology, 2003, (169), 135–140.]

stimulation produces cannabinoid-mediated analgesia, accompanied by a marked increase in the release of anandamide, suggesting that endogenous anandamide may contribute to this analgesic effect. Similar to the involvement of the basal ganglia in movement and periaqueductal gray in pain, the effects of cannabinoids on reward-related brain structures involve disinhibitory effects. Δ^9-THC and synthetic cannabinoids increase the neuronal firing of dopamine neurons in the ventral tegmental area, which can be blocked by CB_1 receptor antagonists. The inhibition of GABAergic inhibitory inputs to dopaminergic neurons may increase the firing rate of ventral tegmental area neurons.

CB_1 receptor knockout mouse studies have confirmed a critical role for the CB_1 receptor in the behavioral effects of cannabinoids. CB_1 knockout mice exhibit no analgesia and no locomotor activity when given Δ^9-THC. They also do not intravenously self-administer the CB_1 receptor agonist WIN 55,212–2. When these mice are chronically treated with

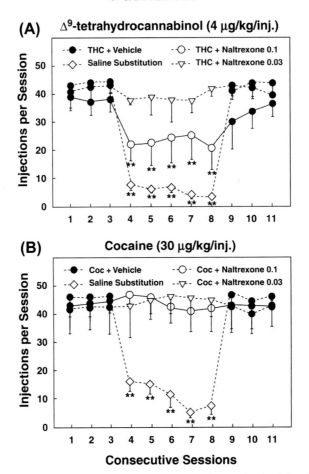

FIGURE 8.20 Effects of 0.03 and 0.1 mg/kg naltrexone on responding maintained by (A) Δ^9-THC and (B) cocaine (Coc) in monkeys over consecutive sessions and extinction of self-administration behavior by substitution of saline injections for injections of (A) Δ^9-THC or (B) cocaine. The number of injections per session during Δ^9-THC (4 µg/kg/inj) and cocaine (30 µg/kg/inj) self-administration sessions after pretreatment with vehicle (sessions 1–3 and 9–11) or naltrexone (sessions 4–8) is shown. The number of injections per session during self-administration sessions when saline was substituted for Δ^9-THC or cocaine (sessions 4–8) is also shown. The data represent the mean number of injections per session from four (Δ^9-THC) and three (cocaine) monkeys. **$p < 0.01$, compared with the last Δ^9-THC session before naltrexone pretreatment or saline substitution (session 3). *These data show that low doses of naltrexone blunt intravenous Δ^9-THC self-administration in squirrel monkeys but do not block intravenous cocaine self-administration, suggesting that the release of opioid peptides in the brain contributes to the reinforcing effects of Δ^9-THC. [Taken with permission from Justinova Z, Tanda G, Munzar P, Goldberg SR. The opioid antagonist naltrexone reduces the reinforcing effects of Δ^9-tetrahydrocannabinol (THC) in squirrel monkeys. Psychopharmacology, 2004, (173), 186–194.]*

Δ^9-THC, they present no cannabinoid withdrawal when administered a CB_1 receptor antagonist (Figure 8.23). Other studies have found that anandamide and some synthetic cannabinoids retain their activity in CB_1 knockout mice, suggesting that anandamide may act on other receptors aside from CB_1 and CB_2. One hypothesis is that the effects of anandamide may be mediated by the vanilloid receptor. The vanilloid receptor is a prominent member of the transient receptor potential vanilloid-1 ion channel family. This receptor

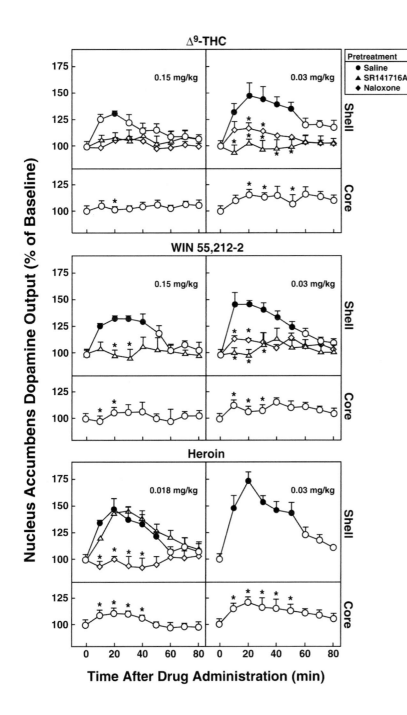

FIGURE 8.21 **Effect of intravenous Δ⁹-THC, WIN 55,212–2, and heroin on dialysate dopamine in the shell (upper panels) and core (lower panels) of the nucleus accumbens.** Rats were pretreated with saline (circles), the CB₁ receptor antagonist SR141716A (triangles; 1 mg/kg, s.c.), or the opioid receptor antagonist naloxone (diamonds; 0.1 mg/kg, i.p.). Solid symbols: $p < 0.05$ compared to baseline values. *$p < 0.05$, compared with corresponding value obtained in the shell of saline-pretreated controls. *These data show that Δ⁹-THC, a synthetic cannabinoid, and heroin all preferentially increase the release of dopamine in the nucleus accumbens shell measured by in vivo microdialysis. The cannabinoid CB₁ receptor antagonist SR141716 and opioid receptor antagonist naloxone blocked the cannabinoid-induced increase in the release of dopamine, suggesting a role for endogenous opioid peptides in the dopamine-releasing effects of cannabinoids. [Taken with permission from Tanda G, Pontieri FE, Di Chiara G. Cannabinoid and heroin activation of mesolimbic dopamine transmission by a common μ¹ opioid receptor mechanism. Science, 1997, (276), 2048–2050.]*

Neurochemical Neurocircuits in Drug Reward Cannabinoids

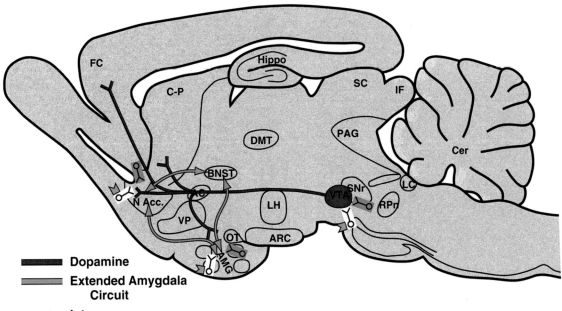

Dopamine

Extended Amygdala Circuit

o—< **Interneurons**

o—■< **Opioid Peptides**

M **Cannabinoid Receptors**

FIGURE 8.22   **Sagittal section through a rodent brain that illustrates the pathways and receptor systems implicated in the acute reinforcing actions of cannabinoids.**   Cannabinoids activate cannabinoid CB_1 receptors in the ventral tegmental area, nucleus accumbens, and amygdala via direct actions on interneurons. Cannabinoids facilitate the release of dopamine in the nucleus accumbens via an action either in the ventral tegmental area or nucleus accumbens but are also hypothesized to activate elements independent of the dopamine system. Endogenous cannabinoids may interact with postsynaptic elements in the nucleus accumbens that involve dopamine and opioid peptide systems. The blue arrows represent the interactions within the extended amygdala system. AC, anterior commissure; AMG, amygdala; ARC, arcuate nucleus; BNST, bed nucleus of the stria terminalis; Cer, cerebellum; C-P, caudate putamen; DMT, dorsomedial thalamus; FC, frontal cortex; Hippo, hippocampus; IF, inferior colliculus; LC, locus coeruleus; LH, lateral hypothalamus; N Acc., nucleus accumbens; OT, olfactory tract; PAG, periaqueductal gray; RPn, reticular pontine nucleus; SC, superior colliculus; SNr, substantia nigra pars reticulata; VP, ventral pallidum; VTA, ventral tegmental area. *[Taken with permission from Koob GF, Le Moal M. Neurobiology of Addiction. Academic Press, London, 2006.]*

can be activated by anandamide at concentrations 10 to 20 times higher than those that activate the CB_1 receptor.

Supporting the pharmacological studies with cannabinoid receptor antagonists, CB_1 knockout mouse studies have shown significant interactions between the reinforcing and dependence-producing effects of opioids and the cannabinoid system. Morphine-induced conditioned place preference, intravenous morphine self-administration, and morphine-induced dopamine release in the nucleus accumbens are all eliminated in CB_1 knockout mice. Δ^9-THC-induced conditioned place

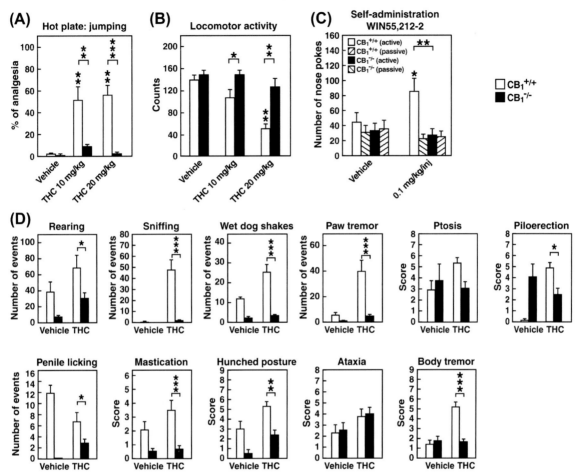

FIGURE 8.23 **Central effects of cannabinoids in mice with (+/+) and without (−/−) CB$_1$ receptors.** An intraperitoneal injection of Δ^9-THC (or vehicle alone) was given 20 min before the measurements. (A) Latency of escape jumping in the hot-plate test. (B) Spontaneous locomotor activity (number of photocell counts within 10 min). (C) Self-administration of the CB$_1$ receptor agonist WIN 55,212–2. (D) Δ^9-THC withdrawal signs. *These data show that constitutive knockout of the cannabinoid CB$_1$ receptor (animals born without a CB$_1$ receptor) block the analgesic, locomotor-activating, reinforcing, and dependence-inducing effects of cannabinoids. [Taken with permission from Ledent C, Valverde O, Cossu G, Petitet F, Aubert JF, Beslot F, Bohme GA, Imperato A, Pedrazzini T, Roques BP, Vassart G, Fratta W, Parmentier M. Unresponsiveness to cannabinoids and reduced addictive effects of opiates in CB^1 receptor knockout mice. Science, 1999, (283), 401–404.]*

preference is blocked in μ opioid receptor knockout mice, and Δ^9-THC-induced conditioned place aversions are blocked in κ opioid receptor knockout mice. However, such cross-talk between the opioid and cannabinoid systems does not extend to measures of analgesia. Opioid-induced antinociception is not modified in CB$_1$ knockout mice, and the antinociception produced by Δ^9-THC is not modified in opioid knockout mice. Knockout studies have provided additional evidence that cannabinoid systems are involved in the reinforcing actions of other drugs of abuse, including alcohol and nicotine.

The role of endogenous cannabinoid systems in drug dependence in general is supported by opioid-cannabinoid interactions. Administration of the CB_1 receptor antagonist SR141716A blocked morphine self-administration in mice and heroin self-administration in rats. Acute administration of SR141716A blocked the expression of morphine-induced conditioned place preference.

Withdrawal/Negative Affect Stage

Neurobiological Mechanisms of Tolerance

Chronic treatment with Δ^9-THC in rodents results in tolerance to its acute behavioral effects, such as analgesia, motor inhibition, and the memory-disruptive effects of cannabis. Such tolerance depends on the dose, duration of treatment, species, and dependent variable measured. For example, tolerance to antinociception and motor inhibition occurs with 3–7 days of treatment, but tolerance to the memory-impairing effects can take weeks. There is significant consensus that the mechanism of such tolerance is pharmacodynamic and not pharmacokinetic (see Chapter 2 for definitions). Biochemical measures show that chronic exposure to Δ^9-THC produces time-dependent and region-specific downregulation and desensitization of brain cannabinoid receptors, as measured by receptor binding and cannabinoid-induced GTPγS binding. GTPγS is guanine 5'-O-[γ-thio]triphosphate, a G-protein-activating analog of guanosine triphosphate used in G-protein binding studies. These effects were most pronounced in the hippocampus and less dramatic in the basal ganglia. Such receptor-mediated changes could at least partially account for the different time courses and degrees of tolerance to the behavioral effects of repeated cannabis administration. Similar downregulation of brain cannabinoid CB_1 receptors was observed in human subjects who chronically smoked cannabis, measured with positron emission tomography. The downregulation correlated with the number of years of cannabis smoking and was selective to cortical brain regions. CB_1 receptor density returned to normal levels after approximately 4 weeks of continuously monitored abstinence from cannabis in a secure research unit (for further reading, see Hirvonen et al., 2012).

Neurobiological Mechanisms of Withdrawal

In preclinical animal studies, cannabinoid withdrawal syndromes have been described in both rats and mice. Although some somatic signs have been observed during spontaneous withdrawal from cannabinoids, most studies have precipitated withdrawal using a CB_1 antagonist (see Chapter 3 for a description of precipitated drug withdrawal). The most characteristic somatic signs of withdrawal in rodents include a combination of the withdrawal signs observed in opioid and sedative-hypnotic (alcohol) withdrawal. In rats, these various somatic withdrawal signs include wet-dog shakes (this is exactly what it sounds like), scratching, facial rubbing, ptosis, mastication, hunched posture, and ataxia. In mice exposed to chronic Δ^9-THC administration, administration of the CB_1 receptor antagonist SR14716A produced a robust withdrawal syndrome. The withdrawal signs in mice include wet-dog shakes, facial rubbing, ptosis, hunched posture, front paw tremor, piloerection, and ataxia (these signs are also common in opioid withdrawal).

Precipitated cannabinoid withdrawal also has some motivational characteristics. Precipitated Δ^9-THC withdrawal causes anxiety-like effects in animal models of anxiety. Spontaneous withdrawal from an acute injection of Δ^9-THC can produce an elevation in brain reward thresholds (Figure 8.24). Administration of the CB_1 receptor antagonist SR141716A in rats that received long-term cannabinoid agonist treatment (HU-210) resulted in anxiety-like responses in the defensive withdrawal test, in which the time that elapsed to exit a small enclosure and enter a larger space is measured in rodents. Notably, however, acute Δ^9-THC administration itself can be considered

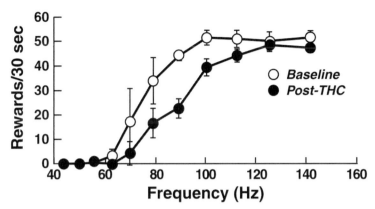

FIGURE 8.24 **Diminished brain stimu-lation reward (elevated reward thresh-olds) during withdrawal from an acute 1.0 mg/kg dose of Δ^9-THC in rats.** With-drawal from Δ^9-THC significantly shifted the reward function to the right. *These data show that acute withdrawal from THC can also produce "dysphoric-like" responses in animals measured by brain stimulation reward. Notice this is a rate-frequency measure of reward thresholds (see* Chapter 3). *[Taken with permission from Gardner EL, Vorel SR. Cannabinoid transmission and reward-related events.* Neu-robiology of Disease, *1998, (5), 502–533.]*

aversive in rodents, reflected by acute canna-binoid-induced conditioned place aversions at moderate to high doses.

Neurobiological mechanisms that may be involved in the motivational withdrawal syndrome include decreased activity in the mesocorticolimbic dopamine system and activation of brain corticotropin-releasing factor (CRF) systems in the extended amyg-dala. Precipitated withdrawal from chronic cannabinoids decreases the firing of ventral tegmental dopamine neurons and decreases extracellular dopamine levels in the nucleus accumbens (Figure 8.25). Precipitated with-drawal increases extracellular levels of CRF in the central nucleus of the amygdala, and the anxiogenic-like effects of precipitated Δ^9-THC withdrawal are blocked by a CRF receptor antagonist (Figure 8.26).

The CB_1 receptor antagonist SR141716A can precipitate both somatic and motivational opioid withdrawal in morphine-dependent rats. Naloxone-precipitated opioid withdrawal is also decreased in CB_1 knockout mice. The cannabinoid withdrawal syndrome is also decreased in μ opioid receptor knockout mice and preproenkephalin knockout mice. This interaction is also bidirectional, in which the opioid antagonist naloxone induces partial cannabinoid withdrawal in rats treated chroni-cally with the synthetic CB_1 agonist HU-210 (Figure 8.27). This appears to be an interac-tion with μ opioid receptors. μ Opioid receptor

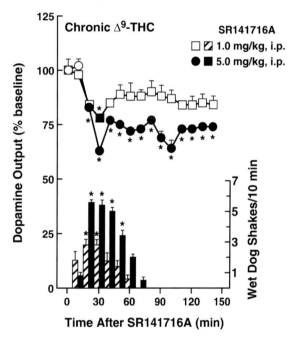

FIGURE 8.25 **Time course of the effects of administra-tion of the CB_1 cannabinoid receptor antagonist SR141716A on dopamine output in dialysate samples from the nucleus accumbens shell and wet-dog shakes in rats chronically treated with Δ^9-THC.** The bars represent the number of wet-dog shakes observed every 10 min after SR141716A adminis-tration. *$p < 0.05$, compared with the corresponding time point in chronic saline-injected rats challenged with SR141716A. *These data show that precipitated withdrawal from chronic Δ^9-THC decreased the release of dopamine in the nucleus accumbens measured by in vivo microdialysis. This is similar to the effects seen with withdrawal from all drugs of abuse and represents a common element of drug dependence (see* Chapters 1 and 2). *[Taken with permission from Tanda G, Loddo P, Di Chiara G, Dependence of mesolimbic dopamine transmission on delta9-tetrahydrocannabi-nol,* European Journal of Pharmacology, *1999, (376), 23–26.].*

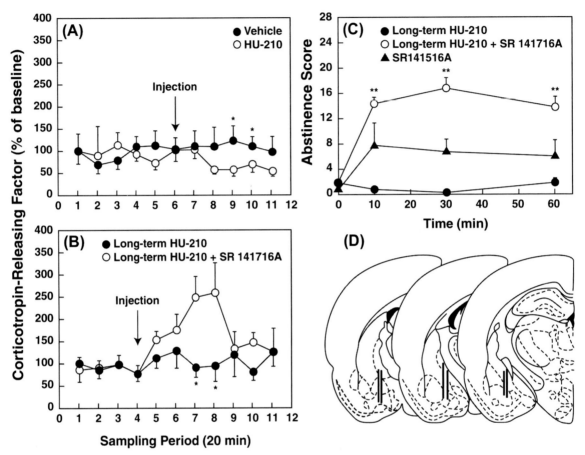

FIGURE 8.26 (A) Effects of a single injection of the cannabinoid receptor agonist HU-210 (100 mg/kg) in rats on cor-
ticotropin-releasing factor (CRF) release from the central nucleus of the amygdala. HU-210 lowered CRF release. Vehicle
injections did not alter CRF release. Administration of the CB_1 receptor antagonist SR141716A did not modify CRF release.
(B) Effects of SR141716A (3 mg/kg) on CRF release from the central nucleus of the amygdala in animals pretreated with
HU-210 (100 mg/kg) for 14 days. Cannabinoid withdrawal induced by SR141716A was associated with increased CRF release.
Vehicle injections did not alter CRF release. (C) Mean of summed cannabinoid withdrawal scores 0, 10, 30, and 60 min after
SR141716A injection in rats treated with HU-210 or its vehicle for 14 days. SR141716A induced a mild behavioral syndrome in
drug-naive rats that received long-term pretreatment with vehicle (SR141716A) and a clear withdrawal syndrome in animals
pretreated with HU-210 (long-term HU-210 + SR141716A). Rats pretreated with the cannabinoid (long-term HU-210) that
received vehicle on the test day did not exhibit withdrawal signs. Drug-naive control animals that received vehicle injections
were indistinguishable from the long-term HU-210 treatment group, and cannabinoid-naive rats did not exhibit observable changes in behavior after a single injection of HU-210. (D) Anatomical location of the microdialysis probes in animals
subjected to SR141716A-induced cannabinoid withdrawal. *These data show an increase in CRF release in the central nucleus of
the amygdala during precipitated withdrawal measured by in vivo microdialysis. Notice that the increase in CRF release in the central
nucleus of the amygdala represents another common element of drug dependence (see Chapters 1 and 2). [Taken with permission from
Rodriguez de Fonseca F, Carrera MRA, Navarro M, Koob GF, Weiss F. Activation of corticotropin-releasing factor in the limbic system
during cannabinoid withdrawal. Science, 1997, (276), 2050–2054.]*

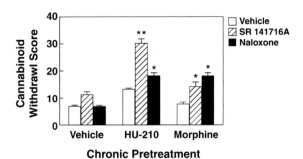

FIGURE 8.27 Naloxone administration (1 mg/kg, i.p.) induced a partial cannabinoid withdrawal syndrome in male rats chronically exposed to either the cannabinoid receptor agonist HU-210 (100 μg/kg for 14 days) or morphine (two 75 mg morphine pellets implanted subcutaneously for 72 h). The CB_1 receptor antagonist SR141716A (3 mg/kg) induced a partial cannabinoid withdrawal syndrome in morphine-dependent animals. *$p<0.05$, **$p<0.01$, significant differences from saline-treated animals ($n = 9 - 15$ per group). *[Taken with permission from Navarro M, Carrera MRA, Fratta W, Valverde O, Cossu G, Fattore L, Chowen JA, Gomez R, Del Arco I, Villanua MA, Maldonado R, Koob GF, Rodriguez de Fonseca F. Functional interaction between opioid and cannabinoid receptors in drug self-administration.* Journal of Neuroscience, *2001, 21: 5344-5350.] These data show that caanabinoid withdrawal can be precipitated by opioid receptor antagonists in cannabinoid-dependent rats, and opioid withdrawal can be precipitated by cannabinoid receptor antagonists in opioid-dependent rats. These results suggest some "cross-talk" in the neuro-adaptations between the endogenous cannabinoid and endogenous opioid peptide systems during the chronic activation of their respective receptors.*

knockout mice chronically treated with Δ^9-THC also show blunted Δ^9-THC-precipitated withdrawal. In summary, endogenous opioid peptides derived from preproenkephalin appear to be important for the Δ^9-THC withdrawal syndrome, and a certain level of endogenous cannabinoid tone appears to contribute to opioid dependence.

Preoccupation/Anticipation Stage

Neurobiological Mechanisms – Cellular and Molecular

As described in the other chapters and Chapter 3, animal models of reinstatement have been used to support hypotheses about the neural substrates of relapse. Treatments that trigger the reinstatement of drug seeking can indicate the likely neural substrates of "craving." Little work has been done with cannabinoids in the reinstatement model. One study involved rats previously trained to intravenously self-administer the synthetic cannabinoid receptor agonist WIN 55,212–2 under a fixed-ratio 1 schedule of reinforcement and

found that intraperitoneal priming injections of a previously self-administered CB_1 receptor agonist reinstated cannabinoid-seeking behavior following extinction. Cues paired with WIN 55,212–2 self-administration can also reinstate cannabinoid seeking. The selective CB_1 receptor antagonist SR 141716A completely prevented cannabinoid-seeking behavior triggered by WIN 55,212–2, but this antagonist did not reinstate responding when administered alone. The opioid receptor agonist heroin facilitates cannabinoid-seeking behavior, and the opioid receptor antagonist naloxone blocks the cannabinoid-induced reinstatement of cannabinoid-seeking behavior. Such results suggest an endogenous opioid contribution to cannabinoid reinstatement.

Cannabinoids can produce reinstatement of drug seeking for other drugs of abuse. Systemic injections of cannabinoids can reinstate cocaine, alcohol, nicotine, and heroin seeking. A CB_1 receptor antagonist blocks the reinstatement of drug seeking in response to cocaine and cocaine-associated cues, nicotine, alcohol, and heroin.

SUMMARY

Marijuana is a dry, shredded green or brown mixture of flowers, stems, seeds and leaves of the hemp plant *Cannabis*. Cannabinoids were originally defined as the phytocannabinoids contained in *Cannabis*. As with opiates, later definitions were more inclusive, defining cannabinoids as "all ligands of the cannabinoid receptor and related compounds including endogenous ligands of the receptors and a large number of synthetic cannabinoid analogs" (Grotenhermen F. Pharmacokinetics and pharmacodynamics of cannabinoids. *Clinical Pharmacokinetics*, 2003, (42), 327–360.).

Preparations of marijuana have a rich history in terms of medical use and myth. The fiber of the plant is used for rope, and the psychoactive varieties of the plant are used for both their medicinal and intoxicating effects. Marijuana contains more than 60 different cannabinoids, but the primary active ingredient is Δ^9-THC. Cannabinoids have two accepted medical uses in the United States. Dronabinol (Marinol; the pure isomer of Δ^9-THC) and nabilone (Cesamet; a synthetic analog of THC) are approved for use in refractory nausea and vomiting associated with cancer chemotherapy and appetite loss in HIV/AIDS patients with anorexia. Many potential medical uses of cannabis preparations are being considered in the United States, including the amelioration of spasticity caused by spinal cord injury and multiple sclerosis, analgesia treatment for asthma, the treatment of glaucoma, and use in the treatment of movement disorders, including dystonias, dyskinesias, and tardive dyskinesia.

Marijuana is also the most commonly used illicit drug in the United States. It produces intoxicating effects when ingested, usually by inhalation, including euphoria and mood swings characterized by initial feelings of "happiness" or sudden talkativeness, a dreaming or lolling state, and general activation and hyperactivity. Higher doses are associated with psychedelic-like effects, such as an increased sensitivity to sound and a keener appreciation of rhythm and timing. The perception of time is often slowed, with an exaggeration of the sense of time. Perceptions of space may be broadened, and near objects may appear distant. Intoxication is commonly associated with visual "hallucination-like" effects that are mostly illusionary transformations of the outer world.

Following ingestion, Δ^9-THC has a peculiar distribution in the body, initially sequestering in vascularized tissue and later in fat-rich tissues. It has a long terminal half-life of approximately 30 h, but its metabolites can be measured in urine for weeks after ingestion. The pathological effects of intoxication or chronic high-dose use include an impaired ability to drive while intoxicated, cardiovascular risks for people with pre-existing cardiac problems, anxiety, panic reactions, impairment in executive function, impairment in the development of executive function, exacerbation of schizophrenic-like symptoms in individuals who are vulnerable to schizophrenia (with some evidence that Δ^9-THC can precipitate schizophrenic-like syndromes), and a possible causal role in the vulnerability to schizophrenia. Marijuana smoke may also have the same potential toxicity as cigarette smoke with regard to lung function.

Marijuana produces a substance use disorder (DSM-5 criteria) or Substance Dependence (DSM-IV criteria) with many characteristics similar to other drugs of abuse. Tolerance develops to the intoxicating and physiological effects, and a withdrawal syndrome has been defined in both humans and animals. In humans, the most common symptoms associated with cannabis withdrawal are decreased appetite and weight loss, irritability, nervousness, anxiety, anger, aggression, restlessness, and sleep disturbances. Most of the DSM-IV criteria for Substance Use Disorder were met by individuals diagnosed with Substance Dependence on cannabis. Preoccupation with obtaining and using marijuana is represented by the persistent presence of marijuana in the individual's daily living and choices of activities. Compulsivity is represented by continued use despite marijuana-related consequences. Relapse or the propensity to relapse is reflected by a return to marijuana use after a period of abstinence and may provide confirmation of the suspected diagnosis.

The behavioral mechanism of action of cannabinoids is hypothesized to include perceptual disinhibition of both external and internal cues or states without motivational disinhibition. This perceptual disinhibition can be pleasant or unpleasant depending on internal and external contexts. The discovery of cannabinoid CB_1 and CB_2 receptors and high-potency ligands in the brain led to the identification of anandamide and 2-AG. These endocannabinoids act as retrograde neuromodulators in the central nervous system and regulate brain excitability through local actions on presynaptic GABA and glutamate neurons. In animals, Δ^9-THC and other cannabinoids have reinforcing properties in models of brain stimulation reward, conditioned place preference, and self-administration. The acute reinforcing effects of cannabinoids involve the mesocorticolimbic dopamine and opioid peptide systems in the ventral tegmental area and basal forebrain. Similarly to alcohol and opioids, the disinhibition of specific GABAergic and glutamatergic systems may facilitate the activation of reward neurotransmitters associated with the acute reinforcing effects of cannabinoids.

Genetic studies have shown that knockout of the CB_1 receptor blocks the acute reinforcing and dependence-inducing effects of cannabinoids and blunts some of the effects of opioids, suggesting cross-talk between the opioid and cannabinoid systems. Cannabinoids that act through the CB_1 receptor inhibit adenylate cyclase, which in turn inhibits phosphokinase A, leading to the activation of inwardly rectifying potassium channels and inhibition of P/Q-type voltage-dependent calcium channels. This combined inhibition leads to a presynaptic action at all levels of the brain motivational systems.

In the *withdrawal/negative affect* stage of the addiction cycle, tolerance is observed in animals, and both somatic and motivational withdrawal syndromes have been observed. Decreases in mesocorticolimbic dopamine activity are associated with the motivational effects of cannabinoid withdrawal. Acute withdrawal from cannabinoids is associated with CRF activation in the extended amygdala, similar to other drugs of abuse.

In the *preoccupation/anticipation* stage, there are limited preclinical data, but cannabinoids can elicit drug-primed reinstatement in relapse models, not only for cannabinoids, but also for other drugs of abuse. This reinstatement can be blocked by CB_1 receptor antagonists and opioid receptor antagonists.

The explosion of research in the cannabinoid field will most certainly provide further insights into the neurobiology of cannabinoid addiction and the role of the endogenous cannabinoids in normal adaptive function.

Suggested Reading

Asbridge, M., Hayden, J.A., Cartwright, J.L., 2012. Acute cannabis consumption and motor vehicle collision risk: systematic review of observational studies and meta-analysis. British Medical Journal 344, e536.

Bergamaschi, M.M., Crippa, J.A., 2013. Why should cannabis be considered doping in sports? Frontiers in Psychiatry 4, 32.

Fergusson, D.M., Boden, J.M., Horwood, L.J., 2006. Cannabis use and other illicit drug use: testing the cannabis gateway hypothesis. Addiction 101, 556–569.

Freund, T.F., Katona, I., Piomelli, D., 2003. Role of endogenous cannabinoids in synaptic signaling. Physiol. Rev. 83, 1017–1066.

Frytak, S., Moertel, C.G., Rubin, J., 1984. Metabolic studies of delta-9-tetrahydrocannabinol in cancer patients. Cancer Treatment Reports 68, 1427–1431.

Haney, M., Bisaga, A., Foltin, R.W., 2003. Interaction between naltrexone and oral THC in heavy marijuana smokers. Psychopharmacology 166, 77–85.

Hirvonen, J., Goodwin, R.S., Li, C.T., Terry, G.E., Zoghbi, S.S., Morse, C., Pike, V.W., Volkow, N.D., Huestis, M.A., Innis, R.B., 2012. Reversible and regionally selective down-regulation of brain cannabinoid CB1 receptors in chronic daily cannabis smokers. Mol. Psychiatry. 17, 642–649.

Huestis, M.A., Henningfield, J.E., Cone, E.J., 1992. Blood cannabinoids: I: Absorption of THC and formation of 11-OH-THC and THCCOOH during and after smoking marijuana. J. Analyt. Toxicol. 16, 276–282.

Kandel, D.B., 1975. Stages in adolescent involvement in drug use. Science 190, 912–914.

Li, H.L., 1974b. An archaeological and historical account of cannabis in China. Economic Botany 28, 437–448.

Li, H.L., 1974a. The origin and use of cannabis in Eastern Asia: linguistic-cultural implications. Economic Botany 28, 293–301.

McGlothlin, W.H., West, L.J., 1968. The marihuana problem: an overview. Am. J. Psychiatry. 125, 126–134.

McGrath, J., Welham, J., Scott, J., Varghese, D., Degenhardt, L., Hayatbakhsh, M.R., Alati, R., Williams, G.M., Bor, W., Najman, J.M., 2010. Association between cannabis use and psychosis-related outcomes using sibling pair analysis in a cohort of young adults. Arch. Gen. Psychiatry. 67, 440–447.

Musshoff, F., Madea, B., Kernbach-Wighton, G., Bicker, W., Kneisel, S., Hutter, M., Auwärter, V., 2013. Driving under the influence of synthetic cannabinoids ("Spice"): a case series. Int. J. Legal. Med. 128, 59–64.

Ohlsson, A., Lindgren, J.E., Wahlen, A., Agurell, S., Hollister, L.E., Gillespie, H.K., 1980. Plasma delta-9 tetrahydrocannabinol concentrations and clinical effects after oral and intravenous administration and smoking. Clin. Pharmacol. Therapeut. 28, 409–416.

Seely, K.A., Lapoint, J., Moran, J.H., Fattore, L., 2012. Spice drugs are more than harmless herbal blends: a review of the pharmacology and toxicology of synthetic cannabinoids. Prog. Neuropsychopharmacol. Biol. Psychiatry. 39, 234–243.

Stott, C.G., White, L., Wright, S., Wilbraham, D., Guy, G.W., 2013. A phase I study to assess the single and multiple dose pharmacokinetics of THC/CBD oromucosal spray. Eur. J. Clin. Pharmacol. 69, 1135–1147.

Timpone, J.G., Wright, D.J., Li, N., Egorin, M.J., Enama, M.E., Mayers, J., Galetto, G., 1997. The safety and pharmacokinetics of single-agent and combination therapy with megestrol acetate and dronabinol for the treatment of HIV wasting syndrome. AIDS Research and Human Retroviruses 13, 305–315.

Medications for the Treatment of Addiction – A Neurobiological Perspective

CONCEPTUAL APPROACH FOR UNDERSTANDING CURRENT AND FUTURE MEDICATIONS DEVELOPMENT

As noted in Chapter 1, an important goal of current neurobiological research is to understand the molecular, neuropharmacological, and neurocircuitry changes that mediate the transition from occasional, controlled drug use to the loss of behavioral control over drug seeking and drug taking that defines chronic addiction. The hypothesis elaborated here is that a combination of validated animal models of addiction, neurobiological targets derived from such models, and the translation to and from the clinical domain provide a framework for developing pharmacotherapeutics for addiction. The existing treatments for addiction that are applied to existing animal models and human laboratory models can provide an evolving Rosetta Stone to accelerate the translation of future novel targets to medications for the treatment of addiction (Box 9.1, Figure 9.1; for further reading, see Koob et al., 2009).

A key element of this approach is to prevent rigidity in the process such that animal models predict only what they have already created. Several points of the Rosetta Stone approach speak to this issue. First, as noted in Chapter 3, no single animal or human laboratory model exists for all aspects of addiction. Instead, the models emulate different *components* of addiction, some of which are still evolving. Second, the process of validation is perceived as dynamic, with changes being discovered and implemented at both ends. New targets from neurobiology will feed forward through the system, and new medications will feed backward through the system, regardless of whether these medications are derived from the feed-forward process (e.g., naltrexone, acamprosate, varenicline), clinical experience (e.g., gabapentin), or serendipity. Third, using face validity of symptoms or components of the addiction cycle, new animal and human laboratory models are regularly coming online from basic research (for example, the animal model of compulsivity/drug seeking in the context of aversive consequences or the human model of imaging in the context of cue-induced imagery). Notably, to accomplish the iterative process described above, the procedures must be initiated to make the drug available for human administration. This requires a series of steps known as the four phases of clinical trials (Box 9.2). To initiate human studies for efficacy, Phase I trials must be completed. Human laboratory

---

BOX 9.1

WHAT IS THE ROSETTA STONE?

The Rosetta Stone is an ancient Egyptian stone tablet inscribed with a decree issued at Memphis in 196 B.C. on behalf of King Ptolemy V. The tablet was found in 1799 near Rashîd in Egypt by a French soldier, Pierre-François Bouchard, a member of the French expedition to Egypt led by Napoleon. The decree is repeated in three scripts of three different languages: Ancient Egyptian hieroglyphs, Demotic script, and Ancient Greek. Thus, this tablet provided the key to the modern understanding of Egyptian hieroglyphs by translating the Greek. The British defeated the French in 1801, and the stone was delivered to the British Museum in 1802 where it can be observed today. For the present chapter, the argument is that the actions of medications that are known to be effective in treating alcoholism will be tested on animal models to validate the animal models or provide reverse translation, similar to how the Rosetta Stone provided a translation for hieroglyphics.

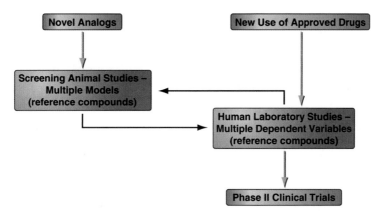

FIGURE 9.1   **A critical aspect of the present hypothesis is the proposed dynamic feedback from the animal model and clinical components not only to provide converging evidence for identification of treatments for drug addiction likely to succeed in clinical trials, but also to facilitate further development of animal and human models.** These data ultimately may provide a rational basis for combination therapies such that multiple components of the addiction cycle can be treated by a given pharmacological strategy. *[Taken with permission from Koob GF, Lloyd GK, Mason BJ. Development of pharmacotherapies for drug addiction: a Rosetta Stone approach.* Nature *Reviews Drug Discovery, 2009, (8), 500–515.]*

BOX 9.2

PHASES OF CLINICAL TRIALS

A *clinical trial* can be defined as "a prospective study comparing the effect and value of intervention(s) against a control in human beings" (Friedman LM, Furberg CD, DeMets DL. *Fundamentals of Clinical Trials*, Springer, New York, 2010). A *prospective study* means that subjects will be followed forward in time, although they may be followed from different starting points. Each subject is enrolled at their own starting date and followed for a specified duration of time. All clinical trials include intervention and control groups to which the intervention is compared. Often this is a placebo group. If the subjects are randomly assigned to groups and the investigators do not know which subjects received which treatment, then this is considered a randomized, double-blind, placebo-controlled trial. There are four phases of pharmaceutical clinical trials:

Phase I: Largely pharmacological studies, examination of drug tolerance, metabolism, drug interactions, pharmacokinetics, and maximum tolerated dose.

Phase II: Therapeutic efficacy studies, examination of different doses and measures of outcome.

Phase III: Therapeutic confirmation studies, demonstration of clinical use and safety profile.

Phase IV: Therapeutic use studies, examination of broad and special populations, and identification of uncommon adverse events.

studies for proof-of-principle (or proof-of-concept) require an approved Investigational New Drug (IND) application from the US Food and Drug Administration (Box 9.3). Human laboratory studies are considered Phase IIa studies.

Stages of the Addiction Cycle – Animal Models

The three stages of addiction conceptualized in Chapter 1 – *binge/intoxication, withdrawal/negative affect*, and *preoccupation/anticipation* – also have value for understanding the medications currently used in the treatment of addiction and in developing future medications (Figures 9.2–9.4). The different animal models that are used to study the neurobiology of addiction can be superimposed on these three stages, which are conceptualized as feeding into each other, becoming more intense, and ultimately leading to the pathological state known as addiction. Animal models for medications development for the *binge/intoxication* stage of the addiction cycle incorporate the construct of drug reinforcement and include drug and alcohol self-administration (Table 9.1). For the *withdrawal/negative affect* stage, animal models exist for the somatic signs of withdrawal for virtually all drugs of abuse. However, more relevant for addiction are the animal models of components of the motivational signs of withdrawal and the negative reinforcing

---

BOX 9.3

INVESTIGATIONAL NEW DRUG APPLICATION

Several aspects of an Investigational New Drug (IND) application are unique for drugs being developed for the treatment of addiction. One unique aspect is that the pharmaceutical industry is likely to have other indications for a drug that may be of significant value to addiction. Such a situation has both advantages and disadvantages. The disadvantage is obvious – addiction trials could be seen as counterproductive to the main commercial goal and thus be delayed or eliminated from development. Nevertheless, a reliable mechanism for generating INDs is to have an investigator initiate an IND application on a drug that already has another indication. Approval for studies on addiction is relatively straightforward if the drug is approved for other indications as long as the dose range required for addiction treatment is the same as that for the approved medication. This process will also work for drugs approved outside of the United States. A key element and critical point for medication development is submitting an IND application to the US FDA (Food and Drug Administration) (or its equivalent in other countries) so that the drug can be tested in humans. The International Commission on Harmonization (ICH) developed strict regulations and requirements that have been mandated by the FDA for the testing of a substance (drug) for a previously unapproved therapeutic indication by an investigator. ICH guidelines have also been incorporated by regulatory agencies in most other countries, resulting in a high degree of consistency in the requirements for chemistry, manufacturing, control, safety, and toxicology prior to testing the drug in humans. In the US, the application for the initial clinical testing of a compound by an individual is governed by the sponsor-investigator submission of an IND application. The data that must be supplied, in addition to the proposed clinical trial protocol and information on the investigators, include detailed information about the chemistry (i.e., synthesis, formulation, stability), toxicology, pharmacology, and prior human studies.

Existing and Future Medications for Addiction:
Binge/Intoxication Stage

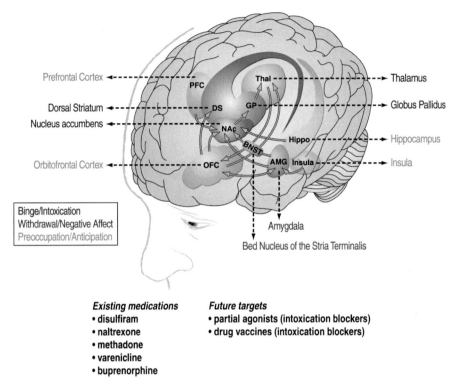

FIGURE 9.2 **Neural circuitry associated with the binge/intoxication stage of the addiction cycle, the drugs that are currently in use for treatment focused on this stage, and the targets identified in this review relevant to this stage**. In the *binge/intoxication* stage, reinforcing effects of drugs may engage associative mechanisms and reward neurotransmitters in the nucleus accumbens shell and core and then engage stimulus-response habits that depend on the dorsal striatum. Green/blue arrows, glutamatergic projections; Orange arrows, dopaminergic projections; Pink arrows, GABAergic projections; AMG, amygdala; BNST, bed nucleus of the stria terminalis; DS, dorsal striatum; GP, globus pallidus; Hippo, hippocampus; NAc, nucleus accumbens; OFC, orbitofrontal cortex; PFC, prefrontal cortex; Thal, thalamus. *[Modified with permission from Koob GF, Everitt BJ, Robbins TW. Reward, motivation, and addiction. In: Squire LG, Berg D, Bloom FE, Du Lac S, Ghosh A, Spitzer N (eds) Fundamental Neuroscience, 3rd edition. Academic Press, Amsterdam, 2008, pp. 987–1016.]*

effects of dependence that are beginning to be used to explore how the nervous system adapts to drug use. These adaptations include anxiety-like responses, conditioned place aversion, elevated reward thresholds, and withdrawal-induced increases in drug self-administration. For the *preoccupation/anticipation* stage, the models include drug-, cue-, and stress-induced reinstatement of drug seeking behavior. Animal models of craving can also include the conditioned rewarding effects of drugs of abuse, measures of the conditioned aversive effects of withdrawal, and signs and symptoms of protracted abstinence (see Chapter 3 for details of the animal models).

Overall Neurocircuitry of Addiction

A critical issue for the development of treatments for addiction is that relevant targets

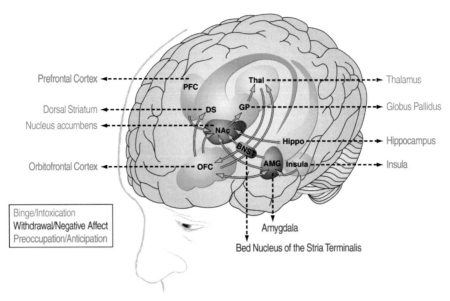

Existing and Future Medications for Addiction: Withdrawal/Negative Affect Stage

Existing medications
- methadone
- nicotine patch
- buprenorphine
- varenicline

Future targets
- GABA modulators (homeostatic resetters)
- CRF$_1$ antagonists (stress reducers)
- κ opioid antagonists (dysphoria reducer)

FIGURE 9.3 **Neural circuitry associated with the withdrawal/negative affect stage of the addiction cycle, the drugs that are currently in use for treatment focused on this stage, and the targets identified in this review relevant to this stage.** In the *withdrawal/negative affect* stage, the negative emotional state of withdrawal may engage the activation of the extended amygdala. The extended amygdala is composed of several basal forebrain structures, including the bed nucleus of the stria terminalis, central nucleus of the amygdala, and possibly the medial portion (or shell) of the nucleus accumbens. A major neurotransmitter in the extended amygdala is corticotropin-releasing factor, projecting to the brainstem where noradrenergic neurons provide a major projection reciprocally to the extended amygdala. Green/blue arrows, glutamatergic projections; Orange arrows, dopaminergic projections; Pink arrows, GABAergic projections; AMG, amygdala; BNST, bed nucleus of the stria terminalis; DS, dorsal striatum; GP, globus pallidus; Hippo, hippocampus; NAc, nucleus accumbens; OFC, orbitofrontal cortex; PFC, prefrontal cortex; Thal, thalamus. *[Modified with permission from Koob GF, Everitt BJ, Robbins TW. Reward, motivation, and addiction. In: Squire LG, Berg D, Bloom FE, Du Lac S, Ghosh A, Spitzer N (eds) Fundamental Neuroscience, 3rd edition. Academic Press, Amsterdam, 2008, pp. 987–1016.]*

should be based on an empirical foundation of the neurobiology of addiction (see Chapter 2). Three neurobiological circuits have been identified that have value for the study of the neurobiological changes associated with the development and persistence of drug dependence (Figures 9.2–9.4). As outlined in detail in Chapter 2, the acute reinforcing effects of drugs of abuse that comprise the *binge/intoxication*

stage most likely involve actions on ventral striatal/extended amygdala reward systems and inputs from the midbrain, hippocampus, amygdala, and frontal cortex. In contrast, the symptoms of acute withdrawal, such as negative affect and increased anxiety, associated with the *withdrawal/negative affect* stage most likely involve decreases in the function of ventral striatal reward systems and recruitment of

Existing and Future Medications for Addiction:
Preoccupation/Anticipation "Craving" Stage

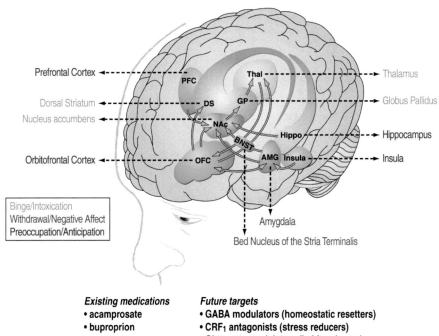

Existing medications
- acamprosate
- buproprion

Future targets
- GABA modulators (homeostatic resetters)
- CRF$_1$ antagonists (stress reducers)
- Glutamate modulators (habit reducers)

FIGURE 9.4   **Neural circuitry associated with the preoccupation/anticipation stage of the addiction cycle, the drugs that are currently in use for treatment focused on this stage, and the targets identified in this review relevant to this stage.** This stage involves the processing of conditioned reinforcement in the basolateral amygdala and the processing of contextual information by the hippocampus. Executive control depends on the prefrontal cortex and includes the representation of contingencies, the representation of outcomes, and their value and subjective states (i.e., craving and, presumably, feelings) associated with drugs. The subjective effect called drug craving in humans involves activation of the orbital and anterior cingulate cortex and temporal lobe, including the amygdala, in functional imaging studies. Green/blue arrows, glutamatergic projections; Orange arrows, dopaminergic projections; Pink arrows, GABAergic projections. AMG, amygdala; BNST, bed nucleus of the stria terminalis; DS, dorsal striatum; GP, globus pallidus; Hippo, hippocampus; NAc, nucleus accumbens; OFC, orbitofrontal cortex; PFC, prefrontal cortex; Thal, thalamus. [*Modified with permission from Koob GF, Everitt BJ, Robbins TW. Reward, motivation, and addiction. In: Squire LG, Berg D, Bloom FE, Du Lac S, Ghosh A, Spitzer N (eds) Fundamental Neuroscience, 3rd edition. Academic Press, Amsterdam, 2008, pp. 987–1016.*]

the extended amygdala brain stress neurocircuitry. The *preoccupation/anticipation* (craving) stage involves key afferent projections to the extended amygdala and nucleus accumbens, specifically from the prefrontal cortex, insula, basolateral amygdala, and hippocampus. Compulsive drug-seeking behavior engages ventral striatal–ventral–pallidal–thalamic–cortical loops that may then engage dorsal striatal–pallidal–thalamic cortical loops, both of which are

exaggerated by concomitant decreased reward function, increased brain stress function, and decreased executive function.

As discussed in Chapter 2, activation of the circuitry related to the origin and terminal regions of the mesocorticolimbic dopamine system, including dopamine and opioid peptides, are a key component of the neurobiology of the positive reinforcing effects of drugs associated with the *binge/intoxication* stage of the addiction

TABLE 9.1   Animal and Human Laboratory Models of the Different Stages of the Addiction Cycle.

Stage of Addiction Cycle	Animal Models	Human Laboratory Models
Binge/Intoxication	• drug/alcohol self-administration • conditioned place preference • intracranial self-stimulation • increased motivation for self-administration in dependent animals	• self-administration in dependent subjects • impulsivity
Withdrawal/Negative Affect	• anxiety-like responses • conditioned place aversion • elevated reward thresholds • withdrawal-induced increased in drug self-administration	• acute withdrawal • self-medication
Preoccupation/Anticipation	• drug-induced reinstatement • cue-induced reinstatement • stress-induced reinstatement	• drug reinstatement • cue reactivity • emotional reactivity • stress-induced craving • resistance to relapse • cue-induced brain imaging responses

From Koob et al., 2009.

cycle. The neural substrates and neuropharmacological mechanisms of the negative motivational effects of drug withdrawal associated with the *withdrawal/negative* affect stage of the addiction cycle involve disruptions of the same neural systems implicated in the positive reinforcing effects of drugs and recruitment of the brain stress systems. Common responses during acute withdrawal from all major drugs of abuse include decreased dopaminergic activity, an activated hypothalamic-pituitary-adrenal axis stress response, and an activated brain stress response with activated amygdala corticotropin-releasing factor (CRF). However, repeated cycles of addiction lead to a blunted hypothalamic-pituitary-adrenal response and a sensitized extrahypothalamic CRF stress system response in the amygdala. The *preoccupation/anticipation* (craving) stage involves key glutamatergic projections

to the extended amygdala and nucleus accumbens, specifically from the prefrontal cortex (for drug-induced reinstatement), basolateral amygdala (for cue-induced reinstatement), and hippocampus (for context-induced reinstatement; for details, see Chapter 2; for further reading, see Koob and Volkow, 2010).

EFFECTS OF KNOWN MEDICATIONS ON ANIMAL MODELS OF ADDICTION – REVERSE VALIDITY (ROSETTA STONE APPROACH)

Seven medications are currently on the market in the United States for the treatment of addiction, including (in chronological order of US approval) disulfiram (Antabuse), methadone (Dolophine), nicotine substitution (gum, lozenge, patch), naltrexone (ReVia, Vivitrol), bupropion (Zyban), buprenorphine (Subutex, Suboxone), acamprosate (Campral), and varenicline (Chantix; Figures 9.2–9.4, Tables 9.2–9.4). One validation procedure has been termed the "Rosetta Stone" approach (or "reverse validity" approach). Drugs that are known to be effective in human clinical studies can be used to validate animal models, and human laboratory models can provide a means of refining such models.

Drugs Currently on the Market for the Treatment of Addiction – Preclinical Background

Alcohol

- *Disulfiram (Antabuse).* Disulfiram is an inhibitor of aldehyde dehydrogenase and is used in the treatment of alcoholism to suppress drinking and prevent relapse. Disulfiram has a variable therapeutic effect, but it can be effective under conditions of compliance. In animal studies, disulfiram decreases alcohol intake, but tolerance develops to the suppression with chronic intake. Disulfiram also has anxiogenic-like effects. Both characteristics are possibly relevant for its therapeutic use.
- *Acamprosate (Campral).* Acamprosate is a modulator of hyperglutamatergic function either through an action on *N*-methyl-D-aspartate (NMDA) receptors or through an action on metabotropic glutamate receptors. The preclinical data that led to the clinical studies on acamprosate began with a series of studies in Europe on the effects of acamprosate on excessive drinking in rats. Acamprosate injected chronically decreased alcohol drinking in rats that were selectively bred for excessive drinking and decreased alcohol drinking in

dependent rats. Acamprosate also reverses the hyperglutamatergic state produced by alcohol withdrawal. Acamprosate was then shown to selectively block the increased alcohol drinking associated with withdrawal and alcohol deprivation. Although at high doses acamprosate had effects on baseline drinking in general, the excessive drinking associated with dependence and withdrawal was much more sensitive to the effects of acamprosate (for further reading, see Littleton et al., 2007).

- *Nalmefene (Selincro).* Nalmefene is an orally active opioid antagonist with high affinity for both μ and κ opioid receptors. It was shown to decrease heavy drinking in individuals with alcoholism in a double-blind, placebo-controlled clinical trial. It is now marketed in parts of Europe for the treatment of alcoholism. Moreover, the efficacy of nalmefene led to preclinical studies that showed greater efficacy in dependent than nondependent animals, thus increasing interest in dynorphin/κ opioid targets for the treatment of alcoholism (see dynorphin discussion below). In human studies, nalmefene has been tested on patients who were instructed to take their pills only on days they felt like they were going to drink; thus, treatment was aimed at curbing heavy drinking on an "as needed basis." Nalmefene received approval for reducing alcohol consumption in alcohol dependence in the European Union in 2013 and is already marketed in some countries in Europe, including Norway, Finland, and Poland. Nalmefene has not been approved for use in the United States.
- *Baclofen (Lioresal).* Preclinical studies show that baclofen can block alcohol self-administration and alcohol seeking in animal models. Baclofen has also been shown to block cocaine and heroin seeking in animals and block nicotine, cocaine, and morphine-induced dopamine release in the shell of the nucleus accumbens. Baclofen is

TABLE 9.2 Medications Currently on the Market for Drug Abuse Treatment for the *Binge/Intoxication* Stage of the Addiction Cycle.

Generic Name	Trade Name	Indication	FDA Approval	Description
disulfiram	Antabuse	alcohol addiction	1954	• Disulfiram is an acetaldehyde dehydrogenase inhibitor used to prevent relapse in detoxified alcoholics. Disulfiram at average therapeutic doses of 250 mg/day (not to exceed 500 mg/day) blocks acetaldehyde dehydrogenase. • Disulfiram produces an aversive reaction if the subject drinks with adequate blood levels of disulfiram, presumably due to increased acetaldehyde in the blood stream which is similar to the intense flush reaction of Asians known to have a deletion of one or two alleles of the *ALDH2* gene.
naltrexone	ReVia Vivitrol Vivitrol	alcohol addiction opioid addiction	1994 2005 2010	• Naltrexone is a competitive opioid antagonist that has oral bioavailability and binds to the μ, δ, and κ opioid receptors, with a higher affinity for the μ receptor than for the δ or κ receptor. • Naltrexone decreases heavy drinking in alcoholics and prevents relapses to heavy drinking at doses of 50 mg/day. Naltrexone has more efficacy when combined with associated behavioral treatments, particularly cognitive behavioral therapy. • Naltrexone blocks μ opioid actions and as such blocks the rewarding (euphoric) effects of opioid self-administration in humans.
varenicline	Chantix	nicotine addiction	2006	• Varenicline is a partial α4β2 nicotinic acetylcholine receptor agonist used for detoxification and treatment of nicotine addiction. Doses of 1 mg twice per day doubled abstinence rates in 12 week trials. • Varenicline has been associated with a number of reports of adverse effects related to suicidal ideation. As a result, the use of Chantix is no longer accepted by the Federal Aviation Administration for aeromedical certification purposes.
buprenorphine	Subutex Suboxone	opioid addiction	2002	• Buprenorphine is an oripavine derivative that is considered a partial agonist at μ receptors, partial agonist at nociceptin receptors, and antagonist at κ receptors. • Multiple controlled studies have shown that maintenance therapy with buprenorphine is an effective treatment for opioid dependence at doses of 16–24 mg/day (maximum 32 mg/day). • Buprenorphine can be prescribed as a sublingual tablet or film consisting of buprenorphine (Subutex) or as a sublingual tablet or film consisting of buprenorphine with naloxone (Suboxone). The addition of naloxone limits diversion because naloxone is inactive when taken orally, but if the preparation is diverted to intravenous use, then naloxone will block the effects of buprenorphine.

From Koob et al., 2009.

TABLE 9.3   Medications Currently on the Market for Drug Abuse Treatment for the *Withdrawal/Negative Affect* Stage of the Addiction Cycle.

Generic Name	Trade Name	Indication	FDA Approval	Description
methadone	Dolophine	opioid addiction	1972	• Methadone, a long-acting opioid, was developed as a substitution treatment for opioid addiction because of its properties of being orally active with a long half-life. Methadone also has become the standard medication for opioid detoxification. • Methadone is effective in reducing illicit opioid use at doses of 80–120 mg/day.
buprenorphine	Subutex Suboxone	opioid addiction	2002	• Buprenorphine (see Table 9.2).
varenicline	Chantix	nicotine addiction	2006	• Varenicline (see Table 9.2).
nicotine gum/ patch/lozenge	Nicorette Nicoderm Commit	nicotine addiction		• Oral slow release nicotine via nicotine chewing gum (2 or 4 mg) or lozenges or percutaneous administration via the nicotine patch are used for detoxification of nicotine addiction. Both the gum and patch facilitate abstinence as an aid to smoking cessation.

From Koob et al., 2009.

TABLE 9.4   Medications Currently on the Market for Drug Abuse Treatment for the *Preoccupation/Anticipation* Stage of the Addiction Cycle.

Generic Name	Trade Name	Indication	FDA Approval	Description
acamprosate	Campral	alcohol addiction	2004	• Acamprosate is a glutamate receptor modulator used to prevent relapse in detoxified alcoholics. Doses are typically two 333 mg tablets three times per day. • In a US multicenter double-blind, placebo-controlled trial of acamprosate, treatment efficacy was particularly robust in patients who had a clearly identified goal of achieving abstinence before starting treatment.
bupropion	Zyban	nicotine addiction	1997	• Bupropion is an antidepressant with efficacy in smoking cessation that has beneficial effects on protracted abstinence consistent with its antidepressant properties. • Bupropion at doses of 150–300 mg/day effectively doubled abstinence rates after 1 year.

From Koob et al., 2009.

a γ-aminobutyric acid-B (GABA$_B$) receptor agonist that blocks the increase in alcohol self-administration during acute withdrawal in dependent rats at lower doses than those that block alcohol self-administration in nondependent rats, suggesting the increased sensitivity of this system during the development of dependence. Baclofen, a GABA$_B$ agonist, was shown to reduce alcohol craving and intake in some double-blind, placebo-controlled clinical trials but not in others (for further reading, see Ameisen, 2008). Baclofen was recently approved for the treatment of alcoholism in France only. It has not yet been approved for the treatment of alcoholism in Europe as a whole or in the United States. Direct GABA$_B$ receptor agonists such as baclofen are also currently in therapeutic use for the relief of flexor spasms in multiple sclerosis, but they have substantial sedative effects at therapeutic dose ranges.

Alcohol and Opioids

- *Naltrexone (Revia, Vivitrol).* Naltrexone, a competitive opioid antagonist, has high affinity for the μ opioid receptor and is less potent at the δ and κ receptors. Naltrexone has long been known to decrease alcohol consumption in animal models. In an early study, intramuscular administration of naltrexone decreased intravenous alcohol self-administration in rhesus monkeys. Subsequently, naltrexone was shown to decrease alcohol drinking and self-administration in various animal models. Brain sites particularly effective in the actions of opioid antagonists on alcohol self-administration include the nucleus accumbens, central nucleus of the amygdala, and ventral tegmental area. Human studies have suggested that endogenous opioids may be involved in the direct reinforcing effects of alcohol, and opioid antagonists may blunt the reinforcing effects of alcohol and blunt the urge to drink elicited by the presentation of alcohol-related cues in alcohol-dependent subjects. Naltrexone has been shown to reduce craving for alcohol in human laboratory studies, and this effect may be related to its ability to activate the hypothalamic–pituitary–adrenal axis. Similar results have been observed in a rat model of cue-induced reinstatement, in which re-exposure to an olfactory stimulus that signaled the availability of alcohol self-administration produced strong reinstatement of responding after extinction. This reinstatement was blocked by systemic administration of naltrexone (for further reading, see Unterwald, 2008). Naltrexone completely blocks the reinforcing and dependence-inducing effects of opioids in animal models. In an actively opioid-dependent animal (or human), naltrexone will "precipitate" opioid withdrawal (for details, see Chapter 5).

Nicotine

- *Bupropion (Zyban).* Bupropion is also an antidepressant (Wellbutrin) with actions that facilitate dopamine and norepinephrine neurotransmission but not serotonin neurotransmission, and it has efficacy in smoking cessation treatment. Bupropion attenuates nicotine withdrawal in rats and decreases mecamylamine-precipitated signs of withdrawal. Bupropion also dose-dependently attenuates the spontaneous nicotine abstinence syndrome and reverses nicotine withdrawal effects in contextual fear conditioning paradigms. Perhaps directly relevant to its therapeutic use, bupropion attenuates the elevation in brain stimulation reward thresholds (decreased reward) during nicotine withdrawal and blocks mecamylamine-precipitated conditioned place aversions. It also decreases nicotine self-administration, an effect amplified with repeated administration, but it failed to block the cue-induced reinstatement of responding.
- *Varenicline (Chantix).* Varenicline is an α4β2 nicotinic acetylcholine receptor partial

agonist with efficacy in smoking cessation treatment. For details of the role of the α4β2 nicotinic acetylcholine receptor in the effects of nicotine, see Chapter 6. When combined with nicotine, varenicline decreases dopamine release in the nucleus accumbens *in vivo* by itself and has less efficacy than nicotine in stimulating dopamine release. Varenicline partially generalizes to nicotine in drug discrimination studies, consistent with its partial agonist mechanism of action (for further reading, see Koob et al., 2009).

Opioids

- *Methadone (Dolophine).* Methadone is a µ opioid receptor agonist with a long oral half-life in humans (22–30h; racemic mixture used in the clinic). It has been an effective substitution pharmacotherapy used for over 40 years in the treatment of opioid addiction (Box 9.4). Methadone has a much shorter half-life in animals than in humans. Chronic 5 day treatment in nondependent rhesus monkeys had little effect on heroin choice but prevented withdrawal-associated increases in heroin choice. Using a slow-release subcutaneous minipump to mimic the pharmacokinetic profile of humans, methadone also blocked cocaine seeking in rats in the conditioned place preference paradigm, blocked responding on a progressive-ratio schedule of reinforcement, and blocked reinstatement at doses that did not have effects on locomotor activity, food intake, or pain responsivity. Human laboratory studies support the clinical observation that persistent heroin use may be reduced by providing larger methadone maintenance doses, because such doses completely block the subjective effects of heroin and produce greater withdrawal suppression during outpatient periods.

- *Buprenorphine (Subutex, Suboxone).* Buprenorphine is an effective maintenance pharmacotherapy for the treatment of opioid addiction. It is a µ opioid partial agonist, a full δ and κ antagonist, and nociceptin receptor

---

BOX 9.4

WHAT IS SUBSTITUTION OR REPLACEMENT THERAPY?

Substitution or replacement pharmacotherapy is a medical procedure used with opioid drugs to replace a drug of addiction with a longer-acting but less euphoria-inducing opioid, such as methadone or buprenorphine. The main principle behind opioid substitution is that an individual with opioid addiction will be able to regain a normal life and schedule while being treated with a substance that stops the person from experiencing withdrawal symptoms and drug cravings, but the replacement substance does not produce strong euphoria. The individual theoretically shows no compulsive drug seeking, because both withdrawal and craving are blocked by full opioid receptor occupancy of the substitution drug. From the public health perspective, reductions of intravenous opioid use bring significant health benefits, such as a lower incidence of HIV/AIDS and hepatitis C infections, and a lower incidence of all other associated complications, such as legal and psychosocial problems, that result from intravenous drug use. However, there is no reversal of neuroadaptations in the brain, and the individual remains dependent and will manifest withdrawal and severe craving if the substitution drug is abruptly removed.

partial agonist (for further reading, see Cowan, 2007). It has pharmacological properties that provide a good safety profile, low physical dependence, and flexibility in dose scheduling. The finding that buprenorphine dose-dependently decreased heroin intake in heroin-dependent animals is consistent with predictive validity for the self-administration dependence model. Buprenorphine was effective in reducing the self-administration of other drugs of abuse in rats, even when the μ opioid receptor was concurrently blocked, suggesting that κ antagonist and nociceptin agonist activity may be effective in modulating the negative reinforcement associated with dependence (see Chapter 2 for general details of the dynorphin-κ opioid system and addiction). Buprenorphine decreases intravenous heroin self-administration in human laboratory studies. From the perspective of the abuse potential of buprenorphine itself, it has reinforcing, discriminative stimulus, and physical dependence-producing effects, but it has less abuse liability than morphine. Buprenorphine maintains lower breakpoints than full agonists in progressive-ratio self-administration procedures. Withdrawal from buprenorphine is characterized by a mild morphine-like abstinence syndrome in animals and humans. Buprenorphine may suppress or precipitate withdrawal in animals maintained on chronic administration of a μ agonist. Lower doses suppress spontaneous withdrawal signs, and higher doses can precipitate an abstinence syndrome.

NOVEL TARGETS FOR MEDICATION DEVELOPMENT

The premise is that different components of the addiction cycle can be targeted by different medications based on evaluating three pieces of key information:

i) Basic neurobiological mechanisms for the different stages of the addiction cycle,

ii) Information about the actions of known effective medications in the treatment of addiction on animal models of the different stages of the addiction cycle, and

iii) Information derived from clinical studies of known medications for other indications that may overlap with specific components of addiction (Figures 9.2–9.4, Table 9.5).

The following section explores four neurotransmitter systems – dopamine, GABA, CRF, and glutamate – as potential targets for the treatment of addiction. Each of these systems has targets that can restore homeostatically dysregulated reward, stress, or executive function systems via the *binge/intoxication* stage (Figure 9.2), *withdrawal/negative affect* stage (Figure 9.3), and *preoccupation/anticipation* stage (Figure 9.4). From a broad perspective, none of these targets are completely new or novel (GABA, glutamate, or CRF), but they all have the potential for providing novel medications from the validation

TABLE 9.5   Targets for Medications Development Derived from Preclinical Basic Research.

Class	Target
Dopamine receptor partial agonists	D_2 receptor partial agonist (aripiprazole) D_3 receptor partial agonist
Modulators of γ-aminobutyric acid	GABA modulators
Modulators of brain stress systems	CRF$_1$ receptor antagonist κ opioid receptor antagonist neurokinin-1 receptor antagonist
Modulators of glutamate	AMPA receptor antagonist NMDA receptor antagonist metabotropic glutamate receptor agonist glutamate-5 receptor antagonist topiramate

framework elaborated here. Finally, in this section, the innovative drug vaccine approach will be elaborated, which largely involves pharmacokinetically limiting the reinstatement of drug taking.

Partial Receptor Agonists – Dopamine Partial Agonists

The mesocorticolimbic dopamine system projects from the ventral tegmental area to basal forebrain sites, the nucleus accumbens, and the central nucleus of the amygdala and plays a key role in motivation in general. Activation of the mesocorticolimbic dopamine system is important for directing behavior toward salient rewarding stimuli. Mesocorticolimbic dopamine activity appears to be critical for the reinforcing actions of indirect sympathomimetics, such as cocaine and amphetamines, and is involved in the incentive salience actions of other drugs of abuse, such as opioids and alcohol.

Based on the allostatic view of addiction, dopaminergic function is compromised during acute withdrawal from all major drugs of abuse (see Chapter 2). Withdrawal from most major drugs of abuse is also associated with decreases in the firing of dopaminergic neurons in the ventral tegmental area, resulting in blunted dopaminergic responses in human imaging studies during abstinence.

Given the role of dopamine in the acute reinforcing effects of drugs and dysregulated dopamine function during withdrawal, a reasonable hypothesis is that a dopamine partial agonist or functional partial agonist may have efficacy in different components of the addiction cycle. A dopamine partial agonist is a drug that binds to a receptor with high affinity but low efficacy. It also has antagonist properties in situations of high intrinsic activity (when dopamine is flooding the synapse) and agonist properties in situations of low intrinsic activity (when there is a low level of dopamine in the synapse). Hypothetically, it also has fewer side effects than full agonists or full antagonists. Because of its intermediate efficacy, a dopamine partial agonist acts as an agonist in the absence of dopamine and acts as an antagonist in the presence of dopamine. Although this approach is theoretically possible, no dopamine receptor partial agonist has progressed past animal studies to date for the treatment of addiction, but see below for a compound that is being tested in human laboratory trials.

D_1 receptor antagonists competitively block cocaine self-administration in rats. To date, however, little work has been done with D_1 partial agonists. D_2 partial agonists have been shown to reverse psychostimulant withdrawal and block the increase in psychostimulant self-administration associated with extended access. However, for psychostimulant addiction, the effects of D_2 partial agonists have not been sufficiently robust to merit clinical trials because of side effects and a lack of specificity for compulsive use. Dopamine D_2 partial agonists dose-dependently decrease the reinforcing effects of intravenous cocaine and amphetamine self-administration and oral alcohol self-administration in nondependent rats, suggesting a nonspecific reward-reducing action. For alcoholism, OSU-6162 (PNU-96391) is a compound that acts like a partial agonist at both dopamine D_2 receptors and serotonin $5\text{-}HT_{2A}$ receptors. It has been termed a "dopamine stabilizer" and has shown antipsychotic and anti-Parkinsonian effects in animal studies. OSU-6162 decreases voluntary alcohol consumption, compulsive-like alcohol seeking, and withdrawal- and cue-induced alcohol seeking. D_3 antagonists do not block baseline cocaine self-administration, but they do block progressive-ratio responding, a measure that reflects the compulsivity component of cocaine seeking. Additionally, D_3 antagonists block cocaine and alcohol cue-induced reinstatement and have been under consideration for medications for psychostimulant addiction. The hypothesis that dysregulated dopamine tone contributes to the motivational effects of drug withdrawal and reinstatement remains viable, and dopamine modulators with appropriate neuropharmaco-logical and pharmacokinetic profiles may be effective in treating certain aspects of addiction (for further reading, see Steensland et al., 2012).

GABA Modulators

GABA is an inhibitory amino acid neu-rotransmitter that acts by binding one of two broad classes of receptors, $GABA_A$ and $GABA_B$. $GABA_A$ receptor antagonists and inverse ago-nists (drugs that bind to a receptor and pro-duce effects opposite to those of an agonist; in the case of a GABA-gated ion channel, an inverse agonist would cause maximal clos-ing of the ion channel; see Chapters 2 and 6) decrease alcohol self-administration. However, their therapeutic actions are limited by severe side effects that involve significant hyperexcit-ability of the central nervous system. In con-trast, GABA agonists/modulators may block drug-seeking behavior by acting on reward, dependence, or both. GABA modulators that increase GABAergic activity directly or indi-rectly decrease cocaine, heroin, nicotine, and alcohol self-administration in non-dependent and dependent rats. GABA receptor agonists also block alcohol withdrawal in animals and humans and decrease drinking and certain components of craving in human individuals with alcoholism.

Another therapeutic approach is to explore GABA modulators that can *indirectly* facili-tate GABA release. Gabapentin, an amino acid designed as a structural analog of GABA, is an anticonvulsant drug that came into clinical use as an adjunctive therapy in the treatment of human seizures and in the treatment of neuro-pathic pain disorders. Gabapentin selectively inhibits Ca^{2+} influx through voltage-operated Ca^{2+} channels. Gabapentin also increases GABA release. In animal models of alcohol dependence, gabapentin has strikingly different cellular and pharmacological effects in nondependent and alcohol-dependent rats. In nondependent rats, gabapentin facilitates GABAergic transmission in the central nucleus of the amygdala but does not affect alcohol intake. In dependent rats, in contrast, gabapentin decreases GABAergic transmission in the central nucleus of the amyg-dala and reduces excessive alcohol intake. Gaba-pentin also suppresses the anxiogenic-like effects of withdrawal from an acute alcohol injection. One hypothesis to explain these results is that during the development of alcohol dependence, neuroadaptive changes occur in the GABAergic system (see Chapter 6). Gabapentin has been shown to be effective in decreasing craving in human laboratory studies, reversing the physi-ological measures of protracted abstinence and reversing sleep deficits in protracted abstinence. It has also shown efficacy in human double-blind placebo-controlled trials, suggesting a key translation from animals to humans (for further reading, see Mason et al., 2012, 2014).

Modulators of the Brain Stress System

CRF Antagonists

Drugs of abuse are powerful activators of the stress systems, an effect that has important implications for understanding the neurobiol-ogy of dependence and relapse, both through the hypothalamic–pituitary–adrenal axis and exten-sive extrahypothalamic, extra-neuroendocrine CRF systems implicated in behavioral responses to stress.

A common response to acute withdrawal and protracted abstinence from all major drugs of abuse is the manifestation of anxiety-like responses in animal models. During drug withdrawal, extrahypothalamic CRF systems become hyperactive, with an increase in extra-cellular CRF within the central nucleus of the amygdala and bed nucleus of the stria termina-lis in dependent rats. Withdrawal from repeated administration of cocaine, alcohol, nicotine, and cannabinoids produces an anxiogenic-like response in the elevated plus maze and defensive burying test. One or both of these effects can be reversed by the administration of selective CRF_1 receptor antagonists or mixed CRF_1/CRF_2 receptor antagonists (for further reading, see Chapter 6 and Koob et al., 2008).

CRF antagonists block the anxiogenic-like and aversive-like motivational effects of drug withdrawal in animal models of dependence. Systemic injections of small-molecule CRF_1 antagonists also block the increase in alcohol intake in alcohol-dependent rats during acute withdrawal and protracted abstinence but not in nondependent rats. CRF antagonists also selectively block the increase in self-administration associated with extended access to cocaine, nicotine, and heroin. These data suggest an important role for CRF, primarily in the central nucleus of the amygdala, in mediating the increased self-administration associated with drug dependence. Several clinical trials have evaluated the effects of CRF_1 antagonists on anxiety and depression, but either they have generated negative results or the trials were stopped because of side effects (for further reading, see Koob and Zorrilla, 2012). No human laboratory studies or clinical trials have yet been published that explored the effects of CRF antagonists on drug dependence, largely due to the limited availability of CRF antagonists for human studies on addiction.

Non-CRF Targets

Preclinical data suggest that other neurotransmitter systems/neuromodulators in the extended amygdala may be dysregulated during the development of dependence and contribute to the "dark side" of addiction (see Chapter 2). Norepinephrine is dysregulated in alcohol, cocaine, and opioid dependence. Dynorphin is dysregulated in cocaine, opioid, and alcohol dependence. Vasopressin is dysregulated in opioid and alcohol dependence. Hypocretin and substance P are dysregulated in cocaine, opioid,

and alcohol dependence. These are examples from animal models of components of the addiction cycle that are activated during the development of dependence. Norepinephrine/CRF interactions have been hypothesized to contribute to the brain stress activation associated with withdrawal from drugs of abuse, and some anti-addiction-like effects have been observed in animal models (for example, administration of the noradrenergic α_1 receptor antagonist prazosin). Dynorphins are the presumed endogenous ligands for the κ opioid receptor. Dynorphin has long been hypothesized to mediate negative emotional states. κ Opioid receptor agonists produce conditioned place aversions, depression, and dysphoria in humans. Substantial evidence suggests that dynorphin peptide, dynorphin gene expression, and κ opioid receptors are activated in the striatum, ventral striatum (nucleus accumbens), and amygdala during acute and chronic administration of drugs in rats and humans. Activation of the dynorphin systems in the nucleus accumbens then decreases activity in dopamine systems. As a result, the activation of dynorphin systems could contribute to the dysphoric syndrome associated with cocaine dependence. κ Opioid receptor antagonists blunt compulsive-like cocaine self-administration in rats with extended access (for further reading, see Wee and Koob, 2010).

Other neuromodulatory systems may act in opposition to CRF in buffering stress and emotional behavior, which may become future targets for medications development for the treatment of addiction. These include neuropeptide Y, nociceptin, and endocannabinoid receptor agonists, all of which reduce excessive drinking associated with alcohol dependence.

Glutamate Modulators

Glutamate plays multiple roles in the neurobiology of addiction, many of which provide potential targets for medications development.

Glutamate is associated with the neuroplasticity that is important for the incentive salience of cues paired with repeated drug administration, particularly psychostimulants. α-Amino-3-hydroxy-5-methyl-4-isoxazolepropionic acid receptors move to the post-synaptic membrane with repeated cocaine administration and play a key role in facilitating drug seeking, particularly after long periods of abstinence. Another prominent hypothesis is that repeated self-administration of psychostimulants decreases the release of glutamate in key brain circuits associated with the *preoccupation/anticipation* stage of the addiction cycle. Strong evidence suggests that repeated psychostimulant administration in animals decreases the extracellular nonsynaptic glutamate pool in the NAc, removing glutamate tone that normally functions to limit glutamate release. As a result of this decrease in glutamate tone, a challenge injection of a psychostimulant is able to increase nucleus accumbens glutamate levels back to the levels observed in controls. Such an exaggerated response of glutamate to activity in these circuits could convey sensitivity to relapse. For example, the drug-induced reinstatement of drug seeking appears to be mediated by a prefrontal cortex glutamatergic projection to the nucleus accumbens. Cue-induced reinstatement involves glutamatergic projections to the nucleus accumbens from the frontal cortex, basolateral amygdala, and ventral subiculum. Pharmacological agents that modulate glutamate function may play a role in glutamate hypo- or hyperexcitability during protracted abstinence, depending on the drug, and may decrease drug- and cue-induced reinstatement. Various glutamatergic modulators, all of which decrease glutamatergic neurotransmission, including AMPA receptor antagonists, NMDA receptor antagonists, metabotropic glutamate-2/3 receptor agonists, and metabotropic glutamate-5 receptor antagonists, have been shown to block cue-induced reinstatement (for further reading, see Wolf, 2010).

Additional evidence for a potential AMPA/kainate glutamate target in addiction comes from studies of topiramate, an anticonvulsant that blocks AMPA/kainate receptors and allosterically modulates ion channel conductance. Controlled clinical trials have reported decreases in drinking behavior in alcohol dependence and improvements in quality of life, but with significant adverse effects on memory and concentration. Given the side effects associated with direct glutamate receptor antagonists, drugs that indirectly modulate the system may be more logical candidates for medications development.

Immunopharmacotherapy

A novel approach to the pharmacotherapy of addiction is largely pharmacokinetic. Immunopharmacotherapy uses highly specific antibodies to sequester the drug of interest while it is still in the bloodstream, thus preventing the drug from reaching the brain. An antibody-drug complex will prevent the drug from crossing the blood-brain barrier into the brain and thus, by definition, will block the pharmacodynamic actions of the drug. The reinforcing effects of the drug are blocked, and the detrimental side effects on the central nervous system or other organs of the body are blocked.

How does immunopharmacotherapy work? In an active immunization approach, an appropriate antigenic drug protein conjugate is directly administered, which causes immune cell activation, leading to the generation of specific antibodies to the drug protein conjugate. The immune system has not evolved to generate a response for molecules that are less than about 10 kDa, a limit that is well above the molecular weight of any drug of abuse. Thus, small-molecule drugs, such as drugs of abuse, must be linked to a carrier protein to trigger an immune response, and this small molecule part of the vaccine is termed a hapten (Box 9.5). The active immunization approach is able to confer longer-lasting protection through immunological memory with minimal treatment compliance and thus is very cost effective. Nevertheless, active immunization requires some exposure time to generate antibodies before protection is conferred; it is also subject to a significant amount of individual variability.

In passive immunization, administration provides immediate protection through the injection of pre-generated high affinity antibodies, typically of the monoclonal type (Box 9.5). Such an approach to the addiction field has been argued to be particularly relevant in a drug overdose scenario as well as during the critical time points during relapse to addiction. However, in passive immunization, the effects are shorter-lasting, depend on the antibody half-life, and are limited to the amount of antibodies supplied.

Successful active immunization with vaccines in animal models has been reported for cocaine, nicotine, phencyclidine, methamphetamine, and heroin. Two nicotine vaccines have been tested in clinical trials. One of these vaccines, NicVAX, was shown to be safe and well tolerated in Phase I and II clinical trials in both smokers and non-smokers. However, it failed to meet its primary endpoints in two separate Phase III trials, even though approximately one-third of the highest-dose vaccine

---

BOX 9.5

IMMUNOLOGICAL TERMS

Vaccine A biological preparation that is administered to produce or increase immunity, usually to a particular disease. In the case of vaccines for drugs of abuse, the hapten combined with a carrier protein stimulates antibodies to form in the blood that recognize the drug as a foreign object and destroy it.

Hapten A small separable part of an antigen that reacts specifically with an antibody but is incapable of stimulating antibody production except in combination with a carrier protein molecule.

Antigen Any substance that is capable of inducing a specific immune response and reacting with a specific antibody.

B cells A group of white blood cells, known as lymphocytes, which can bind to a specific antigen and produce antibodies to it.

Monoclonal antibody Any of a large number of high-molecular-weight proteins that are normally produced by specialized B cells but derived from a single B cell after stimulation by an antigen and act specifically against the antigen in an immune response.

Adjuvant A substance that is added to a vaccine that enhances the immune response to an antigen.

subjects quit smoking. Another nicotine vaccine, NIC002, met a similar fate. A cocaine vaccine (TA-CD) has produced marginal results in promoting continuous abstinence in humans because of substantial variability in the generation of high antibody titers. Another cocaine vaccine and a heroin vaccine are in different stages of preparation for clinical trials. Despite the failure to date of these clinical candidates to meet their primary endpoints, the results demonstrate the feasibility of a vaccine approach for the treatment of addiction: active immunization using nicotine or cocaine immunoconjugates *can* produce high titers of anti-drug antibodies. However, the magnitude of the immune response to vaccination in humans has been highly variable to date and will need to be addressed in future studies (for further reading, see Brimijoin et al., 2013; Moreno and Janda, 2009).

HUMAN LABORATORY STUDIES

A key element and critical point in medication development is submitting an IND application to the US Food and Drug Administration (FDA), or its equivalent in other countries, so that the drug can be tested in humans (see Box 9.3). However, this process is not unique to the development of drugs to treat addiction; it is a generic process for all new drugs for various indications.

Human laboratory studies provide a means of exploring treatment targets for specific components of the addiction cycle, independent of expensive double-blind, placebo-controlled trials. Using the structure of the addiction cycle outlined in this book, human laboratory studies can provide measures for each of the addiction stages and are hypothesized to have value for predicting potential treatment efficacy in these domains (Tables 9.1, 9.2, and 9.4). Although the predictive validity of human laboratory models remains to be determined, ongoing studies with established medications used for addiction treatment provide another iteration of the Rosetta Stone approach with which to evaluate the

validity of animal models and then use human laboratory models as a springboard for novel medication development (for further reading, see Koob, 2009).

Binge/Intoxication Stage

For the *binge/intoxication* stage of the addiction cycle, self-administration procedures for cocaine, heroin, and marijuana in humans have been established largely using operant responding, in which participants who are dependent on the drug make a behavioral response, such as pressing a key on a computer, to receive a drug. Similar to animal models, heroin self-administration is reduced by all three medications currently approved by the FDA to treat opioid dependence – methadone, naltrexone, and buprenorphine – providing some predictive validity. However, for cocaine, the validity is much less robust. A range of medications has been shown to reduce the subjective effects and craving associated with cocaine but do not decrease cocaine self-administration itself. These results are consistent with data from clinical trials. Of the more than 60 medications tested, none have proven to be reliably effective in clinical trials. To date, little or no work has been done on specific treatments for marijuana self-administration.

Other measures, such as impulsivity, could be considered endophenotypes of the *binge/intoxication* stage and have some potential for predicting drugs with possible efficacy for addiction treatment. Impulsivity likely contributes to increasing the probability of engaging in initial drug taking, and the subsequent drug effects on impulsivity may increase impulsive behaviors that in turn facilitate further drug use, prolonging the binge or even provoking relapse (see below). Various tasks have been used to assess impulsivity, including tasks of delayed discounting (i.e., relative preference for smaller, more immediate rewards over larger, more delayed rewards), tasks of behavioral inhibition (e.g., Stop Task), and attentional measures (i.e., subjects show increased variability in reaction times on a simple reaction time task, reflecting lapses in attention).

Withdrawal/Negative Affect Stage

In the *withdrawal/negative affect* stage, negative reinforcement mechanisms are engaged, rather than positive reinforcement mechanisms. Numerous human laboratory measures of acute withdrawal are available and sensitive to drug substitution. In the laboratory, marijuana withdrawal is alleviated by marijuana smoking or by the administration of oral Δ^9-THC. Cognitive measures could be envisioned as sensitive to the withdrawal effects of drug dependence during acute and protracted abstinence and could be considered another endophenotype of the addiction process that is sensitive to medication screening. Nicotine can improve cognitive processing and reduce negative affect in smokers. The cascade of stress hormone interactions with drugs of abuse, from facilitation of the *binge/intoxication* stage to exaggeration of the *withdrawal/negative affect* stage, and sensitization to stress-induced relapse may all be amenable to human laboratory studies.

Preoccupation/Anticipation Stage

For the *preoccupation/anticipation* stage, three major external factors and two internal factors are hypothesized to contribute to relapse. The external factors include priming doses of drug, drug-associated cues, and stressor exposure. The internal factors include the malaise of protracted abstinence and a state of stress associated with protracted abstinence that contributes to malaise. Several human laboratory procedures have been developed to reflect these aspects of the *preoccupation/anticipation* stage. Drug reinstatement has been developed in human laboratory models, notably in the realm of alcohol and tobacco addiction. Priming-induced drinking

in alcohol-dependent subjects in a bar-like setting was greater than in social drinkers and was selectively decreased in the alcohol-dependent groups by opioid receptor antagonists. Similar results were observed in family history-positive alcohol-dependent individuals who received a priming dose of alcohol and in cigarette smokers who were primed with five cigarettes.

Exposure to alcohol cues, such as the sight or smell of alcoholic beverages, using the cue reactivity paradigm reliably increases the urge to drink alcohol, salivation, and attention to cues. Cue reactivity can also predict treatment outcome and has been validated in some cases by the use of medications that successfully treat alcoholism. For example, naltrexone, but not topiramate, blocked cue reactivity in alcohol-dependent subjects, and nicotine replacement therapy decreased craving associated with smoking cues.

Stress responses, including changes in the activity of the hypothalamic–pituitary–adrenal stress axis and extrahypothalamic brain stress systems, impact all phases of the addiction cycle but may be particularly relevant to the *withdrawal/negative affect* and *preoccupation/anticipation* stages. Stress and stressors have also been associated with relapse and the vulnerability to relapse. Negative affect, stress, and withdrawal-related distress increase drug craving. Both stress and drugs of abuse activate the hypothalamic-pituitary-adrenal axis, but the glucocorticoid steroid hormone response becomes blunted with chronic high-dose drug use. High glucocorticoid tone can then drive the brain stress systems in the amygdala. As noted above, a cascade of stress hormone interactions occurs with drugs of abuse, leading to sensitization of stress-induced relapse. All of these changes may be amenable to studies in the human laboratory setting.

Stress-related responses and stress-induced craving can be elicited in addicted individuals using models of stress-induced responsivity with emotional imagery paradigms. Using such emotional imagery paradigms, individuals who administer higher amounts of cocaine and alcohol each week and recovering alcohol-dependent subjects show greater craving and physiological responses to stressors compared with social drinkers. From a validation perspective, stress-induced cocaine craving in the laboratory can predict the time to cocaine relapse. Similar results have been found in alcohol- and nicotine-dependent subjects.

Another approach to cue reactivity that has been developed for the study of craving in alcoholism during protracted abstinence is exploring the interaction between cue exposure and emotional states during protracted abstinence (for further reading, see Mason et al., 2009). A nontreatment-seeking sample of alcohol-dependent subjects was exposed to affective stimuli that had positive or negative valence and then to a beverage cue but with no opportunity to self-administer alcohol. Cue reactivity was measured using subjective measures of craving, measures of emotional reactivity, and psychophysiological measures, including heart rate, skin conductance, and facial electromyography. Alcohol exposure and both positive and negative emotional cues had the expected effects on subjective and emotional reactivity but fewer effects on psychophysiological measures. Gabapentin significantly decreased subjective craving and affectively evoked craving and improved several measures of sleep quality. These results suggest that cue reactivity, combined with an emotional overlay, may provide a powerful means of evaluating potential medications for addiction treatment. Gabapentin has been subsequently shown to significantly increase rates of abstinence and no heavy drinking in a double-blind placebo-controlled trial (for further reading, see Mason et al., 2013).

From a perspective that is different from studies that investigate how to *precipitate* relapse in humans, researchers can measure the *resistance* to relapse. A model termed "smoking lapse behavior" allows the measurement

of two critical features of relapse: the ability to resist the first cigarette and subsequent smoking behavior (for further reading, see McKee, 2009). Nicotine-dependent subjects are first exposed to stimuli that can precipitate smoking relapse, such as alcohol, stress, and nicotine deprivation, and then their ability to resist smoking when presented with their preferred brand of cigarettes is measured. This model still needs to be validated with existing anti-craving medications, but it provides an intriguing extension of cue reactivity that may be useful as an intermediary step between preclinical animal models and clinical trials.

An evolving area in human laboratory relapse models is the measurement of neural correlates of cues for relapse using brain imaging studies, in which increased functional brain activation elicited by drug-associated cues may predict increased relapse risk. Cue-induced functional activation of the brain can be assessed by measuring changes in cerebral blood flow with positron emission tomography or single-photon emission computed tomography or measuring blood flow combined with functional magnetic resonance imaging. Core regions activated in most studies include the anterior cingulate, orbitofrontal cortex, basolateral amygdala, ventral striatum, and dorsal striatum. Strong cue-induced activation of similar regions, including the ventral striatum, dorsal striatum, medial prefrontal cortex, and anterior cingulate, has been observed in alcohol-dependent subjects who experience multiple relapses. Reduced functional activation of the ventral striatum in response to cues that signal nondrug rewards was observed in individuals with alcoholism, suggesting a shift in the incentive salience of drug-related cues. Thus, imaging studies may provide unique insights into subjects who exhibit the most dramatic functional activation to cues and, by extrapolation, who are more likely to relapse. Future studies can explore pharmacotherapeutic approaches to normalize such cue-induced responses and whether such measures will predict therapeutic efficacy in treatment (for further reading, see Fowler et al., 2007).

INDIVIDUAL DIFFERENCES AND MEDICATION DEVELOPMENT

Widespread attempts are being made to identify genetic markers that may be involved in addiction. However, a more exciting possibility is that single-nucleotide polymorphisms in certain genes in the human population may predict a vulnerability to certain subtypes of excessive drinking syndromes and predict responsiveness to the use of medications in the treatment of alcoholism. Animal and human studies are beginning to exploit this tremendous opportunity.

Genetic association studies have focused on two pathways: one that represents the reward side of addiction (μ opioid peptide system) and one that represents the "dark side" of addiction (CRF brain stress system). The human μ opioid receptor is encoded by the OPRM1 gene and is a candidate for the pharmacogenetic variability of the clinical effects of opioid drugs and clinical effects in addiction of anti-opioid receptor drugs. Mutations in the OPRM1 gene have been found in the promoter, coding regions and intron of the gene. One mutation that has received considerable attention is the 118A>G single-nucleotide polymorphism, which causes an amino acid substitution at position 40 of the μ opioid receptor protein where asparagine is substituted with aspartate (termed Asp40 or the G allele). Normal human subjects with this variant allele have been shown to require almost twice as high a plasma level of morphine to achieve the same analgesic response as subjects with the non-mutated allele. In addition, human subjects with this variant allele may respond more robustly to naltrexone treatment than carriers of the more common 118A allele. Subjects with alcoholism and the 118G allele have been termed those with "endorphin-dependent alcoholism," and subjects with this allele are represented in one-third

of subjects of European ancestry with alcoholism (for further reading, see Heilig et al., 2011).

An association was also found between two single-nucleotide polymorphisms of the CRF_1 receptor gene (crhr1) and binge drinking in adolescent and alcohol-dependent adults. Homozygosity at one of these polymorphisms (rs1876831, C allele) was associated with heavy drinking in relation to stressful life events in adolescents. rs1876831 is located on an intron that can potentially influence the transcription of the CRF_1 receptor gene (Table 9.5; for further reading, see Blomeyer et al., 2008).

CLINICAL TRIALS – UNIQUE CHALLENGES AND OPPORTUNITIES

Double-blind, placebo-controlled trials with random treatment assignment are the accepted standard for determining drug efficacy in addiction, similarly to other disorders (see Box 9.2). However, a number of unique features of the clinical trials for medications for the treatment of addiction need to be mentioned. These include a lack of consensus about clinically relevant outcome measures, admission criteria, and methods for detecting relapse between study visits. Additionally, general issues related to medication compliance, placebo response, and dropout rates present challenges for the design of clinical trials in addiction. Safety and tolerability issues also exist that are specific to addiction, including the potential interaction between alcohol and other substances with the drug under study (for further reading, see Koob et al., 2009).

SUMMARY

Tremendous breakthroughs in the basic neurobiology of addiction provide a framework for medication development that is unparalleled in biological psychiatry. Medications currently on the market for the treatment of addiction open a window on the opportunities to facilitate treatment and provide a means for evaluating future medications. The potential for the development of future medications for the treatment of addiction is significant on a number of fronts. A combination of excellent, validated animal models of addiction and an enormous surge in our understanding of the neurocircuits and neuropharmacological mechanisms involved in the development and maintenance of addiction reveal numerous possible targets. Such targets will be derived from this basic research on addiction, with a focus on the neuroadaptive changes that account for the transition to dependence and vulnerability to relapse, possibly within a genetic context. An interactive, iterative process called the Rosetta Stone approach can be established whereby existing medications are used to validate and improve animal and human laboratory models and then predict viable candidates for novel medications.

The development of medications for the treatment of addiction has been a priority in the United States. Similar efforts in the private sector and other countries are being encouraged. Areas of success include the successful development and validation of pharmacological aids to treatment of addiction (e.g., buprenorphine, naltrexone, varenicline, and acamprosate) and the necessary infrastructure for some aspects of drug development. For example, the National Institute on Drug Abuse (part of the United States National Institutes of Health) has established an extensive clinical trials network (http://www.nida.nih.gov/ctn/; accessed February 18, 2014). Nevertheless, despite the tremendous resources that have been devoted to the development of pharmacotherapies for cocaine addiction, little or no success has yet been reported. The burgeoning use of human laboratory studies and the Rosetta Stone approach to link human and animal studies may yield better success. To aid medication development for addiction, the pharmaceutical industry would need to consider addiction as a disease with a therapeutic drug target that is potentially profitable. Recent success with acamprosate, naltrexone, varenicline, and buprenorphine should provide some indication that expanded directions are merited in the addiction field.

Suggested Reading

Ameisen O. *The end of my addiction: le dernier verre (the last glass).* Sarah Crichton Books, New York.

Blomeyer, D., Treutlein, J., Esser, G., Schmidt, M.H., Schumann, G., Laucht, M., 2008. Interaction between CRHR1 gene and stressful life events predicts adolescent heavy alcohol use. Biol. Psychiatry 63, 146–151.

Brimijoin, S., Shen, X., Orson, F., Kosten, T., 2013. Prospects, promise and problems on the road to effective vaccines and related therapies for substance abuse. Expert Rev. Vaccines 12, 323–332.

Cowan, A., 2007. Buprenorphine: the basic pharmacology revisited. J. Addict. Med. 1, 68–72.

Fowler, J.S., Volkow, N.D., Kassed, C.A., Chang, L., 2007. Imaging the addicted human brain. Sci. Pract. Perspect. 3, 4–16.

Heilig, M., Goldman, D., Berrettini, W., O'Brien, C.P., 2011. Pharmacogenetic approaches to the treatment of alcohol addiction. Nat. Rev. Neurosci. 12, 670–684.

Koob, G.F., 2009. New dimensions in human laboratory models of addiction. Addict. Biol. 14, 1–8.

Koob, G.F., Everitt, B.J., Robbins, T.W., 2008. Reward, motivation, and addiction. In: Squire, L.R., Berg, D., Bloom, F.E., du Lac, S., Ghosh, A., Spitzer, N.C. (Eds) Fundamental Neuroscience, 3rd edition. Amsterdam: Academic Press, pp. 987–1016.

Koob, G.F., Lloyd, G.K., Mason, B.J., 2009. Development of pharmacotherapies for drug addiction: a Rosetta Stone approach. Nat. Rev. Drug Discov. 8, 500–515.

Koob, G.F., Volkow, N.D., 2010. Neurocircuitry of addiction. Neuropsychopharmacol. Rev. 35, 217–238. [erratum: (35), 1051].

Koob, G.F., Zorrilla, E.P., 2012. Update on corticotropin-releasing factor pharmacotherapy for psychiatric disorders: a revisionist view. Neuropsychopharmacol. Rev. 37, 308–309.

Littleton, J.M., 2007. Acamprosate in alcohol dependence: implications of a unique mechanism of action. J. Addict. Med. 1, 115–125.

Mason, B.J., Crean, R., Goodell, V., Light, J.M., Quello, S., Shadan, F., Buffkins, K., Kyle, M., Adusumalli, M., Begovic, A., Rao, S., 2012. A proof-of-concept randomized controlled study of gabapentin: effects on cannabis use, withdrawal and executive function deficits in cannabis-dependent adults. Neuropsychopharmacology 37, 1689–1698.

Mason, B.J., Light, J.M., Williams, L.D., Drobes, D.J., 2009. Proof-of-concept human laboratory study for protracted abstinence in alcohol dependence: effects of gabapentin. Addict. Biol. 14, 73–83.

Mason, B.J., Quello, S., Goodell, V., Shaden, F., Kyle, M., Begovic, A., 2014. Gabapentin treatment for alcohol dependence: a randomized controlled trial. JAMA Intern. Med. 174, 70–77.

McKee, S.A., 2009. Developing human laboratory models of smoking lapse behavior for medication screening. Addict. Biol. 14, 99–107.

Moreno, A.Y., Janda, K.D., 2009. Immunopharmacotherapy: vaccination strategies as a treatment for drug abuse and dependence. Pharmacol. Biochem. Behav. 92, 199–205.

Steensland, P., Fredriksson, I., Holst, S., Feltmann, K., Franck, J., Schilström, B., Carlsson, A., 2012. The monoamine stabilizer (−)-OSU6162 attenuates voluntary ethanol intake and ethanol-induced dopamine output in nucleus accumbens. Biol. Psychiatry 72, 823–831.

Unterwald, E.M., 2008. Naltrexone in the treatment of alcohol dependence. J. Addict. Med. 2, 121–127.

Wee, S., Koob, G.F., 2010. The role of the dynorphin-κ opioid system in the reinforcing effects of drugs of abuse. Psychopharmacology 210, 121–135.

Wolf, M.E., 2010. The Bermuda Triangle of cocaine-induced neuroadaptations. Trends Neurosci. 33, 391–398.

Index

Note: Page numbers followed by f denote figures; t, tables; b, boxes.

Printed in the United States
By Bookmasters